AF737094

Bayesian Models in Health Technology Assessment

Bayesian Models in Health Technology Assessment aims at presenting a thorough and yet accessible description of the philosophy underlying the Bayesian approach to statistical inference, as specifically applied to the process of health technology assessment (HTA). The book is grounded in practical examples, mostly taken from the HTA context and covering a wide range of real problems, typically encountered by modellers in their day-to-day work. All the chapters present methodological details, as well as carefully curated R and JAGS code, which can be used as a template to unlock the potential of Bayesian modelling, specifically in HTA.

- Covers introductory chapters on Bayesian modelling and computation, as well as the basics of the statistical modelling for HTA.
- Discusses a range of modelling topics, including the analysis of individual and aggregated-level data, as well as survival analysis and evidence synthesis.
- Presents further, more advanced modelling tools (such as for missing data, population adjustment methods and Value of Information), which should be increasingly familiar for practioners working in HTA and beyond.

The text is primarily for modellers and practitioners working in the HTA context, regulators and reviewers of reimbursement dossiers and cost-effectiveness analysis. More generally, it aims at drawing the attention of researchers whose background is firmly statistical onto the interesting and high impactful area of HTA. It complements a wide range of undergraduate and graduate programmes in health technology assessment, health and public health economics, as well as academic researchers in the field of statistical modelling for health technology assessment.

Chapman & Hall/CRC Biostatistics Series

Series Editors: Mark Chang, *Boston University, USA*

Likelihood Methods in Survival Analysis
with R Examples
Jun Ma, Malcolm Hudson, and Annabel Webb

Biostatistics for Bioassay
Ann Yellowlees and Matthew Stephenson

Power and Sample Size in R
Catherine M. Crespi

R for Health Technology Assessment
Gianluca Baio, Howard Thom, and Petros Pechlivanoglou

Advanced Statistical Analytics for Health Data Science with SAS and R
Ding-Geng Chen and Jeffrey Wilson

Group Sequential and Adaptive Methods for Clinical Trials
Christopher Jennison and Bruce W. Turnbull

Machine Learning for Microbiome Statistics
Yinglin Xia and Jun Sun

Dose-exposure-response Modeling: Methods and Practical Implementation
Jixian Wang

Comparative Effectiveness and Personalized Medicine Research Using Real-World Data
Thomas P. A. Debray, Tri-Long Nguyen, and Robert W. Platt

Master Protocol Clinical Trials for Evidence Generation
Strategies, Designs, Operations, and Case Studies
Edited by Ruixiao Lu, Jingjing Ye, Chengxing (Cindy) Lu, and William Wang

Does This Treatment Cause That Outcome?
The Science of Estimating a Treatment Effect and Why It Matters
Stephen J. Ruberg

Empirical Likelihood Method in Survival Analysis
With R Implementation, Second Edition
Mai Zhou

Bayesian Models in Health Technology Assessment
Gianluca Baio

For more information about this series, please visit: www.routledge.com/Chapman--Hall-CRC-Biostatistics-Series/book-series/CHBIOSTATIS

Bayesian Models in Health Technology Assessment

Gianluca Baio

CRC Press
Taylor & Francis Group
Boca Raton London New York

CRC Press is an imprint of the
Taylor & Francis Group, an **informa** business
A CHAPMAN & HALL BOOK

First edition published 2027
by CRC Press
2385 NW Executive Center Drive, Suite 320, Boca Raton FL 33431

and by CRC Press
4 Park Square, Milton Park, Abingdon, Oxon, OX14 4RN

CRC Press is an imprint of Taylor & Francis Group, LLC

© 2027 Gianluca Baio

Reasonable efforts have been made to publish reliable data and information, but the author and publisher cannot assume responsibility for the validity of all materials or the consequences of their use. The authors and publishers have attempted to trace the copyright holders of all material reproduced in this publication and apologize to copyright holders if permission to publish in this form has not been obtained. If any copyright material has not been acknowledged please write and let us know so we may rectify in any future reprint.

Except as permitted under U.S. Copyright Law, no part of this book may be reprinted, reproduced, transmitted, or utilized in any form by any electronic, mechanical, or other means, now known or hereafter invented, including photocopying, microfilming, and recording, or in any information storage or retrieval system, without written permission from the publishers.

For permission to photocopy or use material electronically from this work, access www.copyright.com or contact the Copyright Clearance Center, Inc. (CCC), 222 Rosewood Drive, Danvers, MA 01923, 978-750-8400. For works that are not available on CCC please contact mpkbookspermissions@tandf.co.uk

For Product Safety Concerns and Information please contact our EU representative GPSR@taylorandfrancis.com. Taylor & Francis Verlag GmbH, Kaufingerstraße 24, 80331 München, Germany.

Trademark notice: Product or corporate names may be trademarks or registered trademarks and are used only for identification and explanation without intent to infringe.

ISBN: 978-1-041-29738-3 (hbk)
ISBN: 978-1-041-29751-2 (pbk)
ISBN: 978-1-003-77105-0 (ebk)

DOI: 10.1201/9781003771050

Typeset in LMRoman
by KnowledgeWorks Global Ltd.

Publisher's note: This book has been prepared from camera-ready copy provided by the authors.

To all the little, random things that have brought me to right here, right now

Contents

Preface

Plan of the book (read carefully!)

In many ways, this is a book of two halves: on the one hand, we focus on the philosophy and practice of Bayesian modelling from a very statistical point of view and, to some extent, the content could be used by readers who do not really have a direct interest in healthcare applications. On the other hand, we are concerned with the general topic of "health technology assessment" (HTA – see below and in Chapter 4 for more details about our framing and definition of this term) as underpinned by Bayesian modelling. Consequently, it is difficult to clearly separate the two components (Bayesian modelling for statistical analysis vs HTA) and in reality we tend to mix them, throughout.

This book is also framed into the concerted effort of bringing the use of R front-and-centre in the HTA community (Baio et al., 2025b). In particular, we are staunch proponents of a workflow in which suitable statistical tools are used to perform the basic components of the economic evaluation, in HTA. The focus on Bayesian modelling ties up nicely and directly with this and leverages the ability of R to interact with suitable Bayesian software – we return to this point later.

We start with Part I, which presents the "preliminaries". Here, we focus heavily on the statistical side of things: Chapter 1 first introduces the main philosophical ideas that serve as cornerstone for the Bayesian approach to statistical inference. We present fundamental concepts such as the likelihood function, the probabilistic quantification of current uncertainty through a model for the sampling variability (associated with observable or observed data) and a prior distribution for the unobservable parameters. Then, we start exploring the ways in which information can be encoded in the model and computation can be made for Bayesian analysis and in order to propagate uncertainty in model parameters.

In Chapter 2, we concentrate on the more "proper" Bayesian learning from observed data, in which we combine the two sources of uncertainty/variation into a suitable posterior distribution. We first look into historical and convenient ways to define the existing contextual information (from "vague" and conjugate, to more modern forms of priors, which can regularise the inference, while not exerting undue impact) and we describe how Bayesian computation can be performed for these simpler (and often overly-simplistic!) models. Then, we move towards more general modelling structures, which require more advanced computational tools. Here, we focus on Markov chain Monte Carlo and, specifically, the Gibbs sampling algorithm.

Of course, this is but one of the possible tools that can be used for Bayesian modelling – and others are potentially more modern (notably, Hamiltonian Monte Carlo). We make a conscious choice of concentrating on Gibbs sampling because of the wider context in which we firmly place our book: firstly, most typical problems in HTA are, generally speaking, dealt very efficiently by Gibbs sampling and do not *need* the use of more advanced (and potentially even more efficient) computation tools. Secondly (but closely related), while HTA has generally become much more technically-minded and skilled over the last decade, it still represents a very heterogeneous field, in which researchers from many different backgrounds operate. With this book, we aim at attracting statisticians, or to train non-statisticians to the practice of Bayesian modelling – but crucially, we try to establish a clear workflow, based on the most established and "safe" tools. For this reason, we think that it is particularly important to provide a substantive and relatively technical introduction to the practice of Bayesian modelling.

This idea propagates to Chapter 3, in which we present a somewhat selective summary of the most important existing tools for the actual performance of Bayesian modelling. Again, while many pieces of software exist, we concentrate on `JAGS`, which much as its close relative `OpenBUGS` is specifically designed to run models using Gibbs sampling.

We acknowledge here and in Section 3.1.2 that other choices are possible – to some extent, our view is that software is often a proxy for the level of the technical sophistication of the modeller and thus it is really not important whether *you* decide to use the material described in this book and `JAGS` to learn about how you could run *your* (HTA) models, or whether *you* are confident and comfortable enough to map all the modelling assumptions and code to, say, `Stan`... The ambition we have with this book is to draw the attention of those who are statistically-numerate and to up-skill those who are not just yet, so that they can then make their own informed decision – as long as they do Bayesian modelling, we are happy!...

Chapter 4 is where we, finally, introduce our core application area for Bayesian modelling. Arguably, the reader has to wait for quite a number of pages before being drawn more specifically into the healthcare economic evaluation context. Even then, we acknowledge that we do so using a very statistical perspective and that, perhaps, readers who come from a more "health economics" background may find our presentation of the basics of HTA lacking of more general context. Again, this is a conscious choice because the main objective is for us to ground the application area within a full Bayesian approach. A broader understanding of the intricacies of HTA is certainly required for modellers wanting to enter (and becoming experts of) this field and we do point the reader to well-known and very worthy textbooks and references, mainly from the non-statistical literature.

We then move to Part II, in which we present a number of modelling frameworks that apply to very many specific cases that constitute, in our view, a large majority of those of interest to a typical HTA modeller. We should hasten to say that we do not claim to be able to describe and consider *all* the possible problems that a researcher may encounter in HTA – especially because the very definition of this field is quite broad and may have slightly different meanings, depending on the actual context and background. Nonetheless, it is our view that the modelling presented in Chapters 5–9 constitute what a modeller aiming to work in the field of "cost-effectiveness analysis for healthcare interventions" should absolutely be familiar with.

Chapter 5 gives a very lengthy account of how Bayesian modelling can be used for the specific purpose of economic evaluation, when individual-level data (ILD) are available. Historically, this has been associated with "cost-effectiveness analysis alongside clinical trials" in the wider HTA literature and this has served to create a potential distinction between what was often labelled cost-effectiveness or cost-utility analysis and more general decision-analytic models (which we discuss in Chapters 6, 7 and 9).

We agree that the general cost-effectiveness analysis using ILD and, possibly, in conjunction with a randomised trial is often a very different enterprise than a fully fledged structure used to represent the benefits and the underlying costs of applying a new healthcare intervention, whose consequences are evaluated over the long run and typically way beyond the inevitably limited duration of an experimental trial.

However, we also believe that there is perhaps a wider *statistical* context (as opposed to the pure HTA interpretation), in which the separation of the two is maybe less helpful – the modelling is different, depending on the availability of data and the purpose of the analysis; but many of the statistical features can be linked up and used in a wider aim of "decision-making under uncertainty".

More in details, in Chapter 5 we describe the general Bayesian framework to model jointly suitable individual measures of benefits and costs; we start by using a simplified (and, again, overly-simplistic!) version based on Normality and independence and then incrementally move to more complex (and realistic) structures in which these assumptions are relaxed. We also introduce the important topic of model selection in Section 5.3 – this is not fundamentally linked to the use of ILD and we return to it in later chapters.

Chapter 6 introduces Bayesian modelling for aggregated level data (ALD) and the wider topic of evidence synthesis. This is very prevalent in the decision-analytic context of HTA and one of the most important component of the modellers' work. In this chapter, we concentrate on the background assumptions in terms of *exchangeability* – or in other words, the level of similarity and the amount by which we are comfortable pooling information together from different sources. Again, we describe this through examples and worked/annotated computer code to run the analysis, with specific modelling drawn from the HTA context.

Following naturally from this framework, we move in Chapter 7 to consider indirect treatment comparisons, another ubiquitous topic in cost-effectiveness modelling and one of the cornerstones of HTA. Again, we run through a motivating example, detailing the code and the results of the analysis based on several model specifications and the ability of assessing the validity of several diverse underpinning assumptions (e.g. "fixed" vs "random" effects). Chapter 7 has fundamental connections with Chapter 11, which expands on the main idea of rebalancing the underlying populations with a view of producing unbiased indirect comparisons.

In Chapter 8, we give a detailed introduction to the complexity associated with time-to-event modelling, obviously with a specific Bayesian perspective. This chapter is rather long and does include links with other parts of the book (e.g. Chapter 9 or Chapter 7) – survival analysis typically underpins cancer studies, which in turn are arguably one of the most important areas of HTA, which makes this topic highly prevalent and another "must-know" for the typical modeller.

This is also one of the few places in the book where we deviate from the "standard" Gibbs sampling analysis and focus on R packages that perform Bayesian modelling using Hamiltonian Monte Carlo (HMC). Because of the inevitable idiosyncrasy of survival data, including censoring and the need for extrapolation beyond the observed time-horizon, computation (and particularly within a Bayesian context) can be complex and thus this is one of the few application areas in which HCM proves to be a much more cost-effective tool, in HTA.

The last topic in Part II is Markov models, described in Chapter 9. We divide this chapter in two broad components: first we present the basic structure underlying the definition of multistate (Markov) models, typically, but not exclusively, used in discrete times, in the context of HTA. We use a running example to show a reasonably complex and comprehensive Bayesian analysis, based on a number of data sources (and thus linking back to the topics of Chapter 6) and then present in much detail the code used to produce the full results, feeding the wider economic analysis.

Then, we consider another very prevalent case-use, based on a combination of survival modelling and a specific Markov model structure (the "three-state cancer model" of Section 9.3). In practice, in either case, running the Markov model effectively amounts to applying some sort of matrix algebra, but we distinguish the process of Bayesian modelling necessary to obtain the "engine" that allows the algebra to work.

Part III of the book has a rather distinct feel to it: while for the first two parts, we have used a consistent alternation between theoretical exposition and practical worked out examples, in Part III we target three specific advanced topics, but focus more on the description of the underlying methodologies and less on giving code and examples. The reason for this choice is two-fold: on the one hand, missing data (which we consider in Chapter 10), population adjustment (Chapter 11) and the analysis of the value of information (Chapter 12) all embed fundamental complexity from the methodological and computational point of view. On the other hand, as they are very topical themes, we are fully aware of the existence of very recent high quality literature, often with a very strong Bayesian nature.

We saw little value in completely re-inventing the wheel, when there are either excellent specific chapters or even entire textbooks dealing exactly with these topics – notably Gabrio et al. (2025), Phillippo et al. (2025a) and Heath et al. (2024). Nonetheless, all of these are, in our view, fundamental tools for HTA modellers and thus we decided to treat them as "further modelling", for which we provide a description of the basic problems and methodologies and point to the external references for more details (including on the practice of *doing* them). We also note that all three are fundamental Bayesian tools, which makes them naturally feature in this book.

Finally, we must acknowledge that our intention was never to produce an encyclopaedic account of "all of HTA" (if such thing were even possible...). Therefore, we have made editorial choices not to include chapters on important tools, such as decision trees or discrete event simulations – but also refer interested readers to other very good literature, such as, for example, Green et al. (2025a) or Degeling et al. (2025), to remain within the R ecosystem.

How to use this book

We use "callouts" to format specific parts of the text in blocks. The icon next to the block title differentiates the type of blocks. For example, a "note" block is formatted as the following and it typically contains some general or historical comment.

> **Some title**
>
> Some text

When we want to highlight something related to computer code, we use the following notation

> **Some title**
>
> Some text

while blocks containing advanced or technical comments are formatted as the following.

Some title

Some text

Finally, blocks in which we present notation or information that the reader should be aware of are formatted as the following.

Some title

Some text

When we use computer code, we format it in listing blocks, where comments are prefixed by a "hash" symbol "#", e.g.

```
# This defines a vector and computes the standard deviation
x=c(1,2,3,4,5)
paste0("Standard deviation = ",round(sd(x),2))
```

while output or results are shown as in the following.

```
[1] "Standard deviation = 1.58"
```

Throughout the book, we switch between "theoretical exposition" of the main concepts and "practical examples", in which we run through a specific topic or method using data analysis and `R` code. Examples are clearly signposted using a different font:

Example X.Y: *A title here.* Some text here...

and are concluded by a line spanning three quarters of the page, as the following.

Computer configuration

Throughout the book, we use a number of running examples (all detailed in the List of examples, immediately after this Preface). The vast majority is based on "real" healthcare economic evaluation and showcase the use of Bayesian modelling. The datasets and annotated code are available at the GitHub repository at `https://github.com/giabaio/bmhta-examples`. In the spirit of open access and reproducibility, users can also take advantage of GitHub functionalities and "fork" the repository to further annotate, modify and expand the examples, as well as create a "pull request", so that their changes may be included in the main repository and be helpful for others.

In order to be able to replicate the analyses and run the code, we assume the following computer specification. Firstly and obviously, we need a recent installation of `R` (full details on installation are available from `https://cran.r-project.org/`).

In the vast majority of the chapters, we perform the Bayesian analysis using `JAGS` (full details on the installation are available at the software website: `https://sourceforge.net/projects/mcmc-jags/files/JAGS/4.x/` – see also Chapter 3). In alternative to `JAGS`, the user may decide to use `OpenBUGS` (see this webpage https://www.mrc-bsu.cam.ac.uk/software for more information). By and large, there will not be important differences, although we highlight the main ones in Section 3.3.

For R, we make extensive use of a number of *packages*. In particular, much of the data "wrangling" and plotting happens using the tidyverse facilities (Wickham et al., 2019), including dplyr (Wickham et al., 2023), tibble (Müller and Wickham, 2025) and ggplot2 (Wickham, 2016). Thus, it is probably a good idea to install the whole tidyverse environment, which we can do by typing into a R terminal the following command:

```
install.packages("tidyverse")
```

(this can be a lengthy process, as tidyverse is a collection of several packages).

Another necessary package is the interface between R and JAGS – there are several options, but we use throughout the book the package R2jags (Su and Yajima, 2010), which again can be installed using the basic install.packages("R2jags") command. BCEA is used to perform the post-processing of the modelling output, for health economic evaluation and thus useful and used in several examples.

Similarly, a bespoke package bmhe (which is not available in the main R package repositories – see Example 1.4 for specific installation instructions) is often used to post-process the output of the Bayesian modelling. For survival analysis, in Chapter 8, we use the package survHE and specifically its "add on" survHEhmc (see Section 8.4 for detailed installation instructions), as well as survextrap, both of which are R front-ends for the rstan package, used to run Hamiltonian Monte Carlo (see Section 2.3.3).

When necessary, other packages are clearly signposted in the relevant part of this book.

Acknowledgements

Special thanks go to Anna Heath, Mark Strong, Chris Jackson, Nicky Welton, Howard Thom, Nathan Green, Natalia Kunst and Antonio Remiro Azocar, who have all been involved in various versions (and might be again, in future ones...) of the summer school *Bayesian methods in health economics* (more details can be found at https://gianluca.statistica.it/teaching/summer-school/).

This book draws heavily on the summer school, both in terms of content and examples, as well as the module I have taught at University College London, for the past few years (STAT0019 – Bayesian methods in health economics), although the material is consolidated, streamlined and updated in here. These friends and colleagues have been instrumental in helping me create some of the material presented here. The students in my module have acted as a focus-group and have guided the narrative, as well as the selection and ordering of the topics I decided to include in the final version.

This is my fourth book with CRC and the brilliant team led by the equally brilliant Rob Calver – I briefly considered pitching it to one of their competitors, who had approached me to see if I had anything I was working on, but the experience had been so great the first three times that I simply had to go back "home" and continue working with CRC. And it was a pleasure to do so!

About the author

Gianluca Baio is Professor of Statistics and Health Economics in the Department of Statistical Science at University College London (UK). Gianluca's main interests are in Bayesian statistical modelling for cost effectiveness analysis and decision-making problems in the health systems, hierarchical/multilevel models and causal inference using the decision-theoretic approach. Gianluca leads the Statistics for Health Economic Evaluation research group within the department of Statistical Science and was the co-director of UCL MSc Programme in Health Economics and Decision Science. He is a founding member and former Scientific co-Director of the R-HTA consortium (https://r-hta.org/) and a founding member of the ConVOI (https://www.convoi-group.org/) network. He also served as Secretary (2014-2016) and then Programme Chair (2016-2018) in the Section on Biostatistics and Pharmaceutical Statistics of the International Society for Bayesian Analysis. He collaborates with the UK National Institute for Health and Care Excellence (NICE) as a Scientific Advisor on Health Technology Appraisal projects and has been the 18th Armitage Lecturer in November 2021. His research activity is now (almost) officially dead, since he has become the head of the department of Statistical Science at UCL, in 2021.

List of examples

List of notes

Part I

Preliminaries

1

Introduction to Bayesian reasoning

1.1 Introduction

The main objective of statistical inference is to use observations we make on some data to learn about some unobservable feature of the general population in which we are interested. To do this, we use statistical models to describe the probabilistic mechanism by which (we assume!) the data have arisen.

Symbols, notation, etc.

Although we keep the mathematical sophistication to an accessible level, we do need to use specific symbols and terminology, for the sake of clarity. Generally speaking, statistical notation distinguishes mainly between **observed** or **observable** variables, which we indicate in upper-case Roman letters, e.g. Y, W, T; and *unobservable* parameters, which are indicated using Greek letters, e.g. θ, μ, σ.

When data are *observed* (and thus their realised value is known to us), we usually indicate in lower-case Roman letters, e.g. y, w, t. When we consider a *vector* of variables or parameters, we typeset them in bold, e.g. $\boldsymbol{Y}$ indicates a vector of observable variables. We often describe this fully as $\boldsymbol{Y} = (Y_1, \ldots, Y_n)$, which can be used to indicate that we have a vector of length n. We apply this to parameters too; for example, if a model is indexed by two parameters μ and σ, we write that the parameter vector is $\boldsymbol{\theta} = (\mu, \sigma)$.

As mentioned above, a crucial part of statistical modelling is to associate variables with probability distributions, e.g. to describe uncertainty or sampling variability. We do this using the terminology

$$y \sim \text{Name of the distribution(Name of the parameters)},$$

where the symbol "$\sim$" is read "is distributed as", or more appropriately "is associated with a XXX distribution with parameters YYY". Alternatively, we may write p(Name of variable | Name of parameters) to indicate the probability distribution associated with a variable and indexed by some parameters. An example is

$$p(y \mid \theta, n) = \binom{n}{y} \theta^y (1-\theta)^{(n-y)}.$$

The symbol "|" (read "given" or "conditionally on") is used to indicate that the argument to its left is the main variable of interest, while the argument(s) to its right are used as parameters or known values.

The notation $\Pr(Y = y \mid \theta)$ indicates the probability that the variable Y takes on the value y – so this is a slightly different concept to the probability *distribution* $p(y \mid \theta)$ – the former is a single value, while the latter is an entire distribution.

DOI: 10.1201/9781003771050-1

We usually represent the **data-generating process** (DGP) specifying the sampling variability associated with the data in terms of a parametric probability distribution, $p(y \mid \boldsymbol{\theta})$, where $\boldsymbol{\theta}$ is a (possibly multivariate) parameter, indexing the distribution. For example, we may consider count data, e.g. the total number of deaths in a given period and geographical location and model them using a Poisson distribution

$$y \sim \text{Poisson}(\theta) \qquad \text{with} \qquad p(y \mid \theta) = \frac{\theta^y \exp(-\theta)}{y!}, \tag{1.1}$$

or use a Gamma distribution, defined in terms of a vector of parameters $\boldsymbol{\theta} = (\text{shape} = \nu, \text{rate} = \gamma)$,

$$y \sim \text{Gamma}(\nu, \gamma) \qquad \text{with} \qquad p(y \mid \nu, \gamma) = \frac{\gamma^\nu}{\Gamma(\nu)} y^{\nu-1} \exp(-\gamma y) \tag{1.2}$$

where

$$\Gamma(x) = (x-1)! = (x-1) \times (x-2) \times \cdots \times 2 \times 1, \tag{1.3}$$

to model continuous, skewed data bounded in the interval $(0, \infty)$, e.g. individual-level costs of access to healthcare resources.

Graphically, the DGP can be represented using the language of *directed acyclical graphs* (DAGs); in a DAG, variables are represented as nodes and links between them are represented as arrows. For instance, Figure 1.1 shows an alleged DGP in which the observed data y depend **probabilistically** on a parameter θ. This dependence is expressed through the distribution $p(y \mid \theta)$, which is used to describe the sampling variability for the observable data.

Standard (frequentist and maximum likelihood) procedures fix the working hypotheses and, by deduction, make inference on the observed data. The main consequence of this approach to statistical inference is that the hypotheses, or the features of the DGP (i.e. the parameters), are always assumed as fixed quantities. We generally do not know their value, but to a non-Bayesian, there is no uncertainty about it – the only source of uncertainty in our modelling is due to sampling variability in the data we have observed, or that we might observe in the future.

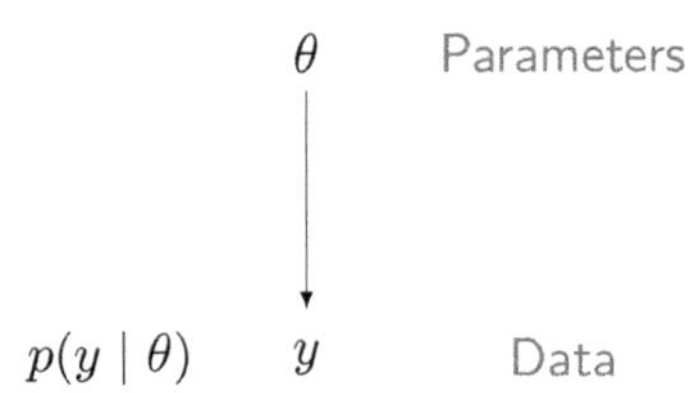

Figure 1.1: A DAG representation of a DGP in which the data y depend probabilistically on a parameter θ, which is used to index the sampling distribution, $p(y \mid \theta)$.

Note 1: We are *not* the same

Often, statistical textbooks tend to conflate the main ideas underpinning the "frequentist" approach to statistical inference (championed among others by Jerzy Neymann and Egon Pearson) with the "likelihood" approach (almost single-handedly devised by Ronald Fisher). The two are in fact quite separate and the history of Statistics is actually full of heated exchanges between frequentists on one side and, mainly, Fisher on the other, to strongly argue over the supremacy of either philosophies[1].

As it happens, Fisher was able to dress up his maximum likelihood theory so as to uphold the basic frequentist features and thus the maximum likelihood estimator is almost universally optimal from a frequentist perspective too. But there are fundamental differences in the two – with the common feature of rejecting the Bayesian philosophy. See Baio (2025) for more discussion of the distinctions in the three major schools of statistical inference, in the context of HTA.

For example, in Figure 1.2a, we show an alleged DGP, in which there are three possible competing hypotheses; the first one assumes that the "true state of the world" is that some parameter Δ (think of it as the difference in effectiveness for a given intervention) is equal to 0%; the second one assumes a small positive effect ($\Delta = 5\%$), while the third one assumes a large positive effect ($\Delta = 10\%$). Under either of these hypotheses, let us assume that there are a number of hypothetical observations we can make – for simplicity we assume a set of discrete outcomes, going from a minor negative result of -5% (indicating that the population given the treatment has slightly worse outcomes than that given the control), to a null outcome (0%), all to way to a very large positive observed effect of $+15\%$.

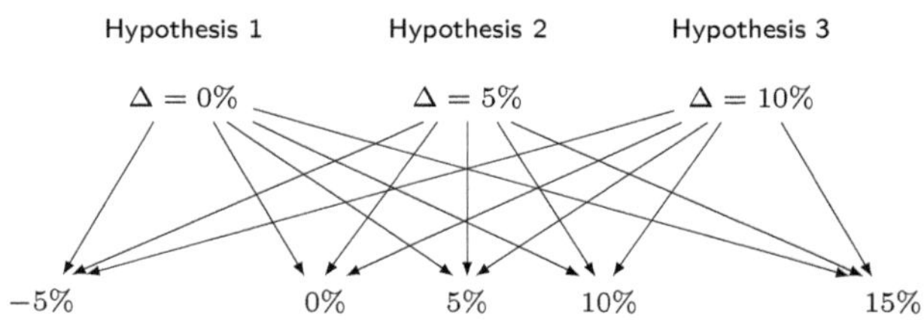

(a) An alleged data-generating process in which we consider three possible hypotheses, or parameter values, say Δ, in the top layer of the graph, which may give rise to one of many possible observed data (bottom layer of the graph).

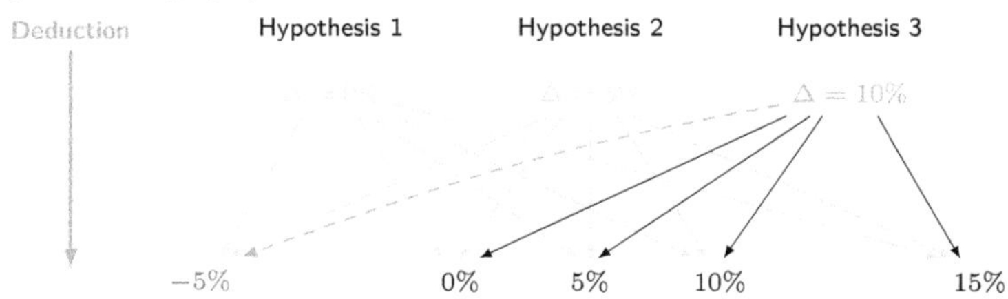

(b) Once the one and only observed data is realised, e.g. the value –5% in panel, we can check the plausibility of each of the hypotheses, for instance, by measuring the likelihood of the observed outcome *conditionally* on a value for Δ (e.g. 10%).

Figure 1.2: The process of deductive inference (adapted from: Goodman, 1999).

[1]Interestingly, when Fisher joined University College London in 1933, a special chair as "Galton Professor of Eugenics" was created in the Department of Eugenics, so as to avoid him being in the then Department of Applied Statistics, which was led by Egon Pearson.

Under a frequentist/maximum likelihood approach, statistical inference is concerned with questions such as

> *If my working hypothesis (e.g. that the true treatment effect is large, say $\Delta = 10\%$) is true, what is the probability of randomly selecting the data that I actually observed (e.g. a difference in outcome of -5%)?*

If this probability is small, then we deduce weak support of the evidence to the hypothesis. In other words, the objective is to assess Pr(Observed data | Hypothesis). In reality (as shown in Figure 1.2b), we cannot observe all possible datasets – say that the one actually realised is -5%. Nonetheless, we use the sampling variability that describes the probability of observing each one of the many possible datasets, under the conditions specified by a given DGP to quantify the weight of the evidence in favour of each competing hypothesis for the DGP. This is directly relevant for standard frequentist/maximum likelihood summaries, e.g. p–values, confidence intervals, etc. Crucially, this process also involves a comparison with data that could have been observed, but have not.

Example 1.1. *Significance testing.* Consider the classical example of significance testing applied to a "two-sample problem", which we may represent using the following distributional assumptions:

$$y_{10}, \ldots, y_{n_0 0} \overset{iid}{\sim} \text{Normal}(\mu_0, \sigma_0^2) \qquad \text{and} \qquad y_{11}, \ldots, y_{n_1 1} \overset{iid}{\sim} \text{Normal}(\mu_1, \sigma_1^2),$$

where, in general,

$$y \sim \text{Normal}(\mu, \sigma) \qquad \Rightarrow \qquad p(y \mid \mu, \sigma) = \frac{1}{\sigma\sqrt{2\pi}} \exp\left(-\frac{1}{2}\left(\frac{y-\mu}{\sigma}\right)^2\right). \tag{1.4}$$

In a case such as this, we may specify a "null" hypothesis as $H_0 : \mu_1 = \mu_0$, or alternatively (and equivalently!) $H_0 : \delta = \mu_1 - \mu_0 = 0$ – i.e. that there is "no treatment effect" at the population level.

Using some basic Normal theory, we can construct an estimator for the difference in the treatment effect $\hat{\delta} = D = \bar{Y}_1 - \bar{Y}_0$ and derive that

$$\begin{aligned} D = \bar{Y}_1 - \bar{Y}_0 &\sim \text{Normal}\left(\mu_D, \sigma_D^2\right) \\ &\sim \text{Normal}\left(\mu_1 - \mu_0, \frac{\sigma_0^2}{n_0} + \frac{\sigma_1^2}{n_1}\right) \end{aligned}$$

and estimating σ_D^2 using the sample variance

$$\begin{aligned} S_D^2 &= \frac{S_0^2}{n_0} + \frac{S_1^2}{n_1} \\ &= \frac{n_0}{n_0 - 1}\sum_{i=1}^{n_0}(Y_{i0} - \bar{Y}_0)^2 + \frac{n_1}{n_1 - 1}\sum_{i=1}^{n_1}(Y_{i1} - \bar{Y}_1)^2 \end{aligned}$$

derive the distribution of the "test statistic"

$$T = \frac{D - \delta}{\sqrt{S_D^2}} \sim \text{t}(0, 1, n-1)$$

where

$$y \sim \text{t}(\mu, \tau, \nu) \quad \Rightarrow \quad p(y \mid \mu, \tau, \nu) = \frac{\Gamma\left(\frac{\nu+1}{2}\right)}{\Gamma\left(\frac{\nu}{2}\right)} \sqrt{\frac{\tau}{\nu\pi}} \left(1 + \frac{\tau}{\nu}(y-\mu)^2\right)^{-\frac{\nu+1}{2}} \tag{1.5}$$

indicates a t distribution with mean μ, precision (a measure of inverse variance) τ and degrees of freedom ν.

Suppose that for the specific case at hand, the sample values and estimates are

$$\begin{aligned} n_0 &= 80; & n_1 &= 78; \\ \bar{y}_0 &= 25.12; & \bar{y}_1 &= 32.58; \\ S_0^2 &= 355.85; & S_1^2 &= 376.88. \end{aligned}$$

Given these numbers, we can compute the observed value for the estimate of the true difference in the two means $d = 7.46$ and the estimate for its variance

$$\begin{aligned} s_D^2 = \frac{s_0^2}{n_0} + \frac{s_1^2}{n_1} &= \frac{355.85}{80} + \frac{376.88}{78} \\ &= 4.45 + 4.83 = 9.28. \end{aligned}$$

Under the null hypothesis, the *observed* test statistic is

$$t = \frac{d - 0}{\sqrt{s_D^2}} = \frac{7.46}{3.05} = 2.45.$$

The fundamental idea underpinning significance testing is that *if* the null hypothesis were true, then we would expect the observed value t of the test statistic T to be fairly "central" in the range of its sampling distribution. In other words, we can use the tail-area probabilities under the sampling distribution $p(t \mid \theta, H_0)$ to find the chance of observing a result "*as extreme as, or even more extreme than*" the one that actually obtained in the current data.

Intuitively, if $t > \text{Med}(T)$, i.e. the observed value of t is "larger than normal", we would be looking at even larger values; conversely, if $t \leq \text{Med}(T)$, "even more extreme" values would be in fact smaller than that observed.

In the present case, we can use R to compute the p–**value** $\Pr(T > t \mid \theta, H_0)$; Figure 1.3 shows this as the grey area to the left of the observed value $t = 2.45$.

```
pt(q=t,df=n-1,lower.tail=FALSE)
```

```
[1] 0.007697083
```

The interpretation of the p–value in terms of assessing the probability of observing something *as extreme as, or even more extreme than* the data actually observed (or, in other words, as a tail-area probability) is clearly a mouthful and a slightly subtle concept. The reason why we need to use such a convoluted phrasing is that, when dealing with continuous data, the sampling distribution does not really represent a probability, but rather a density. So, it is impossible to quantify the strength of the evidence just in correspondence of the observed value for the test statistic.

One criticism associated with this (inevitable!) choice is that the strength of the evidence (or, in other words, whether the observed data are consistent with the working hypothesis) depends on the data actually observed, as well as on data ("even more extreme") that might be – but have not been – observed. In addition to this, by its own nature, it is possible that the same p–value is computed for a very small and a very large study; the conclusion in terms of strength of the evidence would be identical, without distinction of the underlying sample size (Goodman, 1999).

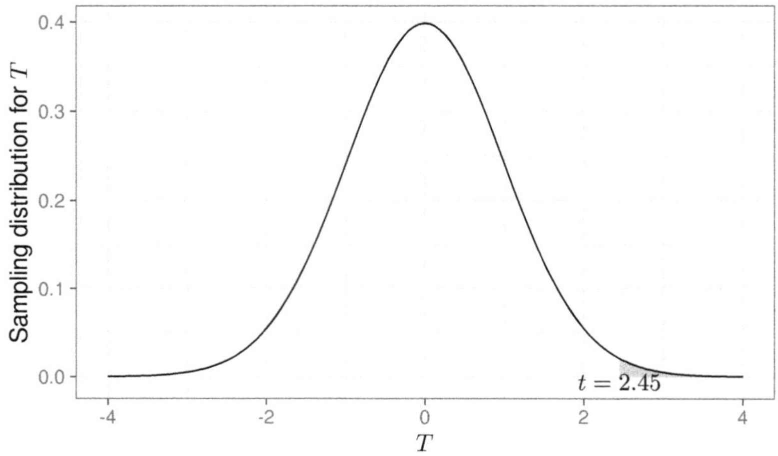

Figure 1.3: The sampling distribution for the statistic T under the null hypothesis, $p(T \mid H_0)$. The shaded area indicates the p–value, $\Pr(T > t = 2.45 \mid H_0) = 0.0077$.

1.2 Bayesian modelling

The Bayesian philosophy proceeds exactly in the opposite direction, i.e. by fixing the value of the observed data and, by induction, making inferences on unobservable hypotheses. Figure 1.4a shows the same DGP described in Figure 1.2a: there are three possible hypotheses that can generate a number of hypothetical observed data. However, from a Bayesian perspective, once the one and only dataset is observed (in this case with a value of -5%, highlighted in Figure 1.4b), there remains no uncertainty over the observations – this is why every other hypothetical outcome is greyed out in Figure 1.4b. The sampling mechanism is relevant to get us there, but once we know what the data are, the only relevant question thus becomes

What is the probability of my working hypothesis, given the data I observed?

If this is less than the probability associated with other competing hypotheses, then we can deduce weak support from the evidence to the hypothesis. This implies that the Bayesian procedure is interested in assessing Pr(Hypothesis | Observed data) and that, crucially, unobserved data have no role in the inference.

Note 2: Where did it all start?

The posthumous work of Reverend Thomas Bayes (1763) is considered the origin of what we now call "Bayesian" approach. However, interestingly, Fienberg (2006) suggests that it was not until the 1950s that the term "Bayesian" came to be used, with Ronald Fisher, one of the most anti-Bayesians of the time, among those potentially credited with the invention of the term (other, perhaps more likely candidates are Dennis Lindley and Irving John Good, who were much more of a Bayesian persuasion...).

As mentioned by Fienberg (2006)

> *...In current statistical language, Bayes' paper introduces a uniform prior distribution on the binomial parameter, θ reasoning by analogy with a "billiard table" and drawing on the form of the marginal distribution of the binomial random variable...*

In fact, quoting Stigler (1982), Fienberg (2006) argues that

> *...Bayes intended his results in a rather more limited way than would modern Bayesians.*

and that the actual development of what we generally refer to as "Bayesian" modelling is perhaps more to do with the later (and, apparently, independent) work of Pierre Simon Laplace (1812) – see also Section 2.2.1.

Bertsch McGrayne (2011) presents an engaging account of the historical impact of Bayesian modelling, including on Alan Turing's work on "cracking the Enigma Code", the complex system of encrypted messages used by the German Army in World War Two, which also led to the foundations of modern computers.

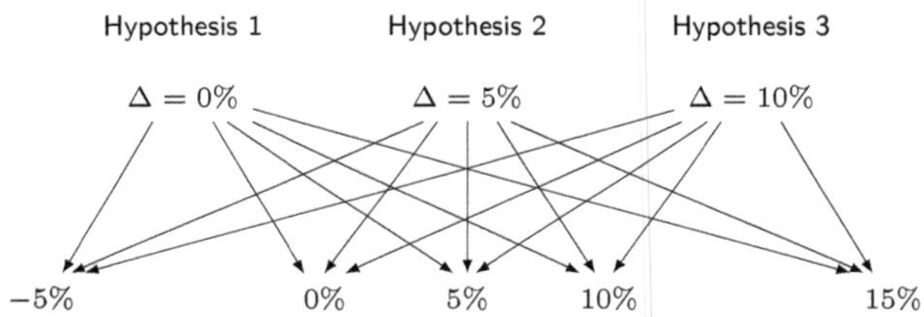

(a) The same alleged data-generating process, which we assume may give rise to possible observed data.

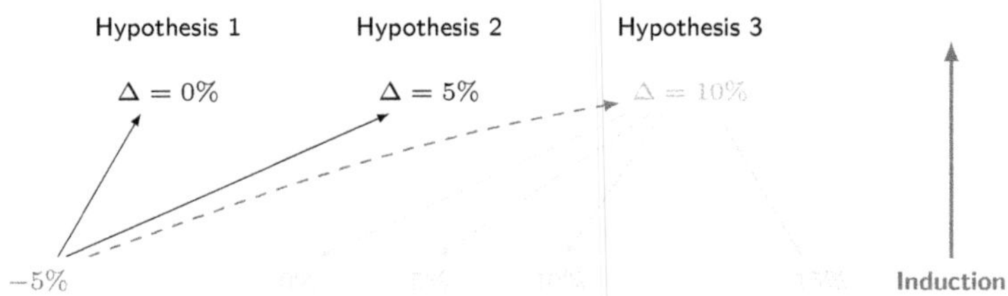

(b) Once the one and only observed data are realised, e.g. the value –5%, there is no more uncertainty about the data; we can use the observed value to update our uncertainty over which DGP is more probably the one that has given rise to the observed data.

Figure 1.4: The process of inductive inference (adapted from: Goodman, 1999).

In a Bayesian context, we need to specify a full probabilistic model that applies to everything over which we have uncertainty – be it *sampling variability* (e.g. the data that we may have observed or that we may be able to observe in the future) or *epistemic uncertainty*, e.g. the parameters of the model (which in fact we are never in a position of observing – the parameters may possess no physical meaning but just be a mathematical construction that helps us define the model!) or some hypothesis that describes the form of the alleged DGP.

In fact, much as in the frequentist/likelihood context, even from a Bayesian perspective it is perfectly possible that parameters may in fact have a "true", underlying, immutable and fixed value; however, because we do not know this value, the Bayesian view is to model this lack of knowledge by associating a suitable probability distribution. This means that, to a

Bayesian, probability is the only language to assess any form of imperfect information or knowledge: there is no need to distinguish between "probability" and "confidence". To be able to work in this context, however, before even seeing the data, we need to identify a suitable probability distribution to describe the overall uncertainty about the data $\boldsymbol{y}$ and the parameters $\boldsymbol{\theta}$, which we can factor as

$$p(\boldsymbol{y}, \boldsymbol{\theta}) = p(\boldsymbol{\theta})p(\boldsymbol{y} \mid \boldsymbol{\theta}) = p(\boldsymbol{y})p(\boldsymbol{\theta} \mid \boldsymbol{y}),$$

from which we can directly derive Bayes' theorem

$$p(\boldsymbol{\theta} \mid \boldsymbol{y}) = \frac{p(\boldsymbol{y} \mid \boldsymbol{\theta})p(\boldsymbol{\theta})}{p(\boldsymbol{y})}. \tag{1.6}$$

The denominator in the right-hand side of Equation 1.6, the marginal distribution for the data

$$p(\boldsymbol{y}) = \int p(\boldsymbol{y} \mid \boldsymbol{\theta})p(\boldsymbol{\theta})d\boldsymbol{\theta}, \tag{1.7}$$

also referred to as *(prior) predictive distribution*, does not depend on $\boldsymbol{\theta}$ and can be seen as a normalising constant, ensuring that the left-hand side integrates to 1 (and so is a proper probability distribution).

For this reason, we can also rewrite Equation 1.6 as

$$p(\boldsymbol{\theta} \mid \boldsymbol{y}) \propto p(\boldsymbol{y} \mid \boldsymbol{\theta})p(\boldsymbol{\theta}) \propto \mathcal{L}(\boldsymbol{\theta} \mid \boldsymbol{y})p(\boldsymbol{\theta}),$$

where $\mathcal{L}(\boldsymbol{\theta} \mid \boldsymbol{y})$ is the *likelihood function* – this is derived from the sampling distribution, but taken as a function of the model parameters, for the fixed, observed value of the data (see Note 3). The posterior distribution is thus proportional to the product of the prior and the likelihood.

Note 3: Likelihood function

Sometimes, statistical texts tend to conflate the concept of *sampling distribution* $p(y \mid \theta)$ with that of *likelihood function* $\mathcal{L}(\theta \mid y)$, because these two functions are mathematically *similar*, since the latter is derived from the former. Nonetheless, they are not quite the same...

Consider, for instance, a model $y \sim \text{Normal}(\mu, \sigma)$, where the sampling distribution is defined as in Equation 1.4. Assume also, for simplicity, that the standard deviation is known and that the only relevant parameter is the mean μ; in this case, the likelihood function is defined with respect to μ only and every term in Equation 1.4 that does not depend on μ should be just dropped, leading to

$$\mathcal{L}(\mu \mid y, \sigma) = \exp\left(-\frac{1}{2\sigma^2}(y-\mu)^2\right)$$

(note that we cannot discard the scaling factor $1/\sigma^2$ inside the exponential, as this changes the shape of the likelihood function and thus affects the main parameter μ).

The likelihood function, in general, does not integrate to 1 (as does any proper sampling distribution) and thus, from a purely mathematical point of view, the two are just *not* the same – there are even more extreme cases in which the data are discrete and the parameter is continuous (see Equations 1.16 and 2.3, for instance).

For these reasons, the phrasing "Normal likelihood" is not really meaningful: the likelihood function derived from a model where the sampling distribution is described by a Normal distribution is just *not* the same as the Normal density. It depends on a different variable (for different known constants) and, in general, it has a different support.

1.2.1 The impact of the prior distribution

Generally speaking, the choice of the prior distribution may exert considerable impact on the inferential process. This is particularly true when the evidence provided by the observed data is non-definitive – examples include cases with limited follow-up or small sample sizes.

On the one hand, this is often seen as a critical part of a Bayesian analysis, because it is unsettling that, despite observing or using the exact same data, two researchers using widely different prior distributions may end up with substantially different inferences. However, on the other hand, this is not entirely surprising, in the case where the information provided by the data is limited – my prior distribution may lead to very different conclusions than yours, simply because we do not have enough in the data to converge towards a common assessment and so where we start from (our contextual background knowledge) does matter and the inference is strongly sensitive to that.

Example 1.2. *Two experts.* Consider a situation in which two experts are called upon to provide information about the population effectiveness of a particular health intervention. The first one (E_1) indicates that, in their considered opinion, the probability that a random individual is cured by receiving that intervention is around 20% and that if they had to provide some kind of range for this, their considered opinion would be between 5% and 40%, approximately.

The second expert (E_2) strongly disagrees and, in their considered opinion, the intervention is much more likely to work; E_2 estimates an average effectiveness around 80% and, if they were forced to provide a range of likely values, they would say something like 60% to 95%.

You, the Bayesian statistician, take this information and manage to translate it into two suitable prior distributions, $p_1(\theta)$ and $p_2(\theta)$. The underlying uncertainty is summarised in the top panel of Figure 1.5, which highlights the very different starting position of the two experts (how you actually map the assumptions to distributions is not important just yet, but we return to this in the next sections).

Imagine that we manage to observe a sample of $n_1 = 10$ individuals, representative of the target population and observe whether the intervention has an effect on them. As it happens, in the sample, $y_1 = 10$ actually have a positive response. You perform a Bayesian analysis and obtain the two posterior distributions in the middle panel of Figure 1.5, with which you revise your uncertainty – again, how you actually obtain the posteriors is not important, for now. As it is possible to see from the middle panel of Figure 1.5, the data do change the prior opinions to rather different extents: E_2 was probably more "calibrated" and their assessment is pretty much in the right "ball-park" as far as this first set of n_1 data is concerned; for E_1, the prior assessment was rather far from the evidence and yet the posterior gets pulled "in the right direction".

With very different prior opinions and little information in the data, the two experts still differ in their judgement, and E_1 is still not convinced that they may be wrong about this (it's probably a man...). To definitively resolve the question, you manage to obtain a very large sample of $n_2 = 200$ people, of which $y_2 = 186$ have a positive response – these new data are much more convincing. You replicate your analysis and produce a new set of posterior

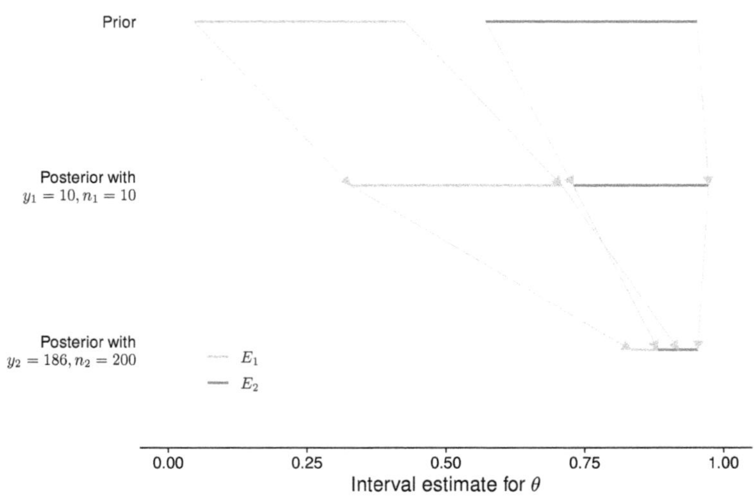

Figure 1.5: Even with very different starting points, the two experts become increasingly aligned in their (posterior) judgement by the effect of increasingly large and definitive evidence from the data.

distributions, shown in the bottom panel of Figure 1.5. Because of the very strong signal provided by the data, now the two experts have effectively coinciding opinions – the two intervals overlap.

As consistent evidence accrues pointing in the same direction, it matters less and less where the two experts were starting from: when modelled rationally through Bayesian updating, the posterior inference tends to coincide, given enough and consistent information coming from the data.

1.2.2 Including contextual information in the prior

As is perhaps obvious from Example 1.2, any form of prior distribution is in fact based on some *background* (contextual) information, available to the experimenter. We may indicate this (possibly qualitative, ideally quantitative) information as $\mathcal{B}$ and thus, the prior distribution should really be described as $p(\theta \mid \mathcal{B})$, which means that if data $\boldsymbol{y}$ become available, our uncertainty will be updated to

$$p(\boldsymbol{\theta} \mid \mathcal{B}, \boldsymbol{y}) = \frac{p(\boldsymbol{\theta} \mid \mathcal{B}) p(\boldsymbol{y} \mid \boldsymbol{\theta})}{p(\boldsymbol{y})}.$$

This notation clarifies that, to a Bayesian, everything is really conditional to whatever is the current state of science. In general, it is possible that $\mathcal{B}$ does contain very little information and therefore $p(\theta \mid \mathcal{B})$ is very vague and subject to a large variance/uncertainty. In that case, it is even more important to present substantial *sensitivity analysis* to assess the impact of choices in how the contextual knowledge is modelled on the inference process – although when the prior is vague, and the amount of information in $\boldsymbol{y}$ is large and consistent, it is

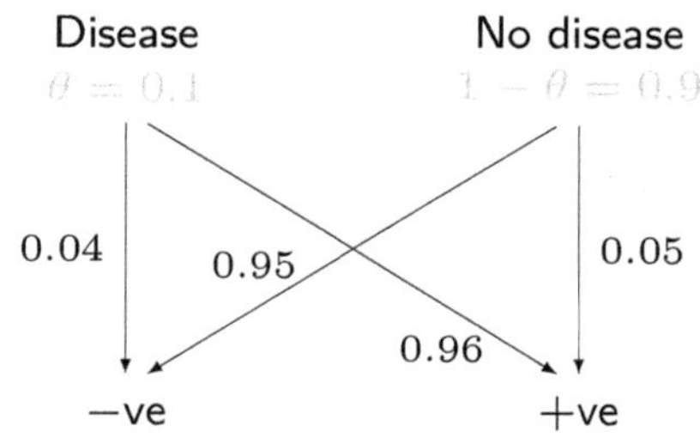

Figure 1.6: The data-generating process for Covid testing. The values of θ and $1 - \theta$ are greyed out to indicate that, in general, we may not know an exact value.

possible that it "supersedes" that included in $\mathcal{B}$ and so, for all intents and purposes, the posterior basically depends on $\boldsymbol{y}$ only (and it sort of "forgets" the input provided by the background, contextual information $\mathcal{B}$, as shown in Example 1.2).

In addition, the notation and discussion above clarify that, from a purely Bayesian perspective, we can *elicit* all sorts of information to construct the prior distribution: we may look at events for which there are masses of existing data and use these to form our prior; or, at the other end of the spectrum, base the prior solely on our subjective knowledge. Both are valid options, to a Bayesian. Whenever possible, of course, we should try and use "hard" evidence to form our prior (e.g. existing studies, registries, literature, etc.).

Notational quirks...

While the discussion above indicates that in reality we should always describe the prior as a conditional distribution, given the background knowledge $p(\theta \mid \mathcal{B})$, almost invariably we favour simplicity over pedantic completeness[2] and just write $p(\theta)$, thus dropping reference to $\mathcal{B}$ altogether.

Example 1.3. *Covid-19 testing.* Imagine that, for a dreadful moment, you are taken back to the Winter of 2020, in the midst of the second Covid-19 pandemic wave. You do not feel very well and so you decide to get tested. Given the evidence and knowledge $\mathcal{B}$ that, by then, was piling up, your doctor is able to consider the situation shown in Figure 1.6.

The assumptions encoded in the DAG are that

1. There is a 96% probability that, if you truly have Covid, your test will be positive.
2. There is a 95% probability that, if you do not have Covid, then you will test negative.

Given these assumptions, if your test comes up negative, there is fairly strong evidence against the hypothesis that the true status is "Disease" – this roughly implies a p–value of 0.04.

But how prevalent is Covid in the population, at the time of your test? Clearly, you should consider this contextual information when assessing the significance (in plain English, rather than in statistical parlance) of this result. One way to do it is to consider Bayes' theorem

[2]The author proudly acknowledges his very pedantic nature, nonetheless.

(adapting Equation 1.6) and combine the information from the data with our contextual knowledge

$$\Pr(\text{Disease} \mid \text{-ve}) = \frac{\Pr(\text{Disease}) \Pr(\text{-ve} \mid \text{Disease})}{\Pr(\text{-ve})},$$

where, by the law of total probabilities (of which Equation 1.7 is a generalisation),

$$\Pr(\text{-ve}) = \Pr(\text{Disease}) \Pr(\text{-ve} \mid \text{Disease}) + \Pr(\text{No disease}) \Pr(\text{-ve} \mid \text{No disease}).$$

Note that, as far as we are considering *events* (rather than random variables), Bayes' theorem is really not controversial at all – it is a simple application of the basic definitions for conditional probabilities, based on Kolmogorov's axioms (which are the cornerstone of the frequentist philosophy of probability too).

For example, suppose that from extensive surveys that were conducted at the time, the doctor is reasonably confident that $\Pr(\text{Disease}) = \theta \approx 0.1$. The evidence from the data alone tells us that the observed result is extremely unlikely under the hypothesis of "Disease"; but this is strongly dependent on the context, as provided by the prior knowledge/epistemic uncertainty, as shown in Figure 1.7.

As is obvious, if we assumed that $\theta = 0$ (which would mean that nobody has Covid, in the reference population), then the negative test would not be very exciting and the posterior probability would also be 0. Similarly, if everyone had Covid, even the negative result would not be able to cheer you up – your posterior probability of having Covid would still be 1, because everyone has it.

For any other possible value of the prior probability of the disease, then there is a gradation and the evidence provided by the negative test moves the prior to a very different posterior – for instance, if 80% of the population had Covid, the fact that you tested negative would still make your probability of having it too at around 14%. In the alleged situation where around 10% of the population has Covid, this means that *your* probability of also being infected, having tested negative, is around 0.0046 – much smaller (and fundamentally different in

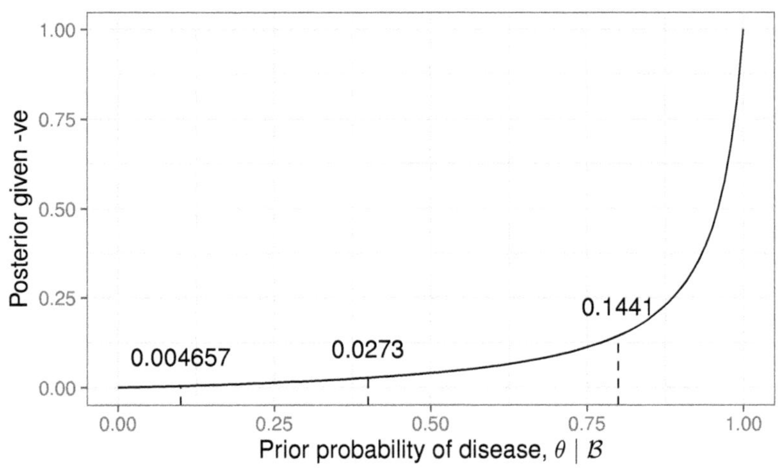

Figure 1.7: The relationship between the 'posterior' probability of disease given the negative result and the 'prior' probability of the disease given current knowledge, considering a range of possible values in [0; 1].

nature!) than the nominal p–value, without direct and explicit reference to the background information.

The discussion above also highlights the *cyclical* nature of Bayesian inference: we start from the contextual knowledge $\mathcal{B}$ to form our current state of uncertainty on some idealised feature of a DGP, $\boldsymbol\theta$, in terms of a prior distribution $p(\boldsymbol\theta \mid \mathcal{B})$. We then observe some data $\boldsymbol y$, which we are willing to assume as conforming with the alleged DGP described by $\boldsymbol\theta$ and use Bayes' theorem to update our state of knowledge to a posterior, which for simplicity we may indicate as $p(\boldsymbol\theta \mid \boldsymbol y)$ – again, dropping for simplicity the initial, background information $\mathcal{B}$, which by now may be much less influential, given the observation of $\boldsymbol y$.

We are not done, though; in fact, the process is only about to start over: this time, our current contextual/background information is described by $p(\boldsymbol\theta \mid \boldsymbol y)$. To put it like Lindley (1972), "*Today's posterior is tomorrow's prior*" and if we observe new data $\boldsymbol y^*$, the process will be repeated to obtain a new, updated posterior

$$p(\boldsymbol\theta \mid \boldsymbol y, \boldsymbol y^*) = \frac{p(\boldsymbol\theta \mid \boldsymbol y)p(\boldsymbol y^* \mid \boldsymbol\theta)}{p(\boldsymbol y^*)}.$$

1.2.3 "Natural"- vs "original"-scale parameters

For all the prominence given to the model parameters, in reality these are merely mathematical constructions that we are willing to "make up" to provide an easier description of a potentially very complicated DGP. In fact, a truly "hard-core" Bayesian would not really put so much emphasis on parameters and the prior/posterior distribution – what they would be really interested in is actually the *predictive* distribution of Equation 1.7.

In general terms, however, when we use a parametric model to describe a sampling distribution and thus a DGP, we make use of a mathematical formulation $p(\boldsymbol y \mid \boldsymbol\theta)$; typically, $\boldsymbol\theta$ represents a vector of **original**-scale parameters – these are used to index the mathematical function $p(\cdot)$. As an example, consider the Gamma distribution of Equation 1.2, which is defined as a function of a shape η and a rate λ. Neither of these parameters has a special physical meaning – they are just quantities we make up to create a functional form that is good enough to describe the DGP we have in mind (a positive, continuous, skewed variable).

In some other cases, the parameters $\boldsymbol\theta$ are much easier to interpret: for instance, in the case of a variable whose sampling distribution is modelled using the Normal distribution of Equation 1.4, the vector of parameters $\boldsymbol\theta = (\mu, \sigma)$ has a very clear and direct interpretation as the mean and the standard deviation. These quantities are original-scale parameters, ensuring that the mathematical properties of the resulting density function align with the assumptions we want to encode (symmetry, unbounded range, continuous support). But they also have the role of **natural**-scale parameters, because they have a direct physical interpretation of which we can make sense.

Interestingly, in essentially all parametric models we encounter, it is possible to relate the original- to the natural-scale parameters: for example, in the Normal case, they coincide, as mentioned above; in the Gamma case, we can use the mathematical properties of the Gamma density and derive that if $y \sim \text{Gamma}(\nu, \gamma)$, then

$$\text{E}[Y] = \mu = \frac{\nu}{\gamma} \qquad \text{and} \qquad \text{Var}[Y] = \sigma^2 = \frac{\nu}{\gamma^2},$$

which implies, using simple algebra, that

$$\gamma = \frac{\mu}{\sigma^2} \qquad \text{and} \qquad \nu = \frac{\mu^2}{\sigma^2}. \tag{1.8}$$

This consideration is very helpful when trying to elicit genuine information $\mathcal{B}$ to form a prior distribution: it may be very awkward to think in terms of shape and rate (of which we would most likely struggle to make sense, from a physical point of view); but it may be much simpler to think in terms of the question

> *What do we know/can we expect as the most likely value for the mean and standard deviation of the variable Y, given current/contextual/background information?*

But if we can derive a relationship such as that of Equation 1.8 (which, in general, we can) between the original- and natural-scale parameters, then we can define a prior for the natural-scale parameters and then derive the implied prior for the original-scale parameters.

1.2.4 Monte Carlo simulation

Mapping a probability distribution from one scale to another is often possible *analytically*, i.e. we can work out the mathematical relationship and determine the exact form of the required distribution for any re-parameterisation in which we are interested. In many other cases, this is either too complicated or even impossible; however, we can still resort to *numerical* approximation – the most popular option is to use *Monte Carlo* simulations.

Inference by simulation

Using simulation methods to perform inferential tasks is *not* a purely Bayesian feature. In a frequentist/maximum likelihood approach, we can still use simulations, e.g. bootstrap (Efron and Tibshirani, 1994) to approximate interval estimates or evaluate the "long-run" properties of specific estimators. This is very popular also in health technology assessment: see Section 4.3.

Arguably, though, in the last 30 years or so, inference by simulations has become ubiquitous especially within a Bayesian context and has fundamentally contributed to its applicability and success.

The main idea is that if we are able to simulate a large number of values from a probability distribution, then we can use these simulations to summarise it; for instance, the mean of a continuous random variable Y defined on the range $\mathcal{Y}$ is computed as the integral

$$\text{E}[Y] = \int_{\mathcal{Y}} yp(y \mid \theta)dy.$$

When this is too complicated, or does not have a closed form solution, or simply we cannot be bothered to sit down and "do the maths"[3], we can approximate this integral by simulating a large number S of values from $p(y \mid \theta)$, say $y^{(1)}, \ldots, y^{(S)}$ and then use these to compute

$$\text{E}[Y] \approx \sum_{s=1}^{S} \frac{y^{(s)}}{S}.$$

[3]This is a luxury we can now enjoy, given that computing power is essentially very cheap. Before the advent of widely available personal computers in the 1980s and 1990s, especially, the "*I can't be bothered to do this integral*" consideration was much less of an option...

Pseudo-random number generator

R has built-in commands to draw pseudo-random numbers – typically these are constructed using the prefix r (for "random") and a string of text describing the distribution (e.g. norm for "Normal", unif for "Uniform", bin for "Binomial", etc.).

The first argument (input) to a call to a rxxxx(...) command is the number of values we want to simulate. Thus, for instance, rnorm(1000,0,6) instructs R to simulate 1000 values from a Normal distribution with mean 0 and standard deviation 6.

In fact, given the sample of Monte Carlo (MC) simulations $y^{(1)}, \ldots, y^{(S)}$, we can use them to summarise *any* feature of the underlying distribution, in the form of a given function $g(y)$ – provided we have enough simulations, so as to reduce the approximation error. For instance, we can use the sample (simulated) quantiles to give an indication of interval estimates, as the following R code demonstrates.

```
# Simulates a sample of S values from y ~ Normal(0,1)
S=100000
y=rnorm(S,0,1)

# Computes the 2.5%  and 97.5% quantile; these are the points y_{0.025} and
# y_{0.975} such that Pr(Y<=y_{0.025})=0.025 and Pr(Y<=y_{0.975})=0.975
quantile(y,c(0.025,0.975))
```

```
     2.5%     97.5%
-1.969646  1.970057
```

The accuracy (or the "Monte Carlo error") of the estimate depends, obviously, on the sample size, as highlighted in Figure 1.8: if we only sample $S = 10$ values from a Normal(0, 1), then the approximation to the analytic quantiles (−1.959964 and 1.959964) is pretty coarse, due to the sampling variability intrinsic in the process. However, increasingly large MC samples get closer and closer to the "true" values – in many circumstances, 1000 MC samples are enough, but this varies and the choice of the number of simulations usually requires some care (see Section 2.3.2). Having a running series of results, as in Figure 1.8 is often very helpful to assess the "stability" of the simulation process – when continuing to increase S does not vary substantially the overall estimate, we can be fairly confident about the results.

Back to the example introduced in Section 1.2.3, if, perhaps using some background knowledge about the likely ranges of the mean and standard deviation for the underlying variable, we set the priors on the natural-scale as $\mu \sim \text{log-Normal}(5.2, 0.2)$ and $\sigma \sim \text{Exponential}(0.35)$, where, in general,

$$y \sim \text{log-Normal}(\eta, \lambda) \qquad \Rightarrow \qquad p(y \mid \eta, \lambda) = \frac{1}{y\sqrt{2\pi\lambda^2}} \exp\left(-\frac{(\log y - \eta)^2}{2\lambda^2}\right) \tag{1.9}$$

and

$$y \sim \text{Exponential}(\theta) \qquad \Rightarrow \qquad p(y \mid \theta) = \theta \exp\left(-\theta y\right), \tag{1.10}$$

we can then use MC simulation to derive the implied priors on the original-scale parameters (η, λ), for instance using the following R code.

```
# Loads relevant packages
library(tibble)  # management of datasets
library(ggplot2) # graphs
```

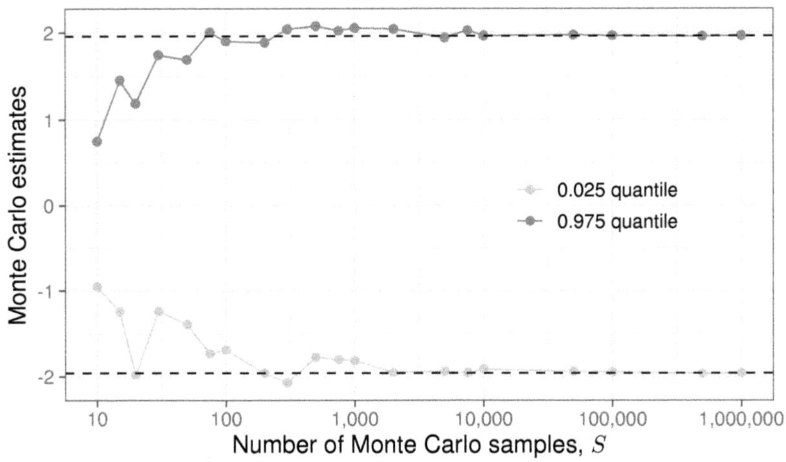

Figure 1.8: Monte Carlo approximation of the 2.5% and 97.5% percentiles of a Normal(0,1) distribution. Increasing number of MC samples improves the accuracy and, effectively, reduces the approximation error to virtually nothing. The dashed horizontal lines indicate the analytic values for the 2.5% and the 97.5% quantiles of the standard Normal distribution.

```
# Simulate values from the prior on the *natural* parameters
mu=rlnorm(10000,5.2,.2)
sigma=rexp(10000,.35)

# Transform the prior for the *original scale* parameters
gamma=sqrt(mu/sigma^2)
nu=mu*gamma

# Plots the resulting prior for eta and lambda
tibble(nu) |> ggplot(aes(nu)) + geom_density()
tibble(gamma) |> ggplot(aes(gamma)) + geom_density()
```

Piping and tidyverse

The code above is fairly simple, but includes a couple of important features that are used throughout the book. In particular, the function `tibble` (from its namesake package, Müller and Wickham, 2025) can be used to construct a modern version of a data frame – in this case we store the variables `nu` and `gamma` using this format.

In the code above (and again throughout the book) we also use the "native pipe" operator `|>`, which applies the code to its right to the object defined to its left – i.e. `x |> mean()` is equivalent to `mean(x)`.

Finally, we use the package `ggplot2` (Wickham, 2016) and its functions `ggplot()` and `geom_density()` to generate the plots shown in Figure 1.9.

Packages such as `dplyr` (Wickham et al., 2023), `tibble` and `ggplot2` are part of the `tidyverse` (Wickham et al., 2019), a collection of tools designed for data science, all built around the principles of tidy data and a consistent, user-friendly syntax.

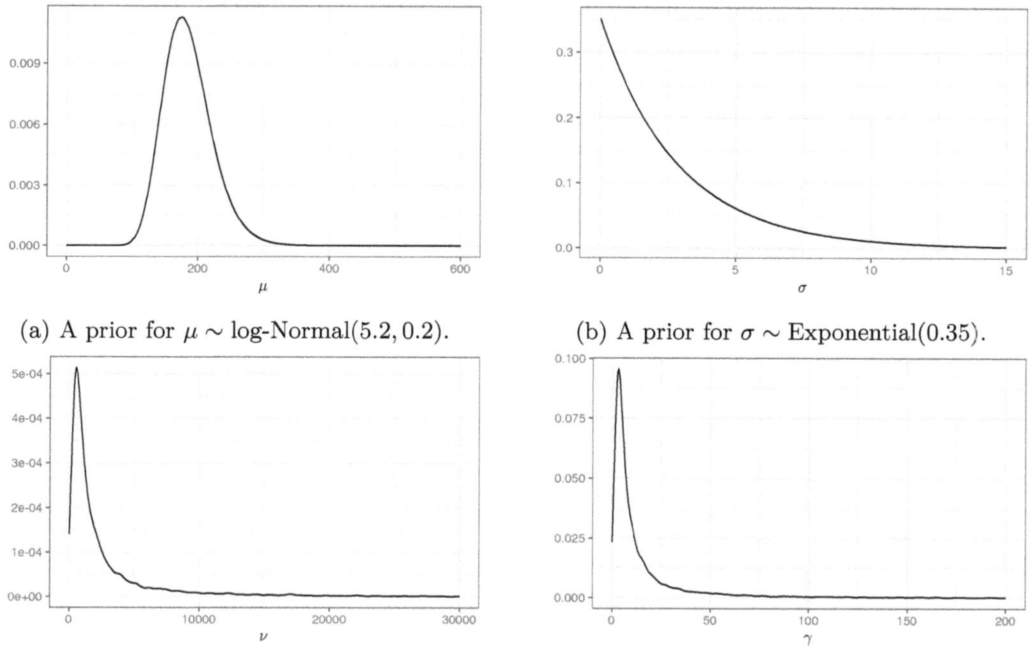

(a) A prior for $\mu \sim \text{log-Normal}(5.2, 0.2)$.

(b) A prior for $\sigma \sim \text{Exponential}(0.35)$.

(c) The implied prior for $\nu = \mu\gamma$.

(d) The implied prior for $\gamma = \sqrt{\frac{\mu}{\sigma^2}}$.

Figure 1.9: Deriving (prior) distributions on different scales, using Monte Carlo simulations.

> Installing and loading `tidyverse` allows the user to access all of these packages, which can however also be installed and loaded independently, as we do in the code above.

In a sense, it does not matter what the resulting prior is for ν and γ – we want the contextual information to make sense on the scale that we can think about in the first instance (μ, σ). In fact, we probably do not know the close form of the resulting prior for (ν, γ), but we do not need this, as long as we can sample from $p(\nu)$ and $p(\gamma)$, which we can, using MC simulations.

Example 1.4. *Drug (adapted and expanded from Spiegelhalter et al., 2004).* Consider a drug that is being developed to reduce back pain. Even before we get to see any data from actual experimentation, we may have some contextual, background evidence $\mathcal{B}$ to inform our "guess" at the drug's effectiveness, indicated as θ, i.e. the probability that a random individual taking the drug manages to control their back pain. We may use expert opinion (e.g. the team of experimenters' knowledge about the biology and pharmacodynamics of the molecule being tested), but also "hard" evidence, for instance obtained from population registers looking at the performance of existing drugs based on the same active principle, or small/pilot studies conducted by the company who are developing the drug.

For example, imagine that the experimenters are convinced that this particular drug is likely to be effective in combating back pain within a 20% to 60% range. The role of the statistician is to map this particular prior *information* into a suitable prior *distribution*.

We could interpret the prior information that "*most of the probability mass lies between 0.2 and 0.6*" by assuming that this basically identifies a symmetrical interval around the mean of the distribution, including something like 95% of the mass to mean "most of the probability". Then, using some basic Normal theory, at least approximately, we can reasonably assume that

$$\mu - 2\sigma = 0.2; \qquad \mu + 2\sigma = 0.6; \qquad \text{and} \qquad \mu = \frac{0.6 + 0.2}{2} = 0.4,$$

from which we can derive $\sigma = 0.1$.

There are of course many ways to encode this knowledge into a suitable prior distribution for θ. Just as an example, we may start by considering a probability model that fits the physical properties of the parameter of interest: because θ represents a probability (the proportion of people who will be relieved from back pain if taking the drug), then we know that it must take on values in the interval $[0; 1]$.

This consideration can help us select a suitable model – in this case, a natural candidate is the Beta distribution, which is defined in the range $(0, 1)$ by a density

$$p(\theta \mid a, b) = \frac{\Gamma(a+b)}{\Gamma(a)\Gamma(b)}\, \theta^{a-1}(1-\theta)^{b-1}, \tag{1.11}$$

where the mean and the variance are defined as

$$\mu = \frac{a}{a+b} \qquad \text{and} \qquad \sigma^2 = \frac{ab}{(a+b)^2(a+b+1)}. \tag{1.12}$$

Back-solving for a, b, we can derive

$$a = \mu\left(\frac{(1-\mu)\mu}{\sigma^2} - 1\right) \qquad \text{and} \qquad b = (1-\mu)\left(\frac{(1-\mu)\mu}{\sigma^2} - 1\right). \tag{1.13}$$

Setting $\mu = 0.4$ and $\sigma = 0.1$ and plugging these values in Equation 1.13 yields $a = 9.2$ and $b = 13.8$. In other words, at least approximately, a Beta$(a = 9.2, b = 13.8)$ implies that most of its mass is included in the interval $[0.2; 0.6]$ and that the mean is around 0.4. We can check this using Monte Carlo simulation, as with the following R code.

```
# Defines the number of simulations
nsim = 10000

# Then defines the prior distribution for theta
alpha = 9.2
beta = 13.8
theta = rbeta(n=nsim, shape1=alpha, shape2=beta)
```

The package bmhe (which is available from the GitHub repository at https://github.com/giabaio/bmhe_utils) provides a number of utility functions to process the output of Bayesian simulations. To install the package (which we will use throughout the book), it is possible to use either of the following commands:

```
# Installs the package 'remotes', that can be used to download packages
# off a GitHub repository (only need to run this command once)
install.packages(remotes)
# Uses 'remotes' to install the package from GitHub
remotes::install_github("giabaio/bmhe_utils")
```

```
# Or via the alternative repository at https://giabaio.r-universe.dev/
install.packages(
  "bmhe",
  repos=c("https://giabaio.r-universe.dev","https://cloud.r-project.org")
)
```

Note 4: Exposing functions and installing packages in `R`

In `R`, the easiest way to "expose" a function from a package, say `pkg`, is simply to load the package in the workspace, which we can do by typing `library(pkg)` on the `R` terminal (assuming of course that `pkg` is installed on the machine we are using, as done in the code shown in the previous section). This ensures that all the functions made available by `pkg` can be called and used in the curent `R` session.

In the code above, we use the alternative `R` notation `pkg::func()`, which means "use the function `func()` from the package `pkg`, without directly loading it. Thus, again assuming that `pkg` is already installed on the user's machine, this command allows to use the function `func()` but gives no direct access to all the other functions that are part of `pkg`.

In particular, the code above instructs `R` to install the package `bmhe` using the function `install_github()` from the package `remotes` (Csárdi et al., 2024). On the one hand, this is very handy because it allows the user to install packages directly from a GitHub repository. However, on the other hand, using the alternative route via the `r-universe` repository allows the flexibility of simply running basic `R` commands such as `install.packages()` and `update.packages()` to integrate this process and management in the normal workflow and thus, for this reason, we recommend it.

Once `bmhe` is installed, we can then use its function `stats()` to summarise the prior distribution

```
# Produces summary statistics for the prior
bmhe::stats(theta)
```

```
      mean         sd       2.5%     median      97.5%
0.40314978 0.09979373 0.21729833 0.40024981 0.60306573
```

and we can also visualise the prior in the form of a histogram, as in Figure 1.10.

As we can see both visually and numerically, most of the mass is between around 20% and 60% (we already knew this – it was the reason why we set up this particular Beta prior). We can also specify prior probabilities associated to specific cut-off points: for example, it may be clinically relevant to report $\Pr(\theta > 0.5)$, which we can easily compute using the simulations from the prior, stored in the vector `theta`:

```
sum(theta>0.5)/length(theta)
```

```
[1] 0.1742
```

(note the use of the built-in function `length()` to characterise the number of values included in the vector `theta`, which is of course identical to the variable `nsim`).

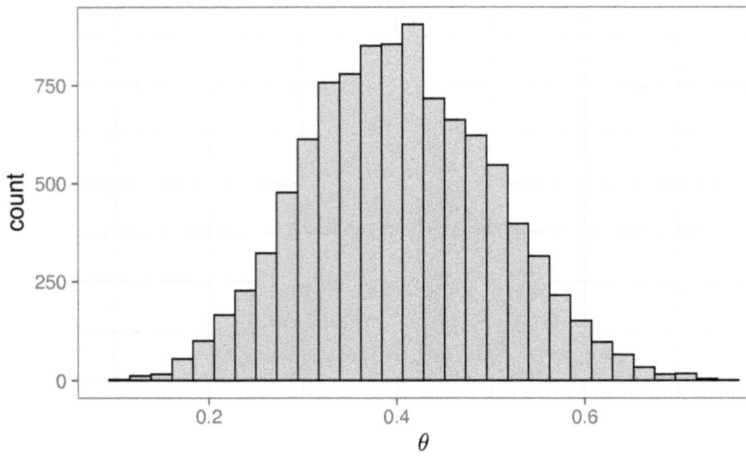

Figure 1.10: A histogram describing the Monte Carlo simulations from a Beta(9.2, 13.8) distribution. As is possible to see, the distribution is roughly speaking centred around 0.4 and most values are included in the interval [0.2; 0.6], as required.

1.2.5 Prior information vs prior distribution

As mentioned in Example 1.4, there is a fundamental distinction between the unique prior *information* that is available to us and the many ways in which we can decide to map it onto a prior probability *distribution*.

For example, we may decide to map the fact that "*more or less 95% of the distribution lies between 0.2 and 0.6*" onto a Beta($a = 9.2, b = 13.8$) distribution, as discussed in Example 1.4. Or: we may decide that it is easier for us to work with Normal distributions – of course applying a Normal distribution to describe a variable that is, by definition, constrained in the $[0; 1]$ interval is not fully appropriate. However, we may first transform the original parameter θ to the $(-\infty; \infty)$ range, e.g. using the logit function and then use a suitable Normal distribution to describe our uncertainty on the logit scale:

$$\phi = \text{logit}(\theta) := \log\left(\frac{\theta}{1-\theta}\right) \sim \text{Normal}(m, s).$$

We can use trial-and-error or some simple algebra to derive values for (m, s) so that the resulting distribution effectively matches the available information; for instance, setting

$$\begin{aligned} m &= \text{logit}(\mu) \\ &= \log\left(\frac{0.4}{1-0.4}\right) = -0.405 \end{aligned}$$

and

$$\begin{aligned} s &= \frac{\text{logit}(\mu+2\sigma) - \text{logit}(\mu)}{z_{0.05}} \\ &= \frac{\text{logit}(0.6) - \text{logit}(0.4)}{1.96} = 0.4137, \end{aligned}$$

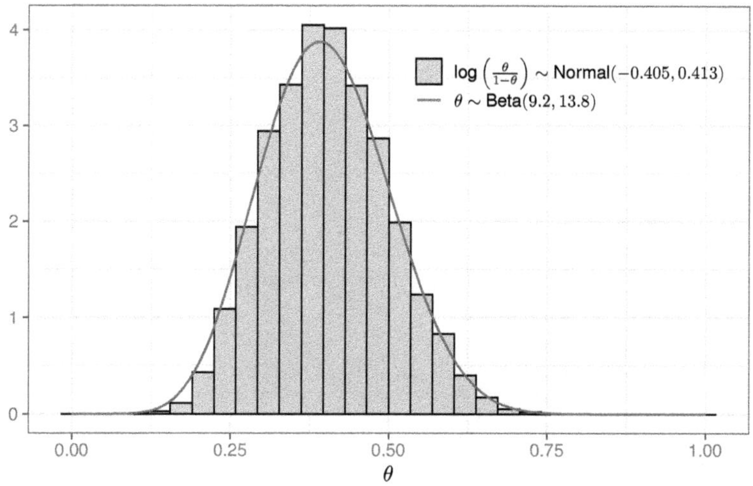

Figure 1.11: The prior *information* indicates that most of the mass for the parameter θ should be contained between 0.2 and 0.6, which can be encoded into two different prior *distributions*: the curve shows a Beta$(9, 2, 13.8)$, while the histogram shows a Normal$(-0.4, 0.413)$ on the logit scale. For all intents and purposes, the two are effectively identical.

where $z_{0.975}$ is the point in a standard Normal distribution leaving 0.975 to its left[4], effectively implies a distribution that, when rescaled to the natural $[0; 1]$ range is, for all intents and purposes, identical with the Beta$(9.2, 13.8)$ prior discussed above (see Figure 1.11). Thus,

$$\phi \sim \text{Normal}(-0.405, 0.4137) \Rightarrow \text{logit}^{-1}(\phi) = \frac{\exp(\phi)}{1 + \exp(\phi)} = \theta \approx \text{Beta}(9.2, 13.8)$$

and we can use either distributional choices (a Normal on the logit scale, or a Beta on the natural scale) to encode the available prior information.

Change of variable

We can actually determine the analytic form of the implied distribution for θ, starting from modelling $\phi = \text{logit}(\theta) \sim \text{Normal}(\mu, \sigma)$, by using a mathematical process, often described as "*change of support variable*" rule.

In general, if $x \sim p_X(x)$ and $y = f(x)$, which obviously implies that $x = f^{-1}(y)$, then we can derive the distribution on the scale of y as

$$\begin{aligned} p_Y(y) &= p_X(x) \left| \frac{\partial f^{-1}(y)}{\partial y} \right| \\ &= p_X\left(f^{-1}(y)\right) \left| \frac{\partial f^{-1}(y)}{\partial y} \right|, \end{aligned} \tag{1.14}$$

where in general the notation $\partial f(x)/\partial x$ indicates the first derivative of a function $f(\cdot)$ with respect to the variable x.

[4]This result derives from basic standard Normal theory and assuming that the interval $[\text{logit}(\mu - 2\sigma); \text{logit}(\mu + 2\sigma)]$ covers 95% of the entire probability mass. See also Example 9.2 for another example of this type of computation.

In the specific case discussed above, we have $\phi \sim \text{Normal}(\mu, \sigma)$ for set values $\mu = -0.405$ and $\sigma = 0.4137$ and

$$\theta = f(\phi) = \frac{\exp(\phi)}{1+\exp(\phi)},$$

which implies that

$$\phi = f^{-1}(\theta) = \log\left(\frac{\theta}{1-\theta}\right) = \log(\theta) - \log(1-\theta)$$

and thus

$$\begin{aligned}\left|\frac{\partial f^{-1}(\theta)}{\partial\theta}\right| &= \left|\frac{\partial \log(\theta) - \log(1-\theta)}{\partial\theta}\right| \\ &= \left|\frac{1}{\theta} + \frac{1}{1-\theta}\right| = \left|\frac{1}{\theta(1-\theta)}\right|.\end{aligned}$$

Applying Equation 1.14, we then get

$$\begin{aligned}p_\theta(\theta) &= p_\phi(f^{-1}(\theta))\left|\frac{1}{\theta(1-\theta)}\right| \\ &= \underbrace{\frac{1}{\sqrt{2\pi}\sigma}\exp\left(-\frac{1}{2}\frac{(\text{logit}(\theta)-\mu)^2}{\sigma^2}\right)}_{\text{Normal density computed at } \phi=\text{logit}(\theta)}\left|\frac{1}{\theta(1-\theta)}\right|, \qquad (1.15)\end{aligned}$$

which we write compactly as $\theta \sim \text{logit-Normal}(\mu, \sigma)$.

We can code this computation up in a small R function

```
dlogitnorm=function(x,mu,sigma) {
  dnorm(log(x/(1-x)),mu,sigma)*abs(1/(x*(1-x)))
}
```

that we can use to determine the value of the logit-Normal density for any input `x` $\in [0; 1]$. Notice that, consistently with Equation 1.15, in the function `dlogitnorm()` the argument `x` is used to compute the Normal density *at its logit*, through the built-in R function `dnorm()`, whose first argument is transformed to `log(x/(1-x))`.

As an example, we can check that running in R the following commands

```
dlogitnorm(0.4,-0.405,0.413)
```

```
[1] 4.024839
```

```
dbeta(0.4,9.2,13.8)
```

```
[1] 3.86089
```

would return near identical values for the density computed at $\theta = 0.4$ for the two models.

More specifically, we can use the custom and built-in functions `dlogitnorm()` and `dbeta()` to compute the densities for a grid of θ values in $[0; 1]$ and then visualise the two resulting distributions, as in Figure 1.12. These are effectively identical (which is obviously aligned with the graph based on the histogram of Figure 1.11).

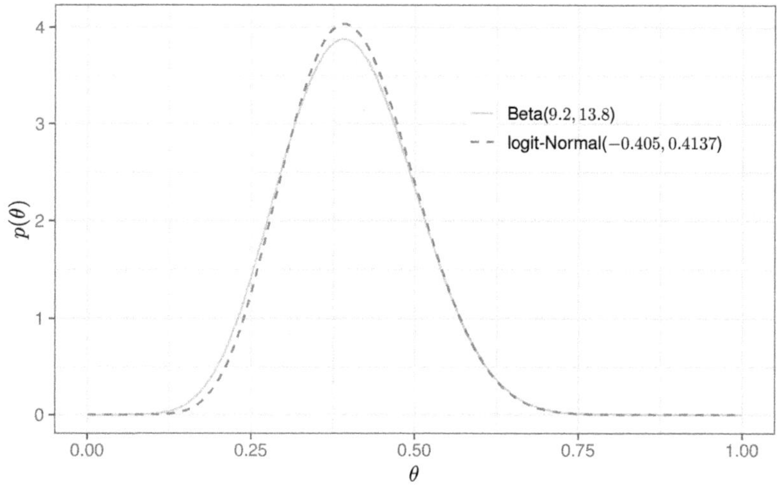

Figure 1.12: Comparison on the Beta and the logit-Normal distributions for θ.

1.2.6 Propagating uncertainty via Monte Carlo simulation ("forward sampling")

One consequence of working within a Bayesian environment is that we can use the prior distribution (which describes our current level of uncertainty on the model inputs, i.e. the parameters) to formally propagate onto the model outcomes, i.e. potentially observable data.

This is relevant, perhaps, at the stage of planning for a new study, when we make assumptions about the alleged DGP *and* the current state of science on its features to determine what we may be reasonably expect to observe if we managed to actually collect relevant data. In a Bayesian context, this effectively amount to estimating the (prior) predictive distribution (see Equation 1.7).

Example 1.5. *Drug (continued): forward sampling.* Consider again the situation described in Example 1.4; we have not obtained any data on actual patients taking the drug, yet; however, we can think of a suitable model to represent the sampling variability that the data would be subject to, if we were able to collect them.

For example, it may be reasonable to consider a possible study in which we observe $n = 20$ individuals suffering of back pain to whom we give the drug (the sample size $n = 20$ is totally arbitrary here and we could, in principle, select any number we can afford to recruit).

Assuming that the main outcome is y, the total number of individuals who, upon taking the drug are relieved from the pain, we can use a Binomial distribution to model the sampling variability. This is defined by the probability distribution

$$p(y \mid \theta) = \left(\begin{array}{c} n \\ y \end{array} \right) \theta^y \, (1-\theta)^{n-y}. \tag{1.16}$$

Starting from the Monte Carlo sample of values from the prior $p(\theta)$, which we have obtained in Example 1.4, we can now simulate `nsim` hypothetical, or "virtual" trials, by sampling `y` from its distribution and propagating "forward" the uncertainty over `theta`.

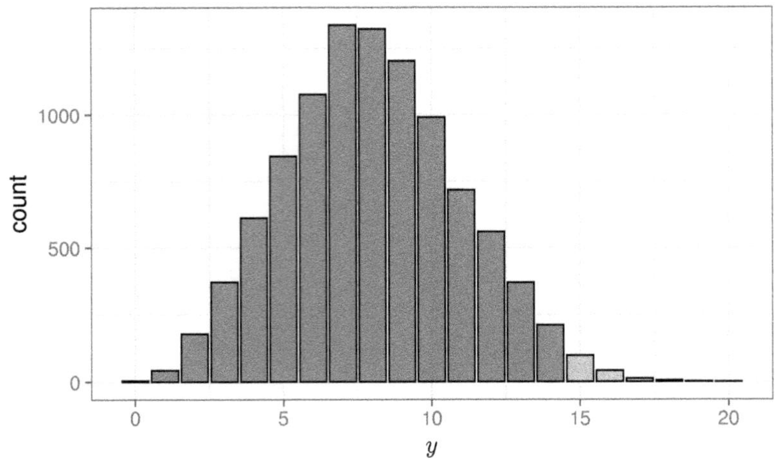

Figure 1.13: The (prior) predictive distribution $p(y)$. The bars in lighter colour indicate the "tail area probability" that the observed results would exceed the threshold set at least 15 successes out of 20 individuals.

```
# Simulates from the (prior) predictive distribution of 'y'
y=rbinom(n=nsim,size=20,prob=theta)
```

(the parameters of the R function `rbinom()` are the number of simulations `n`, the sample size for each experiment, `size` and the probability of success, `prob`). Again, the actual number of simulations is entirely arbitrary; we may choose `nsim`=1000, just to fix the ideas.

This process basically "mixes up" the uncertainty in `theta` (as expressed by the simulations generated above) with the variability inherent to the sampling process for possible values of `y`, generated by the use of the function `rbinom()`. We can also record, for each simulated trial (i.e. each row of the vector `y`), whether the value drawn is greater than a specific threshold (say, 14 successes) in the variable `P.crit`.

```
P.crit=(y>=15)
```

(note that we can define the "strictly greater than 14" condition as either `y>14` or `y>=15`).

The resulting predictive distribution for y can be visualised as in Figure 1.13. The bars in lighter colouring indicate exceedance of the threshold, set at 15 or more successes – this may be derived by clinical or economic considerations (e.g. the trial would actually make sense if at least 15 individuals out of 20 benefitted from the treatment).

We can also use `bmhe::stats()` to give us a numerical summary of the distributions for `y`, `P.crit` and `theta`.

```
# Binds the vectors 'P.crit', 'y' and 'theta' into columns of a matrix
sims = cbind(P.crit,y,theta)
# Runs bmhe::stats to summarise the simulations
bmhe::stats(sims)
```

```
              mean        sd      2.5%    median     97.5%
P.crit 0.0158000 0.1247073 0.0000000 0.0000000  0.000000
y      8.0175000 2.9632873 3.0000000 8.0000000 14.000000
theta  0.4018231 0.1002008 0.2172574 0.3984317  0.603672
```

If we were actually conducting a trial, we would be expecting to observe an average of around 8 patients cured by the drug. It is unlikely that we would see a much bigger result, say above 14, which is the 97.5%-quantile of the distribution for y. Consequently, the value for P_{crit} is, on average, very small (as apparent from Figure 1.13 too).

Obviously, the distribution of θ is the same as in the prior – there is nothing in our set up with which to update it (i.e. we have not yet observed any data) and so our uncertainty about θ cannot be updated, just yet.

1.3 Conclusions

In this chapter we have introduced the philosophical underpinning of Bayesian reasoning and have started to explore how Bayesian computation can include contextual information into the inference. We have started to discuss the mapping of background knowledge and information into a suitable prior distribution and use the process of forward sampling to propagate uncertainty to the model.

In the next chapter, we will look into using observed data to update the current uncertainty over unobserved and unobservable quantities. We will discuss more specifically different ways of defining the prior distributions and explore the basics of Bayesian computation, specifically in terms of Markov Chain Monte Carlo algorithms.

2

Learning from data: Bayesian computation

2.1 Introduction

In Chapter 1 we have considered the main features of Bayesian reasoning and have used Monte Carlo simulations to elicit and manipulate the prior distribution, as well as to propagate the uncertainty in the model parameters onto possible future data, which we have not observed yet, but may be able to do so.

For all intents and purposes, the process of "forward sampling" (see Section 1.2.6) is already fundamentally Bayesian, because it starts with the premise that we are able to map our current epistemic uncertainty on unobservable features of our model through a probability distribution. It is not, however, the full realisation of the Bayesian paradigm, because so far we have not actually used observed data to update our current state of uncertainty on the model parameters – effectively running the process of Bayesian inference from observed data.

To this aim, in this chapter we explore the fundamentals of Bayesian computations as applied to the process of learning from data. We start by considering various choices for the prior distribution; following somewhat the historical patterns that have characterised Bayesian modelling, we start by looking at so-called "vague" priors and the related inferential process. We then consider "conjugate" models, as a slightly less restrictive mode of inference, to then move onto Markov Chain Monte Carlo methods – these have effectively freed up Bayesian computation and rendered it widely applicable, thus constituting a real revolution in statistical modelling.

2.2 Choice of prior distributions

The best way to set a prior distribution is to elicit existing, contextual information (see Section 1.2.2) and to carefully assess the properties of the DGP – for instance, considering whether there is a set of physical properties we need to render with the prior (bounded vs unbounded range, continuous vs discrete, etc.).

In some circumstances, however, we can try and use some "default" priors – these have been historically designed to somehow automate the process of Bayesian inference. They have many merits and should be understood carefully – although, in general, we may be able to do better...

DOI: 10.1201/9781003771050-2

2.2.1 "Vague" priors

To remove some of the sensitivity to the choice of prior (especially in cases where the data do not provide definitive evidence), it is possible to select a distribution that exerts the least amount of impact on the final inference. This type of prior is often referred to as "non-informative" or "vague" and the basic idea is to use a distribution that has a large variance, so as to span more or less uniformly across the entire range of the underlying variable.

A classical example of the use of "vague" priors comes from the work of Pierre Simone Laplace, the French scholar and polymath who is credited to have independently discovered Bayesian modelling (Laplace, 1774, 1812) – see Note 2 in Section 1.2. In one of his many applied contributions, Laplace's research question was about the probability that a new born would be a boy and to investigate this he used data including $y = 241\,945$ females out of $n = 493\,527$ babies born and Christened in Paris between 1745 and 1770, with the following modelling assumptions:

$$\begin{aligned} y &\sim \text{Binomial}(\theta, n) \\ \theta &\sim \text{Uniform}(0, 1) \end{aligned}$$

– note that in general for a variable y and constants (a, b)

$$y \sim \text{Uniform}(a, b) \qquad \Rightarrow \qquad p(y \mid a, b) = \frac{1}{b-a}. \tag{2.1}$$

The choice of a Uniform prior over the entire range of the model parameter θ was justified by Laplace on the grounds that he had no real information and so every possible value for θ should be equally likely (the *principle of insufficient reason*)[1].

More importantly, choosing a Uniform prior simplifies the computation of the posterior, because $p(\theta) = c$ (for some positive constant) and thus

$$p(\theta \mid y) = \frac{p(\theta)p(y \mid \theta)}{p(y)} \propto \frac{c\mathcal{L}(\theta \mid y)}{c\int \mathcal{L}(\theta \mid y)d\theta} \propto \frac{\mathcal{L}(\theta \mid y)}{\int \mathcal{L}(\theta \mid y)d\theta}, \tag{2.2}$$

i.e. the posterior is proportional to the (rescaled) likelihood function, with essentially no impact of the prior distribution. By using a Uniform prior, Laplace was able to compute analytically the posterior distribution, "simply" by solving an integral calculation. For this reason, vague or Uniform priors have been, historically, the first form of Bayesian modelling (because they would allow the full computation of the posterior distribution in a reasonably wide range of applied cases).

Example 2.1. *Drug (continued): Uniform prior.* The analysis of Example 1.5 can be replicated by changing the prior for θ to a Uniform(0,1) distribution, using the following `R` code. This is fundamentally different from the Beta used before, as shown in Figure 2.1.

```
# Constructs a tibble with the density for the Beta and Uniform priors
# and a range of values from 0 to 1 for the x-axis
priors=tibble(
  theta=seq(from=0, to=1, by=.001),
  p1=dbeta(seq(0,1,.001),9.2,13.8),
```

[1]Interestingly, Fienberg (2006) notes that the principle of insufficient reason was not the one guiding Bayes in his original formulation, which was rather based on physical properties of the marginal distribution for the observed data.

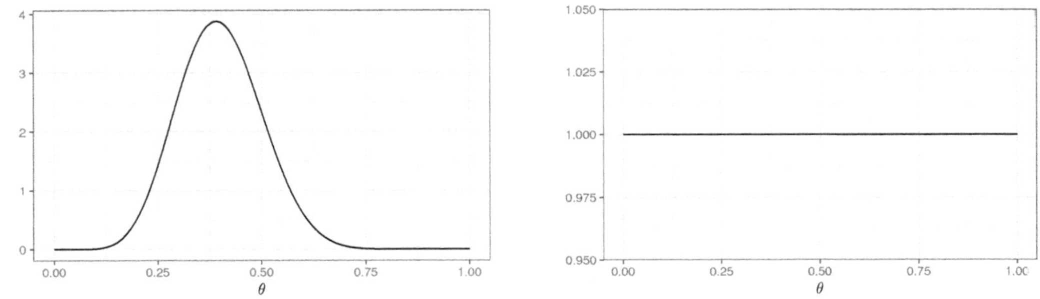

(a) $\theta \sim \text{Beta}(9.2, 13.8)$. (b) $\theta \sim \text{Uniform}(0, 1)$.

Figure 2.1: Two different versions for the prior distribution of θ.

```
  p2=dunif(seq(0,1,.001),0,1)
)
# Plots the densities
priors |> ggplot(aes(theta,p1)) + geom_line()
priors |> ggplot(aes(theta,p2)) + geom_line()
```

Visualising (different choices for) the prior distributions is always a good idea to understand what we are actually implying with the modelling assumptions we use. In this case, the Beta prior would be much more concentrated around the mean of 0.4, while the Uniform would imply a much larger range of plausible values. The latter may be considered as a "lazy" option – we can use it knowing that its natural range (the interval [0,1]) is reasonable for the underlying parameter (because θ is a probability); but we are basically saying that we do not know anything whatsoever about the possibility that the drug is actually good. We most likely have *much* more information than this...

In any case, we can replicate the Monte Carlo analysis using both the Beta and the Uniform prior

```
# Simulates from the two priors for 'theta', Beta(9.2,13.8) and Uniform(0,1)
theta1=rbeta(n=nsim,shape1=9.2,shape2=13.8)
theta2=runif(n=nsim, min=0, max=1)

# MC (forward sampling) simulations of future data 'y1' and 'y2'
y1=rbinom(n=nsim,size=20,prob=theta1)
y2=rbinom(n=nsim,size=20,prob=theta2)
```

and then summarise the resulting distributions for y_1 and y_2 to see what effect the choice of the prior has had.

```
sims = cbind(y1,y2)
bmhe::stats(sims)
```

```
     mean       sd 2.5% median 97.5%
y1 8.0073 2.919949    3      8    14
y2 9.9092 6.063549    0     10    20
```

The most striking result is that the second set of simulations show a much larger variance (and the 95% interval is between 0 and 20 – basically saying that it is very possible that every possible outcome can happen, in the trial, if we actually get money to run it...).

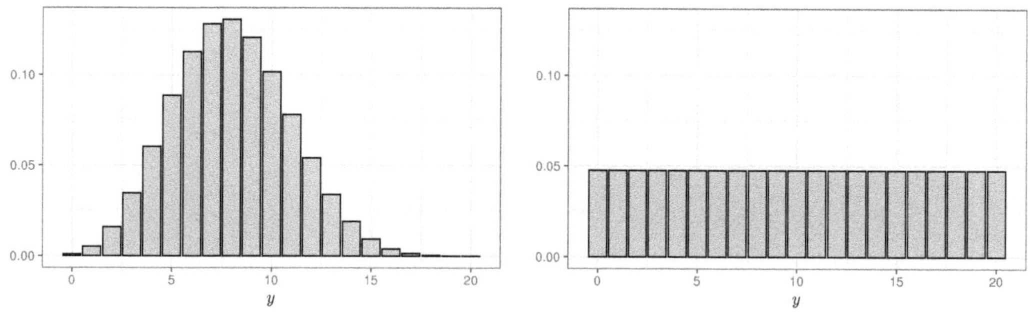

(a) $p(y)$ for Beta(9.2, 13.8) prior. (b) $p(y)$ for Uniform(0, 1) prior.

Figure 2.2: The prior predictive distribution $p(y)$ for the two different choices of priors.

Figure 2.2 shows the resulting prior predictive distributions $p(y) = \int p(y \mid \theta)p(\theta)d\theta$ (see Equation 1.7) for the two choices of priors. While both panels closely resemble the graphs in Figure 2.1, notice that the range along the x–axis is fundamentally different, as the priors are about the parameter θ (which is defined between 0 and 1), while the predictive distributions are about possible future data (which are defined in the range 0 to 20, indicating that none or all of the potential $n = 20$ individuals have a successful outcome from using the drug). In addition, the graphs in Figure 2.1 show the two densities for the continuous variable θ, while those in Figure 2.2 display the probability distributions for the discrete variable y. Figure 2.2a is identical to Figure 1.13, as it represents the exact same analysis.

The advantage of using a Uniform prior is that we can directly perform posterior inference, in the face of actually observed data, with no computational expense. For example, suppose now that we manage to run a pilot study in which we select $n = 20$ patients from a relevant population and give them the drug. Out of these, $y = 15$ are fully relieved from their back pain.

By removing all the terms that do not depend directly on θ from the Binomial sampling distribution of Equation 1.16 we obtain the likelihood function for this model as

$$\mathcal{L}(\theta \mid y) = \theta^y \, (1-\theta)^{n-y}. \tag{2.3}$$

Combining Equation 2.2 (which implies that, using a Uniform prior, the posterior is proportional to the likelihood) with Equation 2.3, we can conclude that

$$p(\theta \mid y, n) \propto \mathcal{L}(\theta \mid y, n) = \theta^y(1-\theta)^{n-y},$$

which is proportional to the kernel of the density for the Beta distribution shown in Equation 1.11. This in turn implies that $\theta \mid y, n \sim \text{Beta}(y+1, n-y+1) = \text{Beta}(16, 6)$ – we return to this point in Section 2.2.2 and Example 2.3.

Figure 2.3 shows a graphical representation of this posterior distribution. The observation of the data effectively drives almost exclusively the inference – we can use Monte Carlo simulations to obtain a sample of observations from the posterior using the following `R` code and then `bmhe` to summarise the results, which are extremely similar to a maximum likelihood analysis, in which the MLE is $\hat{\theta} = 15/20 = 0.75$, with a confidence interval of $[0.509; 0.913]$ – these numbers can be easily obtained using the `R` command `binom.test(x=15,n=20)`.

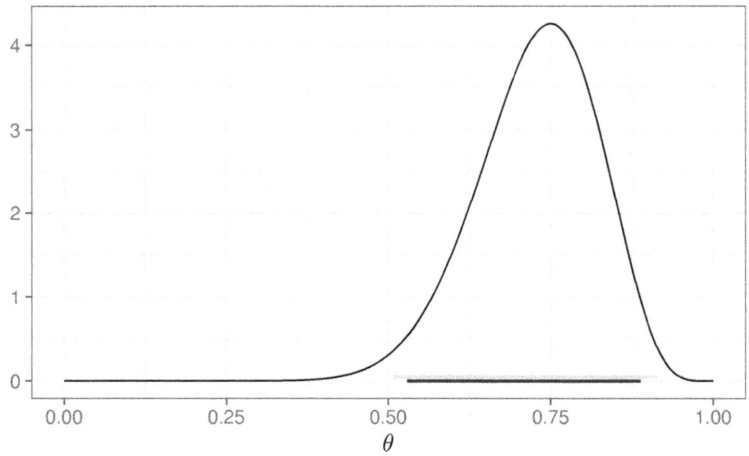

Figure 2.3: Posterior distribution obtained from a Uniform(0,1) prior and with $y = 15$ and $n = 20$. The darker line describes the Bayesian 95% interval, while the lighter line indicates the maximum likelihood estimate for the 95% (confidence) interval.

```
# Sample from the posterior distribution
post=rbeta(10000,15+1,20-15+1)
# Use 'bmhe' to summarise the results
bmhe::stats(post)
```

```
      mean         sd       2.5%     median      97.5%
0.72861422 0.09275955 0.52952955 0.73462481 0.88929082
```

Uniform priors also give us an alternative way of eliciting contextual knowledge and mapping it into suitable distributional assumptions (see Section 1.2.2). We can achieve this by performing a "pretend", thought experiment to derive a suitable current level of uncertainty that we are willing to use in the prior.

The main idea is to think in terms of the alleged DGP and use an "implicit" dataset to update a state of absolute ignorance to a state of (possibly still substantial) uncertainty on the model parameters. In other words, we can start by assuming a "vague" prior to represent the (almost non-existing) background information and construct a model to tune the amount of data we would need to actually observe to modify this prior into a "posterior" that would match a state of uncertainty that we would be comfortable assuming. This updated distribution could then be used as a valid prior before observing any real data.

Example 2.2. *Drug (continued): deriving contextual information via pseudo-data.* Consider again Example 1.4, when we still have not made any observation y on the number of individuals who recover when given the drug, out of the n that we observe. We want to set up a prior distribution $p(\theta)$ to describe our current uncertainty on the model parameter, which represents the probability that a random individual given the drug is relieved by their back-pain.

Let us assume that, to start with, we have no real information about the drug's effectiveness, which we can represent by considering $\theta \mid \mathcal{B} \sim \text{Uniform}(0,1)$ – exactly as in Laplace's original analysis of Section 2.2.1 (notice here that we explicitly condition to the body of background knowledge, $\mathcal{B}$). We know from Equation 2.2 and the analysis in Example 2.1 that $\theta \mid y_O, n_O \sim \text{Beta}(y_O+1, n_O-y_O+1)$, with mean and variance

$$\mu = \frac{y_O+1}{n_O+2} \quad \text{and} \quad \sigma^2 = \frac{(y_O+1)(n_O-y_O+1)}{(n_O+2)^2(n_O+3)}$$

(see Equation 1.12).

We can use trial-and-error and select different values for (y_O, n_O) to calibrate our prior knowledge, as in Figure 2.4. For example, in Figure 2.4a we elicit our prior knowledge in the form of a thought experiment in which we observe $y_O = 8$ successes, out of $n_O = 20$ individuals to whom we give the drug – as is possible to see, this pretty much amounts to the information that around 95% of the prior mass is included in $[0.2; 0.6]$, with a mean of

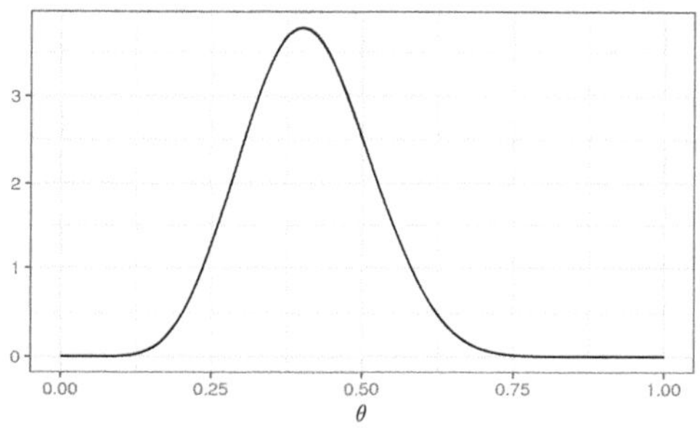

(a) $y_O = 8, n_O = 20$.

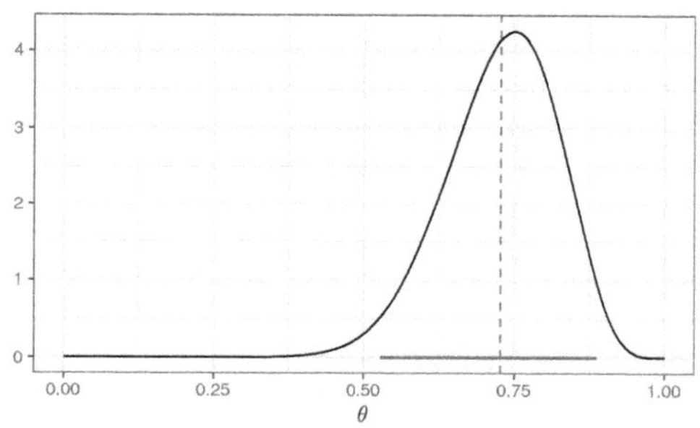

(b) $y_O = 15, n_O = 20$.

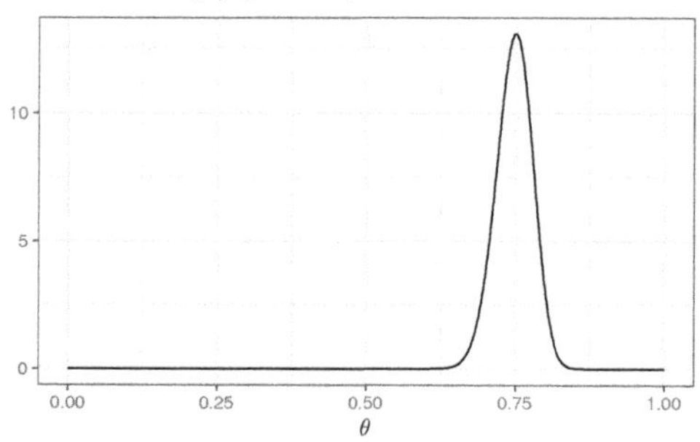

(c) $y_O = 150, n_O = 200$.

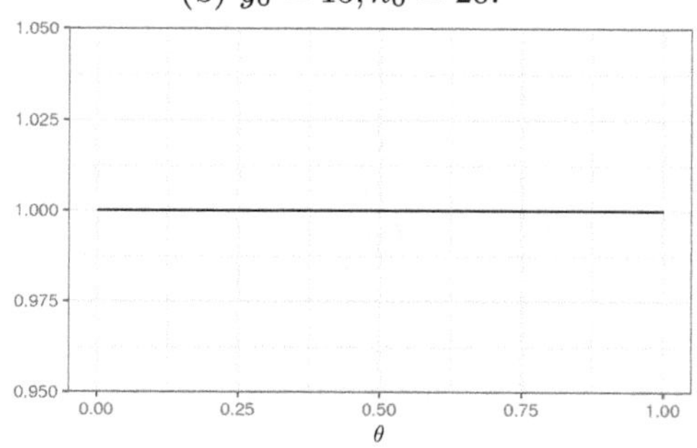

(d) $y_O = 0, n_O = 0$.

Figure 2.4: Starting from a complete level of ignorance in the contextual background $p(\theta \mid \mathcal{B}) \sim \text{Uniform}(0,1)$, we can use "pseudo-data" to tune our level of prior uncertainty, by performing a "pretend" Bayesian analysis and determine a prior $p(\theta)$. In panel (a) we are willing to elicit our level of current uncertainty as if we had observed $n_O = 20$ individuals, of whom $y_O = 8$ have a successful outcome. Panels (b) and (c) show a situation in which we are willing to consider that, on average, we expect a success rate of around 0.75; in panel (b) we have much more uncertainty (and so we use a "pseudo-dataset" of small sample size); in panel (c) we would be much more confident (and thus imagine a "pseudo-dataset" with a sample size 10 times as large). Panel (d) shows the case of "complete ignorance", where we start by knowing nothing and pretend to continue to learn nothing ($y_O = n_O = 0$), leading to, again, a Uniform(0,1) distribution.

around 0.4 and a standard deviation of around 0.1, which we modelled using a Beta(9.2, 13.8) in Example 1.4.

Figures 2.4b and 2.4c show two situations in which we are willing to assume that, on average, we expect a response rate of around 0.75 – the main difference is that in Figure 2.4b we are not very confident about this possibility and thus we consider a "pretend" dataset with a very small sample size ($n_0 = 20$); in Figure 2.4c, while the sample proportion of successes is unchanged (150/200 vs 15/20), the sample size is ten times bigger, indicating that we would be much more confident with this assessment – we effectively would be basing it on a relatively large study in which around 75% of the individuals would have a positive outcome. As a result, the two densities are centred around the same value of 0.75, but the latter has a much smaller variance.

Finally, in Figure 2.4d we show the case in which we elicit the prior information to amount to a study in which we pretend to have observed $y_0 = 0$ successes, out of $n_0 = 0$ trials. This obviously means that we assume we know nothing whatsoever on the drug's effectiveness. Interestingly, when combined with the Uniform(0, 1) prior we have assumed before even thinking of the thought experiment, implies a revised assessment that is still a Uniform(0, 1). In fact, because we know that the posterior given (y_0, n_0) is $\text{Beta}(y_0 + 1, n_0 - y_0 + 1)$, we can derive that

$$\begin{aligned}\text{Beta}(0+1, 0-0+1) &= \text{Beta}(1,1) = \frac{\Gamma(1+1)}{\Gamma(1)\Gamma(1)}\theta^{1-1}(1-\theta)^{1-1} \\ &= 1 = \frac{1}{1-0} = \text{Uniform}(0,1),\end{aligned}$$

recall from Equation 1.3 that $\Gamma(x) = (x-1)! = (x-1) \times (x-2) \times \cdots \times 2 \times 1$ and so $\Gamma(1) = 0! := 1$ and $\Gamma(2) = 1! := 1$. Thus, as is sensible, the thought experiment assuming $y_0 = n_0 = 0$ effectively implies "complete ignorance" and the *non-informative* prior.

While it is sometimes acceptable to imagine a near-complete lack of information in the possible range of likely values for the model parameters, this sort of assumption is often a "lazy" option. In reality, it is very difficult to justify a situation in which we are called to make inference on something about which we claim to know absolutely nothing.

In addition, the nature of the parameter for which we want to elicit a prior distribution may be such as to not conform very well with a Uniform distribution. Consider for example a regression model

$$y_i \sim \text{Normal}(\mu_i, \sigma) \quad \text{with} \quad \mu_i = \beta_0 + \beta_1 x_i,$$

for n observations $(y_i, x_i)_{i=1}^n$. A Bayesian formulation of this model requires setting prior distributions for the parameters $\boldsymbol{\theta} = (\beta_0, \beta_1, \sigma)$.

We may not have (or may want to limit the impact of) any substantial contextual information and so aim at using vague priors. In line with the discussion above, we may spread the prior mass all over the range of the regression coefficients (so as not to favour any specific value)

$$\beta_0, \beta_1 \overset{iid}{\sim} \text{Uniform}(-\infty, \infty).$$

The problem here is that a Uniform distribution defined over the entire $\mathbb{R}$ line has the inconvenient property of not integrating to 1, because

$$\int_{\mathbb{R}} p(\beta_0) d\beta_0 = \int_{\mathbb{R}} c d\beta_0 = \int_{\mathbb{R}} p(\beta_1) d\beta_1 = \int_{\mathbb{R}} c d\beta_1 \to \infty.$$

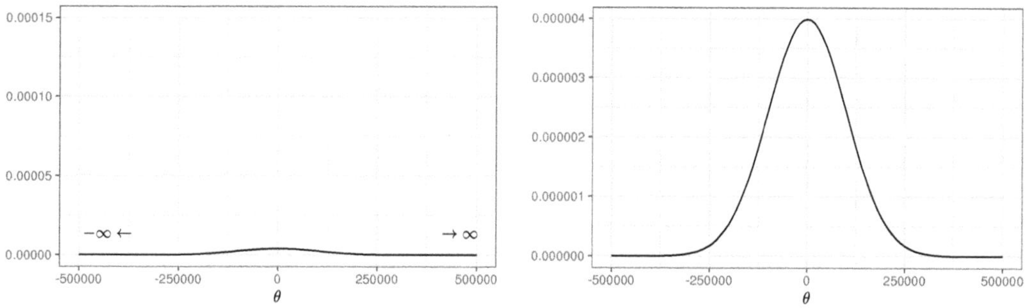

(a) Enlarged y–axis. (b) Zoomed in over the y–axis.

Figure 2.5: A vague Normal prior $\theta \sim \text{Normal}(0, s)$, for a very large value for the standard deviation. For all intents and purposes, this prior spreads the mass all over $\mathbb{R}$, while still being proper, i.e. integrating to 1 over the real line. Panel (a) shows the density with a relatively large y–axis, while panel (b) zooms in over a much smaller range on the y–axis.

This means that a Uniform prior over $\mathbb{R}$ is *not* a proper probability distribution!

In some cases, it is still possible that the process of Bayesian updating transforms an improper prior into a proper posterior, i.e.

$$\int_{\Theta} p(\theta \mid \boldsymbol{y})d\theta = 1 \qquad \text{even if} \qquad \int_{\Theta} p(\theta)d\theta \rightarrow \infty,$$

where Θ is the range of the parameter θ. In general, however, improper priors are worrisome because a) their interpretation is meaningless, since they do not represent a probability distribution; and more importantly, b) the posterior may also remain improper, implying that the entire inferential process is meaningless.

For this reason, when the parameter of interest is unbounded, we may want to express "vagueness" using a different prior – a popular (and sensible) choice is to use a Normal distribution with large variance, i.e. $\theta \sim \text{Normal}(0, s)$, for a large constant standard deviation, s. Figure 2.5 shows such an example (with $s = 100\,000$).

In some cases, it is not a major problem to use such extremely vague Normal priors, e.g. if we have enough data (y_i, x_i) to fit our regression model, which means that the evidence in the likelihood will dominate in forming the posterior. But especially when data are sparse or non-definitive, "lazy" options such as these may lead to unnecessary inefficiencies, or even fundamental bias in our inference. In fact, in effectively every applied problem, we should be able to do better than just assuming that "anything goes": odds ratios are hardly ever bigger than 3 or 4; the scale of a covariate effect can be determined with some level of approximation in a finite interval etc. – all these considerations can be used to determine a "large enough" value for s, without going crazy about it…

i Objective subjectivity

From a purely Bayesian point of view, we would actually never want to limit the impact of contextual information. In fact, we would highlight its use as a defining feature of our analysis.

The idea of "hiding" the subjectivity inherent in a Bayesian modelling is more of a "historically accident" – at a time when frequentism was the dominant philosophical paradigm for probability (roughly speaking, for large part of the 20th century), Bayesians found themselves trying to defend their views by suggesting that subjectivism could be limited by taking appropriate actions in forming the prior, e.g. using vague (or "non-informative") distributions – see also Note 5 below.

At the same time, prominent Bayesian scholars such as Dennis Lindley, Bruno de Finetti and Leonard Jimmie Savage were adamant that subjectivism was a key feature of science and continued to advocate for a "proper" use of the Bayesian machinery in statistical inference, thus taking full stock of any contextual information, whenever available.

2.2.2 Conjugate analysis

Until the mid-1990s, when simulation algorithms adapted from Physics (see Section 2.3 and Section 2.3.1) effectively rendered Bayesian computation feasible for problems of, virtually, any level of complexity, a "conjugate analysis" was the only practical way of running Bayesian modelling.

The main ideas originated in the Bayesian school at the University of Chicago, in the US, with the work of Raiffa and Schlaifer (1961) and build on the recognition that, sometimes, it is possible to exploit the mathematical form of a given prior distribution, which, when combined with the likelihood corresponding to a particular sampling distribution for the data, has the very convenient property that the resulting posterior distribution remains in the same parametric family as the prior.

Technically, a prior distribution $p(\theta)$ is said to be "*conjugate*" to a given likelihood if

$$p(\theta) \in f(\theta; \boldsymbol{a}) \quad \Rightarrow \quad p(\theta \mid y) \propto p(\theta)\mathcal{L}(\theta \mid y) \in f(\theta; \boldsymbol{a}^*), \tag{2.4}$$

where $f(\theta; \boldsymbol{a})$ is a parametric family (e.g. a Beta, or a Gamma), as a function of a set of parameters $\boldsymbol{a}$, e.g. (a, b) in Equation 1.11. Equation 2.4 implies that, under conjugacy, the posterior distribution belongs to the same distributional family as the prior, $f(\cdot)$ – the update only involves the parameters that change from $\boldsymbol{a}$ to $\boldsymbol{a}^*$, by effect of the information contained in the likelihood function.

Sufficient statistics and conjugacy

If a *sufficient statistic* $S(y)$ of fixed dimension exists for a given likelihood function $\mathcal{L}(\theta \mid y)$, then any arbitrarily large data can be summarised fully through it – technically, this can be represented equivalently using either of the following relationships

$$p(y \mid S(y), \theta) = p(y \mid S(y)) \Leftrightarrow y \perp\!\!\!\perp \theta \mid S(y),$$

which also hold when we can express the sampling distribution as

$$p(y \mid \theta) = h(y)g(S(y), \theta), \tag{2.5}$$

for given functions $h(\cdot)$ and $g(\cdot)$.

The sufficient statistic tells us *everything* we need to know about the parameter and thus, conditionally on it, the distribution of the data y is independent on the parameter θ and, in particular, from Equation 2.5 we can see that the data only enter the likelihood through $S(y)$.

Although this concept is grounded in Fisher's likelihood theory (which also fulfils the most important frequentist principles – cfr. Note 1 in Section 1.1), it does play a key role in Bayesian modelling too, because if a sufficient statistic exists for a given model, then we can prove that a conjugate prior distribution also exists (Raiffa and Schlaifer, 1961; DeGroot, 1970).

Consider for example a sample of n independent observations $\boldsymbol{y} = (y_1, \ldots, y_n) \sim \text{Normal}(\mu, \sigma)$, for some fixed value[2] σ. The multivariate form of the sampling distribution is

$$p(\boldsymbol{y} \mid \mu, \sigma) = \left(\frac{1}{2\pi\sigma^2}\right)^{\frac{n}{2}} \exp\left(-\frac{1}{2\sigma^2}\sum_{i=1}^{n}(y_i-\mu)^2\right).$$

If we use some simple algebra to re-write

$$\sum_{i=1}^{n}(y_i-\mu)^2 = n(\mu-\bar{y})^2 + \sum_{i=1}^{n}(y_i-\bar{y})^2,$$

then we can rearrange the sampling distribution as

$$p(\boldsymbol{y} \mid \mu, \sigma) = \left(\frac{1}{2\pi\sigma^2}\right)^{\frac{n}{2}} \exp\left(-\frac{1}{2\sigma^2}\sum_{i=1}^{n}(y_i-\bar{y})^2\right) \exp\left(-\frac{n}{2\sigma^2}(\mu-\bar{y})^2\right). \tag{2.6}$$

The only term in Equation 2.6 that is a function of μ, i.e. the likelihood function for the parameter of interest μ, given the observed data $\boldsymbol{y}$ and the "nuisance" parameter σ, is then

$$\mathcal{L}(\mu \mid \boldsymbol{y}, \sigma) = \exp\left(-\frac{n}{2\sigma^2}(\mu-\bar{y})^2\right), \tag{2.7}$$

which depends on the observed data only through the sample mean $\bar{y}$ and the sample size n – which are thus the two sufficient statistics: all the information contained in the data can be summarised fully through $\boldsymbol{S} = (\bar{y}, n)$.

Interestingly, as a function of μ, Equation 2.7 closely resembles the kernel of a Normal density (see Equation 1.4) and the intuition behind conjugacy is that, if we define a prior based on this form, i.e. in this case $\mu \sim \text{Normal}(m_0, s_0)$ for some set values m_0, s_0 for the mean and standard deviation, then we can compute the posterior distribution as

$$\begin{aligned} p(\mu \mid \boldsymbol{y}, \sigma) &\propto p(\mu \mid m_0, s_0)\mathcal{L}(\mu \mid \boldsymbol{y}, \sigma) \\ &\propto \exp\left(-\frac{1}{2s_0^2}(\mu-m_0)^2\right)\exp\left(-\frac{n}{2\sigma^2}(\mu-\bar{y})^2\right), \end{aligned}$$

which, with some simple algebra, we can re-write as

$$\exp\left(-\frac{1}{2}\left(\frac{1}{s_0^2}+\frac{1}{\sigma^2}\right)\left(\mu-\left(\frac{1}{s_0^2}+\frac{1}{\sigma^2}\right)^{-1}\left(\frac{m_0}{s_0^2}+\frac{n\bar{y}}{\sigma^2}\right)\right)^2\right).$$

This is in turn again the kernel of a Normal density, meaning that the posterior remains in the same parametric family as the prior and is $\mu \mid \boldsymbol{y} \sim \text{Normal}(m_1, s_1)$, with

$$m_1 = s_1^2\left(\frac{m_0}{s_0^2}+\frac{n\bar{y}}{\sigma^2}\right) \quad \text{and} \quad s_1 = \sqrt{\left(\frac{1}{s_0^2}+\frac{n}{\sigma^2}\right)^{-1}}. \tag{2.8}$$

A large number of conjugate models exist for set inferential problems (cfr. Table 3.1 in Lunn et al., 2013 for a list of univariate conjugate models). Examples include

$$\begin{cases} \theta \sim \text{Gamma}(a,b) \\ y_1,\ldots,y_n \mid \theta \overset{iid}{\sim} \text{Poisson}(\theta) \end{cases} \quad \Rightarrow \quad \theta \mid \boldsymbol{y} \sim \text{Gamma}\left(a + \sum_{i=1}^{n} y_i, n+b\right)$$

and

$$\begin{cases} \tau = \dfrac{1}{\sigma^2} \sim \text{Gamma}(a,b) \\ y_1,\ldots,y_n \mid \mu,\sigma \overset{iid}{\sim} \text{Normal}(\mu,\sigma) \end{cases} \Rightarrow \tau \mid \mu, \boldsymbol{y} \sim \text{Gamma}\left(a + \frac{n}{2}, b + \frac{1}{2}\sum_{i=1}^{n}(y_i - \mu)^2\right) \tag{2.9}$$

(note that Equation 2.9 is a posterior distribution considering μ as fixed – see Example 2.7).

Example 2.3. *Drug (continued): conjugate analysis.* If we now model $\theta \sim \text{Beta}(a_0, b_0)$ – say, again, with $a_0 = 9.2$ and $b_0 = 13.8$, given the form of the density for the Beta distribution shown in Equation 1.11, we can write

$$p(\theta \mid a_0, b_0) \propto \theta^{a_0-1}(1-\theta)^{b_0-1}$$

and applying Bayes' theorem, we obtain that

$$\begin{aligned} p(\theta \mid y) &\propto p(\theta)\mathcal{L}(\theta \mid y) \\ &\propto \theta^{a_0-1}(1-\theta)^{b_0-1}\theta^{y}\,(1-\theta)^{n-y} \\ &\propto \theta^{a_0+y-1}(1-\theta)^{b_0+n-y-1} \\ &\propto \theta^{a_1-1}(1-\theta)^{b_1-1} \sim \text{Beta}(a_1,b_1), \end{aligned}$$

with $a_1 = a_0 + y$ and $b_1 = b_0 + n - y$, for the observed $y = 15$ and $n = 20$.

In other words, with these modelling assumptions, a Beta prior is updated to a Beta posterior by the observation of data whose sampling variability can be modelled using a Binomial distribution. The update does not involve the distributional form of the prior (which remains unchanged in the posterior), but only the parameters, which change from (a_0, b_0) to (a_1, b_1), as a function of the values for the observed data. This is obviously very attractive because we do not need any complex computational mechanism to obtain the posterior distribution in closed form.

Figure 2.6 shows the prior, likelihood and resulting posterior using this conjugate analysis. In this case, the posterior results in a "compromise" between what we knew before observing the data and what we now know, after the data have become available. An analysis based on the likelihood function only would perhaps be overly-enthusiastic about the actual drug's effectiveness – we do observe the vast majority of the patient to have a positive outcome.

Of course, it is possible that our prior be badly calibrated: perhaps the new drug is truly magical and thus the information available to us at the point of starting the experimentation bears little relevance and we should base our inference mostly on the data. Then again, generally speaking this surprising result is perhaps more likely to arise because of quirks in our data – perhaps the sample size is not large enough; or may be our patients are selected in a way that is not entirely representative of the underlying population, etc. For this reason,

[2]Assuming that the standard deviation is known without uncertainty is of course a gross, but not entirely uncommon simplification – see for instance Example 1.1.

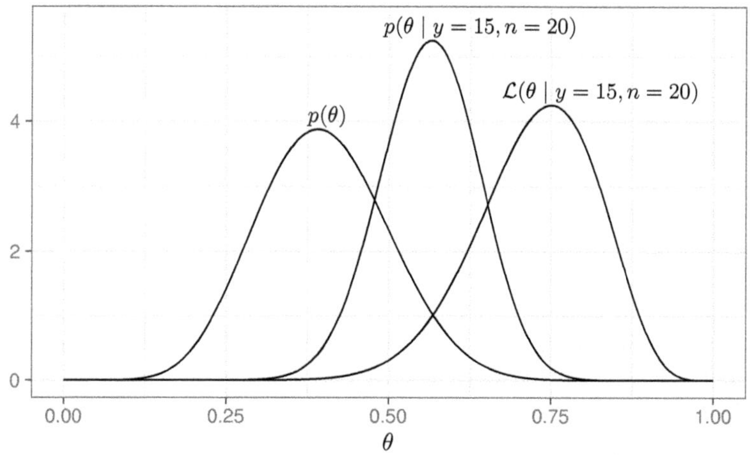

Figure 2.6: The process of Bayesian conjugate analysis for the Beta-Binomial model of the drug's effectiveness.

it makes sense, arguably, to include in our inference every little source of information we may have.

Conjugacy is a very handy property, from the mathematical perspective, but it can also be very restrictive, because it imposes a distributional form for the prior that may be insufficient to model the case at hand. For instance, there is no conjugated prior for a model such as logistic regression. Nevertheless, the computational appeal of conjugacy is sometimes still exploited even in real life, critical applications.

Example 2.4. *Covid vaccine experimentation.* In the wake of the Covid-19 pandemic, several biotechnology and pharmaceutical companies started collaborating on the development of a vaccine, in an unprecedented effort to deliver vital innovation in a short amount of time. The first vaccine to be approved by the US Food and Drug Administration (FDA, the federal agency responsible for ensuring safety of drugs introduced on the market, in the US) in December 2020 was the one developed jointly by German biotech company *BioNTech* and US pharmaceutical giant *Pfizer*. The development of the vaccine was based on a Phase I/II/III multicentre, placebo-controlled trial to evaluate the safety, tolerability, immunogenicity and efficacy of the candidate vaccine.

The Phase II/III study was designed using a Bayesian approach based on the following setup. There are two arms: one is randomised to receive two doses of a placebo, while the active arm receives two doses of the candidate vaccine. The data relevant for the efficacy analysis are the number of individuals who in each arm are confirmed Covid-19 cases, over the total number of individuals randomised to the specific arm. This can be formalised as $y_{\text{plac}} \sim \text{Binomial}(\pi_{\text{plac}}, n_{\text{plac}})$ and $y_{\text{vac}} \sim \text{Binomial}(\pi_{\text{vac}}, n_{\text{vac}})$, respectively. The actual measure of vaccine efficacy is defined as $\text{VE} = \left(1 - \frac{\pi_{\text{vac}}}{\pi_{\text{plac}}}\right)$, assuming a 1:1 allocation ratio in the two arms and thus $n_{\text{plac}} = n_{\text{vac}} = N$.

However, the analysis is based on a reformulation of the problem: the experimenters actually model $y = y_{\text{vac}}$ = number of Covid-19 cases among the individuals in the treatment arm over $n = (y_{\text{vac}} + y_{\text{plac}})$ = the total number of Covid-19 cases in the two arms. This is modelled as $y \sim \text{Binomial}(\theta, n)$, where

$$\begin{aligned}\theta &= \frac{\pi_{\text{vac}}}{\pi_{\text{vac}} + \pi_{\text{plac}}} \\ &= \frac{1 - \text{VE}}{2 - \text{VE}}.\end{aligned} \tag{2.10}$$

The reason for this seemingly overly-complex (and obscure) setup is that it allows the experimenters to only specify one observational model and, crucially, a single prior distribution for the parameter θ – of course, once $p(\theta \mid \text{data})$ is available, using the equation above, it is straightforward (e.g. through Monte Carlo simulation) to obtain directly the posterior distribution for the main parameter of interest $p(\text{VE} \mid \text{data})$.

Sample size calculation

The determination of the sample size calculation is based on a simulation approach. The experimenter looked to determine a sample size large enough to be able to provide a probability exceeding 90% to conclude that VE > 30% with a "high probability" (we note here that the study protocol is vague on the actual threshold selected).

The simulation exercise proceeds in two steps. Firstly, the experimenters make assumptions about some of the features of the "data-generating process". For instance, in the study protocol, they stipulate a "true" vaccine efficacy $\widehat{\text{VE}} = 0.6$ (i.e. a reduction by 40% in the infection rate in the vaccine arm, in comparison to the placebo population). This implies that the "true" proportion of Covid-19 cases in the vaccine arm over the total of cases is

$$\hat{\theta} = \frac{1 - \widehat{\text{VE}}}{2 - \widehat{\text{VE}}} = 0.2857.$$

Using these assumption, we can simulate a large number S (say, 100 000) of potential trial data from the alleged generating process $y^{(s)} \sim \text{Binomial}(\hat{\theta}, n)$, where the superscript (s) indicates the s–th simulated dataset and given a fixed value of the overall number of cases n. Typically, we repeat the simulation for a grid of possible values of n (e.g. $n = [10, 20, 30, 40, 50, 60, 70, \ldots]$).

Once the hypothetical trial data have been generated, the second step consists in analysing them according to the statistical analysis plan defined in the protocol. In this case, the full model specification is required, which involves defining a prior distribution for θ.

For simplicity, the experimenters set a minimally informative Beta prior $\theta \sim \text{Beta}(\alpha_0, \beta_0)$, where the parameters α_0 and β_0 are selected to express the limited amount of information available a priori (recall that θ represents the proportion of Covid-19 cases occurred in the vaccine group). We know from Equation 1.13 that $\text{E}[\theta] = \dfrac{\alpha_0}{\alpha_0 + \beta_0}$. If we fix $\beta_0 = 1$, then we can solve for α_0 so that the prior mean for θ is equal to some pre-specified value – in particular, the experimenters had chosen a threshold of VE = 30% as the minimum level of efficacy they were prepared to entertain. This value can be mapped to the scale of θ as $\dfrac{1 - 0.3}{2 - 0.3} = 0.4117$ and thus solving

$$\frac{\alpha_0}{\alpha_0 + 1} = 0.4117$$

gives $\alpha_0 = 0.700102$.

Because of conjugacy, for each simulated dataset we can easily update the Beta(0.700102, 1) prior to a Beta(α_1, β_1) posterior distribution for θ, where $\alpha_1 = 0.700102 + y^{(s)}$ and $\beta_1 = 1 + n - y^{(s)}$. Moreover, for each simulation s, we can compute *analytically* any tail-area probability from $p(\theta \mid \text{data})$. Once again, we are really interested in $\Pr(\text{VE} > 0.3 \mid \text{data})$, but using the deterministic relationship linking VE to θ, we can re-express this as

$$\begin{aligned}\Pr(\text{VE} > 0.3 \mid \text{data}) &= \Pr\left(\frac{1-2\theta}{1-\theta} > 0.3 \mid \text{data}\right)\\ &= \Pr(\theta < 0.4117 \mid \text{data}),\end{aligned}$$

which can be computed for each simulation s. This produces a large number of simulations that can be used to determine the "power" for a given sample size, as the proportion of times in which this computed probability exceeds a set threshold (i.e. is "large enough" in the phrasing of the study protocol).

The experimenters compute $n = 164$ as the optimal number of total Covid-19 cases that are necessary to be able to ascertain that VE $> 30\%$ with a large probability.

Then, it is necessary to determine the overall sample size (i.e. the total number of individuals to be recruited in the study) so that a total of 164 cases is likely to be observed within the required time frame. Once again, it is necessary to make some assumption about the data-generating process; specifically the experimenters consider a 1.3% illness rate per year in the placebo group. Because the study aims at accruing 164 cases within 6 months, this essentially amounts to assuming that $\pi_{\text{plac}} \approx 0.013/2$ and thus $\pi_{\text{vac}} \approx (\pi_{\text{plac}} \times 0.4)/2$ (recall that we are assuming a 60% vaccine efficacy, or that $\pi_{\text{vac}} = 0.4 \times \pi_{\text{plac}}$).

We can once again resort to simulations to estimate what sample size in each arm N is necessary so that we can expect $y_{\text{vac}} + y_{\text{plac}} \geq 164$ – this returns an optimal sample size of $N = 17\,600$ per group. Finally, considering an attrition rate of 20% (indicating that such proportion of individuals would not generate an evaluable outcome could be observed), the experimenters inflate the sample size to obtain $N^* = \dfrac{N}{0.8} = 21\,999$ per group (or a total of 43 998 individuals).

Data analysis

At the end of the actual study (Polack et al., 2020), there were $y_{\text{vac}} = 8$ and $y_{\text{plac}} = 162$ confirmed Covid-19 cases in the vaccine and the placebo group, respectively. These imply that $y = 8$ and $n = (8 + 162) = 170$. However, there is a slight extra complication: the setup describe above implies the assumption of 1:1 allocation (i.e. $n_{\text{plac}} = n_{\text{vac}}$) – this is crucial to ensure the simple deterministic relationship between VE and θ. In actual fact, the placebo group had a slightly higher number of individuals, by the time of the data analysis (there were 17,411 and 17,511 individuals with valid data in the vaccine and placebo group, respectively). Thus, we need to rescale the observed data, which can be done by considering $y^*_{\text{vac}} = y_{\text{vac}}\dfrac{17\,461}{17\,411} = 8.02297$ and $y^*_{\text{plac}} = y_{\text{plac}}\dfrac{17\,461}{17\,511} = 161.53743$, where $17\,461 = \dfrac{17\,411 + 17\,511}{2}$ and thus $y^* = 8.02297$ and $n^* = 169.5604$.

These data can be used to update the prior distribution Beta(0.700102, 1) into a Beta(8.723072, 162.5374) posterior for θ. Finally, we can rescale this posterior to determine the relevant posterior distribution $p(\text{VE} \mid \text{data})$, for instance using Monte Carlo to simulate a large number S of values $\theta^{(s)} \sim \text{Beta}(8.723072, 162.5374)$ and then computing

$\text{VE}^{(s)} = \dfrac{1-2\theta^{(s)}}{1-\theta^{(s)}}$ and then use these to characterise the uncertainty around the vaccine efficacy.

```
# Sets up the value for the parameters
alpha.0=0.700102
beta.0=1
# Observed data
y=c(8,162)
n=c(17411,17511)
# So needs to reproportion as if the treatment arms had the same
# sample size (to be in line with model assumptions!)
y=y*mean(n)/n
# Now can update the Beta prior with the observed data
alpha.1=alpha.0+y[1]
beta.1=beta.0+y[2]

# Monte Carlo analysis for theta and ve
theta=rbeta(100000,alpha.1,beta.1)
ve=(1-2*theta)/(1-theta)
```

In this case, the posterior distributions $p(\theta \mid \text{data})$ and $p(\text{VE} \mid \text{data})$ can be visualised in Figure 2.7.

We can also use the resulting samples from the posterior distribution to estimate the 95% interval of $[0.9034; 0.9761]$ for the vaccine efficacy, indicating that we expect the vaccine to perform extremely well.

2.2.3 Penalised complexity priors

Simpson et al. (2017) have recently introduced the concept of "penalised complexity" (PC) prior. This is closely related to the principle of using "default" distributional assumptions and the basic idea is that PC priors can be constructed to penalise deviations from (i.e. added complexity in comparison to) the simpler, base model.

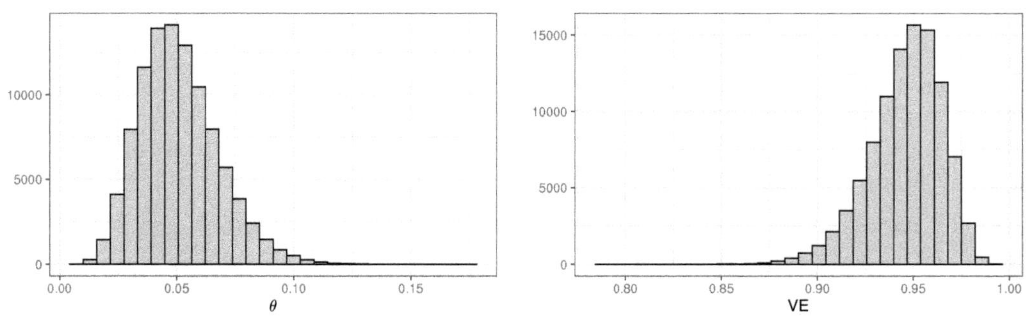

(a) Proportion of Covid-19 cases in the vaccine arm.

(b) Vaccine efficacy.

Figure 2.7: The results of the vaccine experimentation.

PC priors are based on four principles, underlying the features that Simpson et al. (2017) regard as desirable for a prior distribution in order for it to not influence the results unduly (i.e. over and above the impact of the data). The first principle is the philosophical idea of "Occam's razor", which suggests that modelling assumptions that are overly complicated should be discarded in favour of simpler ones, until there is enough support for the more complex version of the model.

The way in which "complexity" is measured in the framework of PC priors is through the Kullback-Leibler divergence (KLD), generically defined as

$$\text{KLD}(f,g) = \int f(x) \log\left(\frac{f(x)}{g(x)}\right) dx,$$

which is a measure of the information lost when some base model g is used as a possibly rough approximation to a more complex model f, which includes some additional parameter ξ.

A scaled version of the KLD, $d(f,g) = \sqrt{2\text{KLD}(f,g)}$, is used as a measure of *distance* between two competing models. Assuming a constant rate of penalisation for increasingly complex models, essentially implies an Exponential distribution on the distance scale, d: $p(d) = \lambda \exp(-\lambda d) \sim \text{Exponential}(\lambda)$ – cfr Equation 1.10; also, this is akin to the consideration that the hazard is constant for an Exponential distribution, in survival modelling (see Chapter 8). Using the calculus rules for the change of support variable (see Equation 1.14), this corresponds to a prior on the parameter ξ, which can be constructed in the form

$$p(\xi) = \lambda e^{-\lambda d(\xi)} \left| \frac{\partial d(\xi)}{\partial \xi} \right|.$$

Simpson et al. (2017) suggest that the parameter λ could be selected so as to control the prior mass in the tail of the resulting distribution for ξ.

Example 2.5. *PC prior for a standard deviation.* Consider for example the two competing models for some data y as a function of a *precision* $\tau = \sigma^{-2}$

$$g(\tau) \sim \text{Normal}(0, \tau = \tau_0 \to \infty) \qquad \text{and} \qquad f(\tau) \sim \text{Normal}(0,\tau), \tau \in (0,\infty).$$

This basically assumes that the "base case" model has $\sigma = 0$ (or equivalently $\tau \to \infty$) – see Chapter 6 for more applications of this concept in the context of hierarchical modelling.

If we parameterise the Normal distribution in Equation 1.4 with mean equal to 0 and in terms of the precision, we then get

$$f = \sqrt{\frac{\tau}{2\pi}} \exp\left(-\frac{\tau}{2}y^2\right) \quad \text{and} \quad g = \sqrt{\frac{\tau_0}{2\pi}} \exp\left(-\frac{\tau_0}{2}y^2\right).$$

Thus

$$\begin{aligned}
\text{KLD}(f,g) &= \int \text{Normal}(0,\tau) \left[\frac{1}{2}\log\left(\frac{\tau}{\tau_0}\right) - \frac{y^2}{2}(\tau - \tau_0)\right] dy \\
&= \frac{1}{2}\log\left(\frac{\tau}{\tau_0}\right) \underbrace{\int \text{Normal}(0,\tau) dy}_{=1} - \frac{1}{2}(\tau-\tau_0) \underbrace{\int y^2\, \text{Normal}(0,\tau) dy}_{=1/\tau} \\
&= \frac{1}{2}\log\left(\frac{\tau}{\tau_0}\right) - \frac{1}{2}\frac{\tau - \tau_0}{\tau} \\
&= \frac{1}{2}\frac{\tau_0}{\tau}\left[1 + \frac{\tau}{\tau_0}\log\left(\frac{\tau}{\tau_0}\right) - \frac{\tau}{\tau_0}\right] \to \frac{1}{2}\frac{\tau_0}{\tau},
\end{aligned}$$

because $\tau_0 \to \infty$. Thus

$$d(\tau) = \sqrt{2\text{KLD}(f,g)} = \sqrt{\frac{\tau_0}{\tau}} = \tau_0^{1/2}\tau^{-1/2} \propto \tau^{-1/2}.$$

Assuming $p(d) = \lambda \exp(-\lambda d)$ then

$$\left|\frac{\partial d(\tau)}{\partial \tau}\right| = \left|-\frac{1}{2}\tau^{-3/2}\right| = \frac{1}{2}\tau^{-3/2} \quad \Rightarrow \quad \begin{aligned} p(\tau) &= \lambda \exp\left[-\lambda d(\tau)\right] \left|\frac{\partial d(\tau)}{\partial \tau}\right| \\ &= \frac{\lambda}{2}\tau^{-3/2} \exp\left(-\lambda \tau^{-1/2}\right) \\ &\sim \text{type-2 Gumbel}\left(a = \frac{1}{2}, b = \lambda\right) \end{aligned}$$

and

$$\left|\frac{\partial \tau}{\partial \sigma}\right| = \left|\frac{\partial \sigma^{-2}}{\partial \sigma}\right| = |-2\sigma^{-3}| = 2\sigma^{-3} \quad \Rightarrow \quad \begin{aligned} p(\sigma) &= \frac{\lambda}{2}\sigma^3 \exp\left(-\lambda\sigma\right) \left|\frac{\partial \tau}{\partial \sigma}\right| \\ &= \lambda \exp(-\lambda\sigma) \sim \text{Exponential}(\lambda). \end{aligned}$$

We can control the amount of information we include in the Exponential prior for σ by modulating the value of the parameter λ. For example, we could set a constraint $\Pr(\sigma > \sigma_0) = \alpha$, in terms of the constants σ_0 and α, which by the properties of the Exponential distribution implies

$$\lambda = -\frac{\log(\alpha)}{\sigma_0}.$$

So, for instance, setting $\alpha = 0.01$ and $\sigma_0 = 1$, we get

$$\Pr(\sigma > 1) = 0.01 \Rightarrow \lambda = -\log(0.01) \approx 4.61$$

and thus the resulting PC prior is $\sigma \sim \text{Exponential}(4.61)$, which is depicted in Figure 2.8b, together with the prior on τ, in Figure 2.8a.

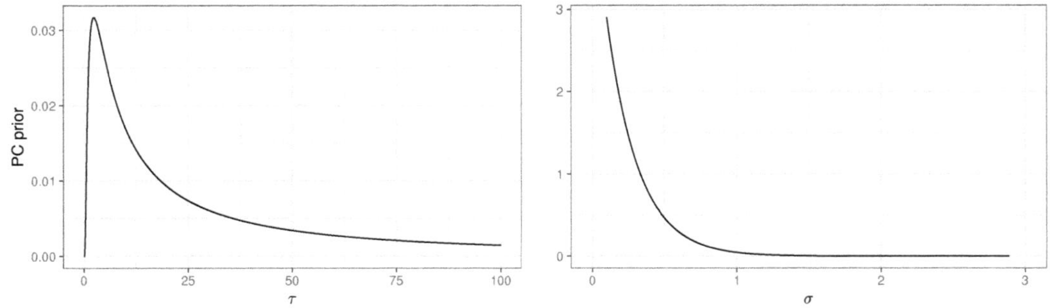

(a) The type-2 Gumbel prior for τ. (b) The resulting Exponential prior for σ.

Figure 2.8: The PC prior for the precision τ and then rescaled for the standard deviation σ, under the constraint $\Pr(\sigma > 1) = 0.01$.

Note 5: Jeffreys' default prior

The idea of using a "default" prior to limit the subjective element of a Bayesian analysis is not new – Jeffreys (1961) provides a comprehensive review of work originating as far back as the 1930s. Jeffreys' work is grounded in the midst of the frequentist domination, when Bayesian modelling was seen as impractical as well as philosophically unsound, because of the subjectivity intrinsic in the analysis. To combat this, he proposed a prior of the form

$$p(\theta) \propto \mathcal{I}(\theta)^{1/2},$$

where

$$\mathcal{I}(\theta) = -\text{E}_{Y\mid\theta}\left[\frac{\partial^2 \log \mathcal{L}(\theta \mid y)}{\partial\theta^2}\right] = \text{E}_{Y\mid\theta}\left[\left(\frac{\partial \log \mathcal{L}(\theta \mid y)}{\partial\theta}\right)^2\right]$$

is the *Fisher information*, a measure of the amount of information that the observable random quantity y carries on the parameter θ.

For example, the likelihood associated with $y \sim \text{Binomial}(\theta, n)$ is as in Equation 2.3; thus

$$\frac{\partial \log \mathcal{L}(\theta \mid y)}{\partial\theta} = \frac{y}{\theta} - \frac{(n-y)}{1-\theta} \quad \Rightarrow \quad \frac{\partial^2 \log \mathcal{L}(\theta \mid y)}{\partial\theta^2} = \frac{y}{\theta^2} + \frac{(n-y)}{(1-\theta)^2}$$

and

$$\begin{aligned} \mathcal{I}(\theta) = -\text{E}_{Y\mid\theta}\left[\frac{\partial^2 \log \mathcal{L}(\theta \mid y)}{\partial\theta^2}\right] &= \frac{n\theta}{\theta^2} + \frac{n-n\theta}{(1-\theta)^2} \\ &= \frac{n}{\theta(1-\theta)}, \end{aligned}$$

which implies

$$p(\theta) \propto \left(\theta^{-1}(1-\theta)^{-1}\right)^{1/2} = \theta^{-1/2}(1-\theta)^{-1/2}.$$

Using the argument discussed in Examples 2.1 and 2.3, we can see that this is the kernel of a Beta(0.5, 0.5).

The main intuition behind Jeffreys' prior is that by using a function of the likelihood, we derive a prior that is guaranteed to bring the least impact on the posterior. In the Binomial case above, we know from the analysis in Example 2.3 that a Beta(0.5, 0.5) is conjugated and so

$$p(\theta \mid y) \propto \text{Beta}(0.5 + y, 0.5 + n - y).$$

Whatever observed value for (y, n), this is essentially saying that the prior adds almost nothing to the information coming from the likelihood, which instead pretty much dominates and informs the shape of the posterior, as is clear from Figure 2.9: whenever the prior and the likelihood are in conflict, the likelihood always "wins" and determines the shape of the posterior in its image. Conversely, when the prior agrees with the likelihood, it acts like a "magnifier" and the posterior has even larger mass in that area.

If we take it at face value, in the Binomial case above, the Jeffreys' prior seems to suggest that we believe that the true underlying value for the population probability θ is either 0 or 1 and everything in between is more unlikely. In reality, Jeffreys' priors are just a beautiful *mathematical* formulation to ensure that whatever observation we end up making, it will be the data to dominate the posterior and that particular form for the prior will truly have minimal impact – in *this* sense they are considered as "non-informative".

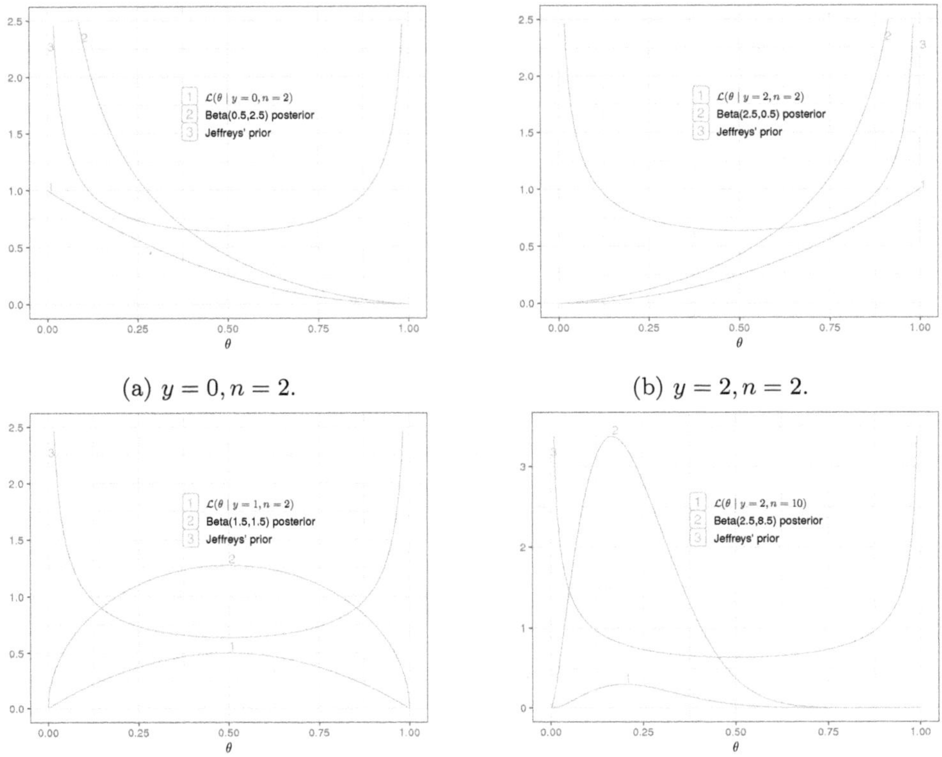

(a) $y = 0, n = 2$. (b) $y = 2, n = 2$.

(c) $y = 1, n = 2$. (d) $y = 2, n = 10$.

Figure 2.9: Jeffreys' prior, the likelihood function and the implied posterior distribution for different observed data in a Binomial experiment.

From the Bayesian *statistical* point of view, arguably they are a bit confusing and counter-intuitive, because, by definition, they completely discard any real and substantive information or belief we elicit in our prior. Back to the Binomial example, if we use Jeffreys' prior, it is *not* true that we are willing to say that we strongly believe in its shape (i.e. that values at either extreme are very likely, but anything in between is extremely not plausible) – we just want to use that to limit the impact of the prior on the posterior.

We return to this point in Note 18 in Chapter 6.

Example 2.6. *PC prior for Binomial parameter.* Another simple example is for binary data recorded for a set of individuals, $y_i \sim \text{Bernoulli}(\theta)$. We can consider as a "base-case" model the simple scenario in which $\theta = 0.5$ and thus set $g = \text{Bernoulli}(\theta_0 = 0.5)$. We want to contrast this with the more flexible (and realistic) case in which θ is unknown and can take on the values in $[0; 1]$, i.e. considering $f = \text{Bernoulli}(\theta)$.

The KLD between two Bernoulli distributions with parameters θ and θ_0, respectively, is

$$\begin{aligned}\text{KLD}(f,g) &= \sum_{y=0}^{1} \theta^y (1-\theta)^{(1-y)} \log\left[\left(\frac{\theta}{\theta_0}\right)^y \left(\frac{1-\theta}{1-\theta_0}\right)^{(1-y)}\right] \\ &= \log\left(\frac{\theta}{\theta_0}\right) \underbrace{\sum_{y=0}^{1} y\theta^y (1-\theta)^{(1-y)}}_{\text{E}_{Y|\theta}[Y]} + \log\left(\frac{1-\theta}{1-\theta_0}\right) \underbrace{\sum_{y=0}^{1} (1-y)\theta^y(1-\theta)^{(1-y)}}_{\text{E}_{Y|\theta}[1-Y]} \\ &= \theta \log\left(\frac{\theta}{\theta_0}\right) + (1-\theta)\log\left(\frac{1-\theta}{1-\theta_0}\right)\end{aligned}$$

and thus

$$d(\theta) = \sqrt{2\theta \log\left(\frac{\theta}{\theta_0}\right) + 2(1-\theta)\log\left(\frac{1-\theta}{1-\theta_0}\right)}.$$

Using simple calculus properties, we can prove that for a generic function $h(x)$, $\dfrac{\partial h(x)^{1/2}}{\partial x} = \dfrac{h'(x)}{2\sqrt{h(x)}}$. Applying this to $d(\theta)$, we can then compute

$$\begin{aligned}\frac{\partial d(\theta)}{\partial \theta} &= \frac{\left[2\theta \log\left(\frac{\theta}{\theta_0}\right) + 2(1-\theta)\log\left(\frac{1-\theta}{1-\theta_0}\right)\right]'}{2d(\theta)} \\ &= \frac{1}{d(\theta)}\left[\log\left(\frac{\theta}{1-\theta}\right) - \log\left(\frac{\theta_0}{1-\theta_0}\right)\right]\end{aligned}$$

and so we can derive the PC prior for θ as

$$p(\theta) = \lambda e^{-\lambda d(\theta)} \left|\frac{1}{d(\theta)}\left[\log\left(\frac{\theta}{1-\theta}\right) - \log\left(\frac{\theta_0}{1-\theta_0}\right)\right]\right|, \tag{2.11}$$

for given baseline probability θ_0 and scaling factor λ.

For example, we can set $\lambda = 1$ and use trial and error and numerical approximation (as in the R code below) to determine that this choice implies that about 22% of the probability mass exceed some arbitrary threshold of 0.75.

```
# Constructs a function with the definition of the PC prior
pc_prior=function(theta,theta0=0.5,lambda=1){
  # theta0 = baseline probability used in g(theta_0) - defaults at 0.5
  # lambda = scaling factor - defaults at 1

  # Computes the PC prior, guarding against singularity at d -> 0, in deriv
  d=sqrt(2*theta*log(theta/theta0) + 2*(1-theta)*log((1-theta)/(1-theta0)))
  deriv=ifelse(
    d<1e-10,1,abs((log(theta)-log(1-theta)-log(theta0)+log(1-theta0))/d)
  )
  lambda*exp(-lambda*d)*deriv
}

# Numerical integration of the function pc_prior()
```

```
# 1. selects a grid of values for theta
theta=seq(0,1,.0001)
# 2. uses the function integrate() to compute Pr(theta>0.5) under the density
# implied by the PC prior defined above. To do so, we select a grid of values
# from 0.5 to (almost) 1, as the integral must go from the value of u to 1...
u=seq(0.5,.9999,.01)
# 3. for each value in u, integrate the PC prior from that value of u up to 1
ints=list()
for (i in 1:length(u)) {
  ints[[i]]=integrate(pc_prior,u[i],1)
}
# 4. as we are only interested in the first element of the object 'cond'
# (named 'value'), we extract these and arrange them in a vector 'probs'
probs=numeric()
for (i in 1:length(ints)) {
  probs[i]=ints[[i]]$value
}
# NB: We could do more efficiently using 'lapply' and 'unlist'
ints=lapply(u,function(x) integrate(pc_prior,x,1))
probs=unlist(lapply(ints, `[[`,1))
# Normalises the probabilities (divide by the overall area under the density)
probs=probs/integrate(pc_prior,0,1)$value

# 5. searches the minimum value less than or equal to the set threshold alpha
alpha=0.22
u[min(which(probs<=alpha))]
```

```
[1] 0.75
```

Note 6: For loops vs apply functions in R

In R, functions such as `lapply()` are essentially glorified `for` loops – in fact, they do run a `for` loop in the background. However, the underlying code often calls `C` routines to do so, which makes the family of `apply()` functions slightly faster than regular `for` loops. They are also more compact and potentially easier to parallelise, which overall may generate more computational efficiency.

In other words, this prior encodes the assumption that we place around 80% chance on the fact that the underlying probability for the observed binary data is below 0.75, while keeping the impact of this prior to a minimum.

This can be appreciated by considering the very high probability associated with the tails of the resulting PC prior – cfr. this with the "standard" vague Uniform(0,1) and Jeffreys' prior, a Beta$(0.5, 0.5)$, in Figure 2.10.

We also include in Figure 2.10 another PC prior, this time computed assuming a baseline probability $\theta_0 = 0.2$ and a scaling factor $\lambda = 2$ – again, trial and error (and R code that can be adapted from the above), can show that this implies $\Pr(\theta > 0.75) \approx 0.04$.

Among other features (and unlike Jeffreys' formulation), PC priors have the advantage of being invariant to reparameterisation even in multivariate cases and provide a principled way of including "minimal information" in the prior for the model parameters.

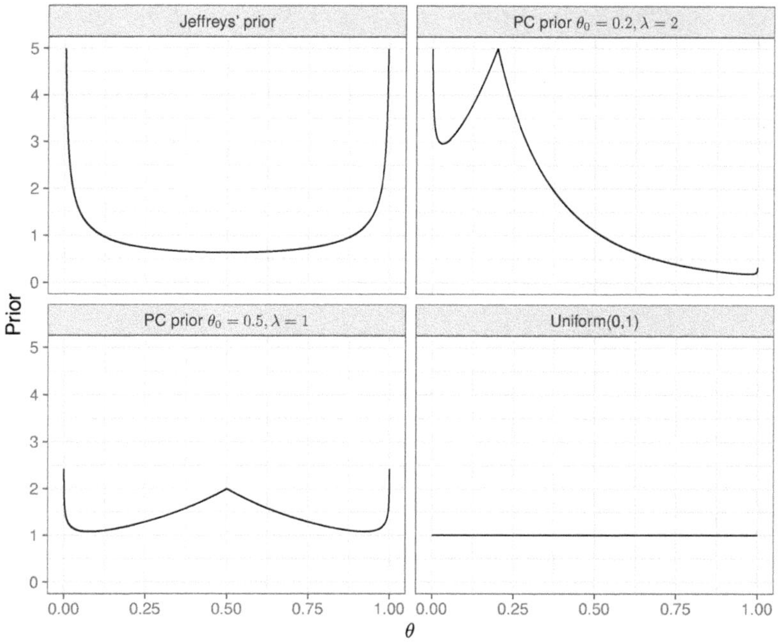

Figure 2.10: Examples of PC prior for the parameter θ, indicating a probability for a Bernoulli experiment, in comparison to the Jeffreys' prior Beta$(0.5, 0.5)$ and a Uniform$(0, 1)$. Assuming a scaling factor $\lambda = 1$ and a baseline probability of $\theta_0 = 0.5$, generates a distribution that implies that we believe that $\Pr(\theta > 0.75) \approx 0.22$. Changing the baseline probability to $\theta_0 = 0.2$ and using a scaling factor $\lambda = 2$ modifies the shape of the resulting PC prior, which now implies $\Pr(\theta > 0.75) \approx 0.04$.

On the other hand, they may not be straightforward to think about and code up (we return to this point in Section 3.4), as well as requiring the specification of a "base case" prior model.

While representing a modern and principled version, as well as also overcoming some of the mathematical and practical limitations of "default" priors, PC priors have the disadvantage that they do not necessarily imply close-form computation of the posterior distribution. In all cases where it is not possible to either write down the posterior analytically, or to approximate it numerically (e.g. through MC simulation), Bayesian modelling has for the longest time remained more or less wishful thinking – until the perfect storm of cheap computing becoming increasingly available and very helpful algorithms borrowed from Physics have been discovered, in the mid-1990s.

2.3 Markov Chain Monte Carlo

Markov Chain Monte Carlo (MCMC) methods are a class of algorithms specifically designed to obtain samples from generic probability distributions (Gilks et al., 1996; Gamerman, 1997;

Robert and Casella, 2004, 2010; Brooks et al., 2011; Gelman et al., 2013; Kruschke, 2015; McElreath, 2015).

To some extent, the first example of MCMC algorithm can be dated back to the 1950s, with what has then become famous as the "Metropolis algorithm" (Metropolis et al., 1953), later compounded by the work of Hastings (1970). The main idea underlying MCMC is that of a *Markov chain*, i.e. a sequence of random variables $Y_0, Y_1, Y_2, \ldots$, for which the distribution of the future state of the process, given the current and the past values, does not depend on the whole history, but only on part of it. In the simplest case, only the immediate past t is relevant for the next state $t+1$:

$$p(y_{t+1} \mid y_0, y_1, \ldots, y_t) = p(y_{t+1} \mid y_t) \tag{2.12}$$

and the process is said to be of "order 1", which we indicate in short as "Markov(1)", but higher order dependence is possible.

To grossly simplify a rather complex methodology, MCMC methods are based on the construction of a Markov chain that converges to the desired target distribution $p(\cdot)$ – this is the distribution from which we want to simulate; in a Bayesian context, this is the unknown posterior distribution of some parameter of interest.

Under rather broad regularity conditions, which are usually met by most practical problems (Gamerman, 1997; Jackman, 2009; Brooks et al., 2011; Kruschke, 2015; McElreath, 2015), after a sufficiently large number of iterations, the chain will forget the initial state and will converge to a unique stationary distribution, which does not depend on t or Y_0. Once convergence is reached, it is possible to calculate any required statistic using Monte Carlo simulations.

i And the rest is history...

Robert and Casella (2011) present a brief history of MCMC in the context of statistical modelling. Interestingly, much of what is now considered landmark work in Statistics has a very firm grounding in other fields, notably Physics, where algorithms (e.g. the "Gibbs sampling" – see Section 2.3.1) were designed, typically to solve a very specific (and often limited) problem.

The seminal paper by Gelfand and Smith (1990) was able to link up the two literatures – recognising that what these algorithms could do was particularly helpful for the problem of Bayesian inference. Alan Gelfand tells the fascinating story of his encounter and subsequent collaboration with Adrian Smith in Carlin and Herring (2015).

2.3.1 Gibbs sampling

One of the most popular MCMC method is the *Gibbs sampling* (Geman and Geman, 1984; Gelfand and Smith, 1990), which can be considered as a specialised version of the Metropolis-Hastings algorithm.

If we assume that the model of interest is characterised by Q parameters, $\boldsymbol\theta = (\theta_1, \theta_2, \ldots, \theta_Q)$, in the Bayesian context the objective is to obtain a representative sample from the *marginal* posterior distribution, given some relevant data $\boldsymbol y$, for all the model parameters: $p(\theta_1 \mid \boldsymbol y)$, $p(\theta_2 \mid \boldsymbol y), \ldots, p(\theta_Q \mid \boldsymbol y)$, which we assume are not analytically available. Note that these are marginal distributions because, for any element of the parameter vector θ_q, they only depend on the observed data $\boldsymbol y$ and not on the remaining parameters $\boldsymbol\theta_{-q} = (\theta_1, \theta_2, \ldots, \theta_{q-1}, \theta_{q+1}, \ldots, \theta_Q)$.

The basic condition to run the Gibbs sampling is the ability to sample from the so-called "*full-conditional*" distributions $p(\theta_1 \mid \boldsymbol{\theta}_{-1}, \boldsymbol{y}), p(\theta_2 \mid \boldsymbol{\theta}_{-2}, \boldsymbol{y}), \ldots, p(\theta_Q \mid \boldsymbol{\theta}_{-Q}, \boldsymbol{y})$ – these are not the target of the Bayesian inference, because they condition on other parameters, as well as the observed data. Nevertheless, they may make life easier, in the end, because they condition on a larger number of variables, i.e. they have more variables to the right of the conditional sign "|".

Schematically, the steps required to perform a MCMC simulation via Gibbs sampling are the following.

1. Define an initial value to be arbitrarily assigned to the parameter of interest $\theta_1^{(0)}, \theta_2^{(0)}, \ldots, \theta_Q^{(0)}$.
2. Sample:
$$\theta_1^{(1)} \sim p(\theta_1 \mid \theta_2^{(0)}, \theta_3^{(0)}, \ldots, \theta_Q^{(0)}, \boldsymbol{y})$$
$$\theta_2^{(1)} \sim p(\theta_2 \mid \theta_1^{(1)}, \theta_3^{(0)}, \ldots, \theta_Q^{(0)}, \boldsymbol{y})$$
$$\ldots$$
$$\theta_Q^{(1)} \sim p(\theta_Q \mid \theta_1^{(1)}, \theta_2^{(1)}, \ldots, \theta_{Q-1}^{(1)}, \boldsymbol{y}).$$
3. Repeat step 2. for S times until convergence is reached (see Section 2.3.2) and produce a sample from the distribution $p(\boldsymbol{\theta} \mid y)$ using Monte Carlo simulations.

We can think of this as a sampling process where we "fix" the value of all the other parameters $\boldsymbol{\theta}_{-q}$ and only sample the remaining one θ_q. The intuition as to why this actually work is that if we were able to do this repeated sampling for ∞ times, we would have a grid for $\boldsymbol{\theta}_{-q}$ with so many values that, effectively, we will have accounted for all the possible configurations in the marginal distribution $p(\theta_q \mid \boldsymbol{y})$.

Effectively, this process **marginalises out** the uncertainty in the other parameters

$$p(\theta_q \mid \boldsymbol{y}) = \int p(\theta_q \mid \boldsymbol{y}, \boldsymbol{\theta}_{-q}) p(\boldsymbol{\theta}_{-q}) d\boldsymbol{\theta}_{-p}.$$

Another way to see this is to think that, more or less,

$$p(\theta_q \mid \boldsymbol{\theta}_{-q}, \boldsymbol{y}) \approx p(\theta_q \mid \boldsymbol{y})$$

and if we have very many values of $\boldsymbol{\theta}_{-q}$, this approximation is pretty good.

Figure 2.11 shows a graphical visualisation of this process, considering a vector of $Q = 2$ parameters $\boldsymbol{\theta} = (\theta_1, \theta_2)$. In Figure 2.11a, we show the "true", underlying target distribution, indicated as $p(\theta_1, \theta_2 \mid y)$ – of course, in practice we do not know this (and that is the reason why we are running the MCMC algorithm in the first place!). We also highlight the initial point $(\theta_1^{(0)}, \theta_2^{(0)})$. As is possible to see, we have (perhaps randomly) chosen a value that is actually quite far from the target distribution.

In Figure 2.11b, we consider the first iteration of the process. First, we fix θ_2 to its current value (the initialisation $\theta_2^{(0)}$) and we simulate from the full conditional $p(\theta_1 \mid y, \theta_2^{(0)})$, depicted as the curve on the x–axis. The simulated value is the point indicated by the cross along the x–axis and we can label it as $\theta_1^{(1)}$. This is the first move from the initialisation point – the arrow going from $(\theta_1^{(0)}, \theta_2^{(0)})$ moving along the x–axis. Then, we fix θ_1 to the new current value $\theta_1^{(1)}$ and simulate a new value for θ_2 from the full conditional $p(\theta_2 \mid y, \theta_1^{(1)})$,

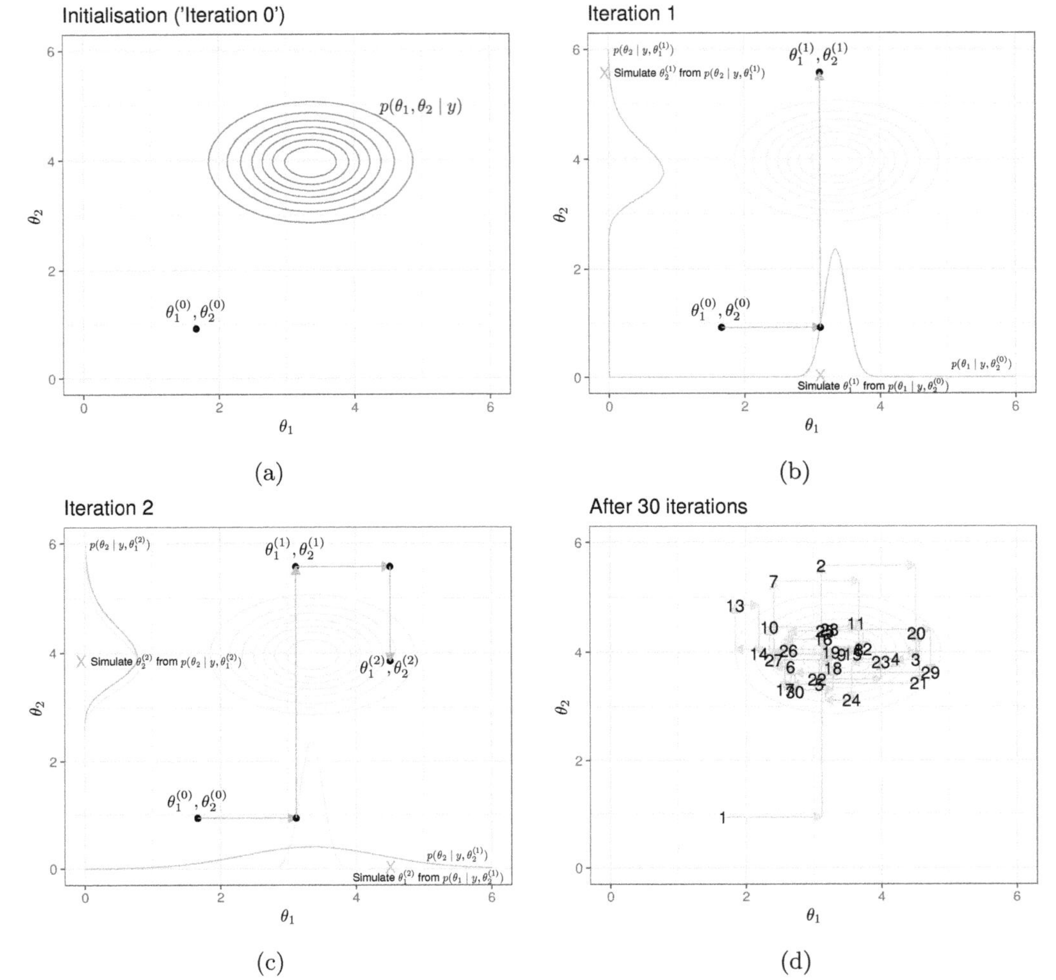

Figure 2.11: The Gibbs sampling algorithm. Starting from initialisation, we can repeatedly sample from the full conditional distributions. After we have run the process for long enough, we start to consistently visit the core part of the parametric space (the "target", posterior distribution) and we can use these simulations to summarise our revised uncertainty.

depicted as the curve along the y–axis. The simulated point $\theta_2^{(1)}$ is again indicated with the cross on the y–axis. With this, we have now completed the first iteration and a full move from $(\theta_1^{(0)}, \theta_2^{(0)})$ to $(\theta_1^{(1)}, \theta_2^{(1)})$.

Figure 2.11c shows the second iteration. We simulate from the current full conditional $p(\theta_1 \mid y, \theta_2^{(1)})$, which again is the curve along the x–axis. Notice that we have greyed out the previous full conditional (which we used at iteration 1); the current distribution has a much wider variance, which is consistent with the fact that the previous one was conditional on a smaller value for θ_2 (this would be obvious, if for instance θ_1 was a location parameter, e.g. a mean and θ_2 was a scale parameter, e.g. a variance – cfr Example 2.7). The new simulated value for θ_1, indicated as $\theta_1^{(2)}$ is again the cross along the x–axis. Then, we compute the new full posterior $p(\theta_2 \mid y, \theta_1^{(2)})$ and use it to draw a random value $\theta_2^{(2)}$, the red cross along the y–axis. Again, we grey out the previous full conditional along the y–axis – that is not relevant anymore, because we are conditioning on a different value for θ_1.

Finally, Figure 2.11d shows the MCMC trajectory for the first 30 iterations. Starting from the point labelled as 1 (the initialisation) all the way to the point labelled as 30. As we can see, while some simulations are outside of the target area, many do cover the part of the parametric space for $\boldsymbol{\theta}$. Depending on the problem, the choice of the initial values may be crucial in getting us to visit consistently the relevant portion of the parametric space – and, crucially, the first batch of iteration may be highly biased, i.e. visit parts of the parametric space that have negligible probability mass under the target (posterior) distribution. We return to these two points in Section 2.3.2.

Example 2.7. *Semi-conjugated model.* Consider the following model:

$$\begin{aligned} \boldsymbol{y} = (y_1, y_2, \ldots, y_n) &\stackrel{iid}{\sim} \text{Normal}(\mu, \sigma^2), \\ \mu &\sim \text{Normal}(\mu_0, \sigma_0^2) \\ \tau = \frac{1}{\sigma^2} &\sim \text{Gamma}(\alpha_0, \beta_0) \end{aligned}$$

Under these assumptions we can *prove* analytically (Gelman et al., 2013) that the full conditional distributions for the two parameters μ and τ are

$$\mu \mid \sigma^2, \boldsymbol{y} \sim \text{Normal}(\mu_1, \sigma_1^2) \qquad \text{with: } \mu_1 = \sigma_1^2\left(\frac{\mu_0}{\sigma_0^2} + \frac{n\bar{y}}{\sigma^2}\right) \qquad \text{and:} \quad \sigma_1^2 = \left(\frac{1}{\sigma_0^2} + \frac{n}{\sigma^2}\right)^{-1}$$

(cfr. Equation 2.8) and

$$\tau \mid \mu, \boldsymbol{y} \sim \text{Gamma}(\alpha_1, \beta_1) \qquad \text{with: } \alpha_1 = \alpha_0 + \frac{n}{2} \quad \text{and:} \quad \beta_1 = \beta_0 + \frac{1}{2}\sum_{i=1}^{n}(y_i - \mu)^2$$

(cfr. Equation 2.9).

Notice that this example does not really require Gibbs sampling or any form of MCMC to estimate the joint posterior distribution for the parameters and, in fact, we could determine the form of the posterior distributions for both $\mu \mid \boldsymbol{y}$ and $\sigma \mid \boldsymbol{y}$. However, because of its specific assumptions it is very helpful because essentially we can determine analytically the full conditional distributions for each parameter (details later). This means that we can directly and repeatedly sample from them (which is a pre-requisite of Gibbs sampling and what software such as `BUGS` do – see Chapter 3).

Notice that the full conditionals are **not** the target distributions for Bayesian inference. What we really want is the marginal posterior distributions $p(\mu \mid \boldsymbol{y})$ and $p(\tau \mid \boldsymbol{y})$, which can be simply obtained from the joint posterior $p(\mu, \tau \mid \boldsymbol{y})$.

Marginalisation

The main intuition here is to do with the basic properties of conditional probabilities. Recall that given two events A and B, then by definition $\Pr(A \mid B) = \dfrac{\Pr(A, B)}{\Pr(B)}$.

Now we can extend this to the case of three events A, B and C, by adding C to the conditioning set (i.e. to the right of the "|" symbol throughout the equation) and get

$\Pr(A \mid B, C) = \dfrac{\Pr(A, B \mid C)}{Pr(B \mid C)}$. If we replace μ for A, σ^2 for B, $\boldsymbol{y}$ for C and a probability distribution $p(\cdot)$ for the probability associated with an event $\Pr(\cdot)$, we can write

$$p(\mu \mid \sigma^2, \boldsymbol{y}) = \frac{p(\mu, \sigma^2 \mid \boldsymbol{y})}{p(\sigma^2 \mid \boldsymbol{y})} \propto p(\mu, \sigma^2 \mid \boldsymbol{y}).$$

Similarly,

$$p(\sigma^2 \mid \mu, \boldsymbol{y}) = \frac{p(\mu, \sigma^2 \mid \boldsymbol{y})}{p(\mu \mid \boldsymbol{y})} \propto p(\mu, \sigma^2 \mid \boldsymbol{y}).$$

We can then see that each full conditional is proportional to the target distribution (i.e. the joint posterior of all the parameters).

Thus, sampling repeatedly from all the full conditionals essentially gives us something that is, broadly speaking, proportional to our target joint posterior distribution. Formal theorems ensure that if we do this long enough, we are guaranteed to actually approximate the target to an arbitrary degree of precision – see also Figure 2.12.

In this case, for each of the two parameters, conditionally on (i.e. given) the other, the posterior is in the same family of the prior – the posterior for $\mu \mid \boldsymbol{y}, \sigma^2$ is still a Normal and the posterior for $\tau \mid \boldsymbol{y}, \mu$ is still a Gamma; what changes is the value of the "hyper-parameters" (i.e. the parameters of these distributions), which move from (μ_0, σ_0^2) to (μ_1, σ_1^2) and from (α_0, β_0) to (α_1, β_1). For this reason, this model is called "semi-conjugated".

These relationships clarify that the (posterior) distribution of the mean μ depends (among other things) on the variance $\sigma^2 = 1/\tau$ as well as that the posterior for the precision τ depends (among other things) on the mean μ. Crucially, *in this example*, this dependence is known in closed form. A very useful implication of this set up is that it means that we can directly determine not just the distributional form of the full conditionals (Normal for the mean and Gamma for the precision), but also the numerical value of the "hyper-parameters" $(\mu_1, \sigma_1^2, \alpha_1, \beta_1)$.

What do we really need to do?

We need to create a routine that can simulate sequentially from these distributions, with the aim of obtaining a sample from the joint posterior distribution $p(\mu, \tau \mid \boldsymbol{y})$. So, once the data $\boldsymbol{y}$ have been observed and we have fixed the values for the parameters of the prior distributions $(\mu_0, \sigma_0^2, \alpha_0, \beta_0)$, we can use for instance R, to simulate from the resulting full conditionals.

At each iteration, we will update sequentially the values of the two parameters: first we update μ by simulating from its full conditional, then we set the value of μ to the one we have just simulated and update the value of τ by randomly drawing from its full conditional. And we repeat this process "until convergence".

Data and fixed quantities

Suppose we have observed a sample of $n = 30$ data points, for example, in R you may input the data onto your workspace using the following command.

```
# Vector of observed data
y = c(
```

```
  1.2697,7.7637,2.2532,3.4557,4.1776,6.4320,-3.6623,7.7567,5.9032,
  7.2671,-2.3447,8.0160,3.5013,2.8495,0.6467,3.2371,5.8573,-3.3749,
  4.1507,4.3092,11.7327,2.6174,9.4942,-2.7639,-1.5859,3.6986,2.4544,
  -0.3294,0.2329,5.2846
)
```

Assume also that you want to set the value of the parameters for the priors as $\mu_0 = 0$, $\sigma_0^2 = 10000$ and $\alpha_0 = \beta_0 = 0.1$. In R we could define these using the following commands.

```
# "Hyper-parameters" (ie parameters for the prior distributions)
mu_0 = 0
sigma2_0 = 10000
alpha_0 = 0.01
beta_0 = 0.01
```

These are of course arbitrary values and we may have more specific knowledge to set them to different numbers.

We may also want to define some "utility" variables, that can be used later on, for instance the sample size and observed sample mean, which we can input in R as in the following code.

```
# Sample size and sample mean of the data
n = length(y)
ybar = mean(y)
```

The actual values of these variables are now stored in the respective R "objects" and can be accessed at any point. For instance, we can simply call the name of the objects to output the sample size and mean.

```
n
```

```
[1] 30
```

```
ybar
```

```
[1] 3.343347
```

Initial values

In order to run the Gibbs sampling algorithm, we need to initialise the Markov chains. This essentially means telling the computer what values should be used at iteration 0 of the process for anything that is a) associated with a probability distribution (i.e. it is not known with absolute certainty); and b) has not been observed.

In this case, the variables that are modelled with a probability distribution but are not observed are μ and τ; $\boldsymbol{y}$ is also associated with a probability distribution, but as it is observed, the MCMC algorithm does not require any further input.

We can do this in R using the following code.

```
# Sets the "seed" (for reproducibility). With this command, you will
# *always* get the exact same output
set.seed(13)
# Initialises the parameters
mu = tau = numeric()
```

```
sigma2 = 1/tau
mu[1] = rnorm(1,0,3)
tau[1] = runif(1,0,3)
sigma2[1] = 1/tau[1]
```

First, we set the "random seed" (in this case to the totally arbitrary value `13`), which ensures replicability of the results. If we run this code on any machine, we will always and invariably obtain the same results.

Then, we define the parameters `mu` and `tau` to be vectors, which in `R` we do by using the `R` built-in command function `numeric()`. Basically, the command `mu = tau = numeric()` instructs `R` to expect these two objects to be vectors of (as yet) unspecified length (if we used the command `x = numeric(5)`, we would define a vector of length 5).

Finally, we set the first value of `mu` and `tau` to be randomly generated, respectively from a Normal(mean $= 0$, sd $= 3$) and a Uniform(0, 3). Again, this is arbitrary and we may decide instead to specify a fixed, set initial point, e.g. `mu[1]=2` and `tau[1]=5` – this would also work, provided the given values are consistent with the probabilistic assumptions made for the underlying variable (thus, for instance, `tau[1]=-5` would simply break the process).

We can check the values that have been selected to initialise your Markov chain by simply typing the name of the variables (or some suitable function thereof).

```
mu
```

```
[1] 1.662981
```

```
sqrt(sigma2)
```

```
[1] 0.9249339
```

Running the Gibbs sampling

Generally speaking, the actual Gibbs sampling is really simple (if the full conditionals are known analytically!) and reduces to code such as the following.

```
# Sets the number of iterations (nsim)
nsim = 1000
# Loops over to sequentially update the parameters
for (i in 2:nsim) {
  # 1. Updates the sd of the full conditional for mu
  sigma_1 = sqrt(1/(1/sigma2_0 + n/sigma2[i-1]))
  # 2. Updates the mean of the full conditional for mu
  mu_1 = (mu_0/sigma2_0 + n*ybar/sigma2[i-1])*sigma_1^2
  # 3. Samples from the updated full conditional for mu
  mu[i] = rnorm(1,mu_1,sigma_1)
  # 4. Updates the 1st parameter of the full conditional for tau
  alpha_1 = alpha_0+n/2
  # 5. Updates the 2nd parameter of the full conditional for tau
  beta_1 = beta_0 + sum((y-mu[i])^2)/2
  # 6. Samples from the updated full conditional for tau
  tau[i] = rgamma(1,alpha_1,beta_1)
  # 7. Re-scales the sampled value on the variance scale
  sigma2[i] = 1/tau[i]
}
```

The code above matches perfectly the mathematical expressions defined for the (updated) parameters of the full posterior distributions. The loop goes from `2` to `nsim` – the first value of the vectors `mu`, `tau` and `sigma2` are filled at initialisation. Note that there is a slight inconsistency in the terminology: usually, we refer the initialisation of the process as "iteration 0" (see for instance in Figure 2.11. However, `R` does not let us index a vector with the number 0, i.e. the first element of a vector is indexed by the number 1. Thus, what we would in general indicate as $\mu^{(0)}$ to highlight the pre-algorithm stage, is actually written as `mu[1]` in the `R` code. Similarly, the updated value for μ at iteration 2 is indicated as $\mu^{(2)}$ if we start from $\mu^{(0)}$, but as `mu[3]` in the `R` code.

Note that the code above produces simulations from the full conditional of the precision τ , which are then rescaled to produce a vector of simulations from the joint posterior distribution for the variance σ^2 . It is of course very easy to also rescale these further to obtain a sample of values from the posterior of the standard deviation σ, for example using the code `sigma=sqrt(sigma2)`. This is a point we have already made in Section 1.2.3.

Once this code has been executed in `R` our output is made by vectors that, if the procedure has worked (i.e. it has converged), are drawn, at least with a very good degree of approximation, from the joint posterior distribution of the parameters.

2.3.2 Diagnostics: checking convergence and autocorrelation

For any MCMC algorithm, we need to make sure that the results we use for the Monte Carlo analysis are indeed representative of the underlying target posterior distribution. Figure 2.11 shows that the starting point may in general be very distant from the target area – of course, we do not know where the true posterior probability is in the parametric space (that is the reason why we run the MCMC procedure in the first place), but we need to account for the possibility that it may take us some time to consistently reach and sample from the core of the target posterior distribution.

Intuitively, if we only have a small number of iterations (say, 15, as in Figure 2.12a), we are not really exploring the range of the two marginal distributions (for θ_1 along the x–axis and for θ_2 along the y–axis). Thus, the simulations from the full conditionals (red crosses along the axes) are *not* a good representation of the posteriors.

However, if we run the process for long enough (in theory, for ∞ times; Figure 2.12b uses 1000 iterations), then we do cover the full range of the parameters and so the samples that we obtain can be used to describe the two posterior distributions (e.g. the histograms on the top and right sides of the plots).

There are perhaps two main implications:

1. The first few simulated values, starting from the initialisation, could be very different from representative samples from the target posterior distribution;
2. We need to select a large enough number of simulations to be reasonably sure that we are, in fact, covering the true target posterior distribution.

2.3.2.1 Burn-in and convergence

Probably the most obvious way to remedy the first issue is to run the MCMC process for long enough, so that we can simply discard the "first few" iterations, as they are potentially

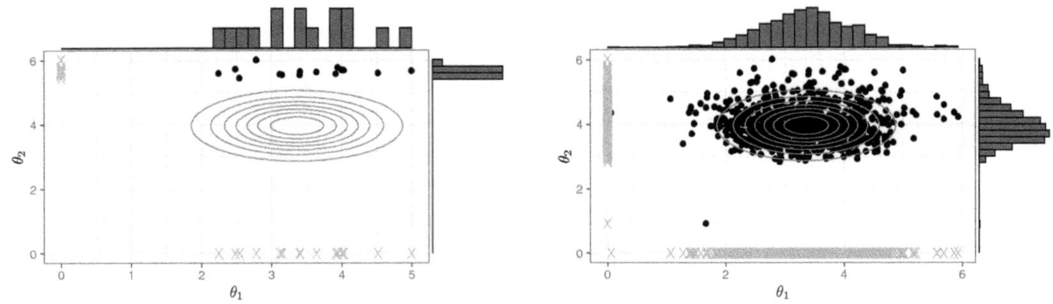

(a) (b)

Figure 2.12: With only a few simulations from the full conditionals as in panel (a), the target area is not covered and so the process has not converged. Increasing the number of simulations from the full conditionals to 1000, as in panel (b), the target area is now fully covered and the process has now reached convergence.

non-representative of the target posterior distribution. This batch of iterations to be discarded is often termed the "burn-in" (or the "warm-up"). Interestingly, this aspect was not immediately understood when the Gibbs sampling algorithm became popular in Statistics, in the mid-1990s.

Of course, as we do not know what the target distribution is, it is also difficult to assess how long should the burn-in be; for this reason, when the problem became clear (and computation became increasingly cheaper), researchers started to suggest running two or more parallel Markov chains, starting from different initial values.

Figure 2.13 shows this graphically. Here, we start Chain 1 (the darker curve) from a very large value for the parameter of interest (close to 200) and Chain 2 (the lighter one) from a value at the opposite end of the spectrum in the likely range of the parameter. For the first 250 iterations or so, the two *traceplots* go their separate way, trying to find the target posterior distribution. At about iteration 250, they start to *consistently* be on top of each other, indicating that they are now visiting the same portion of the parametric space. Eyeballing the traceplot is a relatively easy way of checking convergence, i.e. that irrespective of where we started from, we have now reached the relevant target distribution and are consistently simulating from it.

This process can drive our choice in the burn-in period. If, for instance, in the example of Figure 2.13, we had decided to initially run the MCMC algorithm for 200 iterations, using the two separate chains would allow us to clearly see an obvious lack of convergence, indicating the need to run it for longer.

We can also run more formal diagnostics to check if multiple chains end up in essentially same place. Perhaps one of the most popular is the Brooks-Gelman-Rubin statistic, more often referred to as *Potential Scale Reduction* (PSR), or $\hat{R}$ (Brooks and Gelman, 1998; Gelman and Rubin, 1992). This is based on ratio of between- to within-variances of multiple chains, formally defined as

$$\hat{R} = \sqrt{\frac{1}{W}\left(\frac{n_{sims}-1}{n_{sims}}W + \frac{1}{n_{chains}}B\right)} \tag{2.13}$$

where:

$$W = \mathrm{E}\left[\hat{\sigma}^2_1, \ldots, \hat{\sigma}^2_{n_{chains}}\right] \quad \text{and} \quad B = n_{sims}\,\mathrm{Var}\left[\hat{\mu}_1, \ldots, \hat{\mu}_{n_{chains}}\right]$$

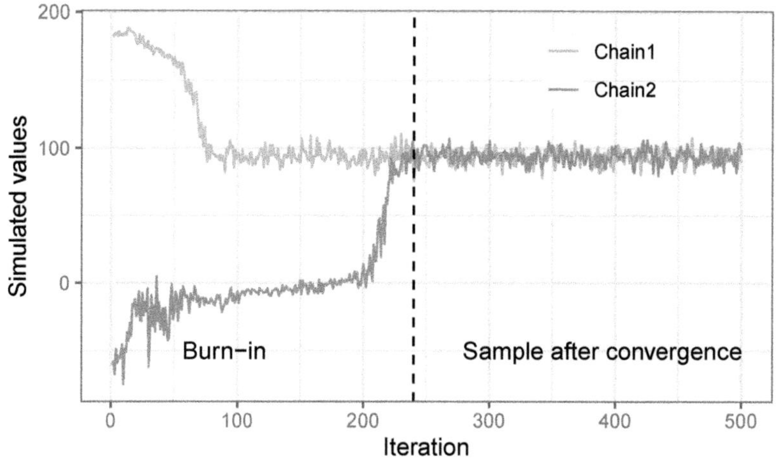

Figure 2.13: To assess convergence, we can start two independent chains from very different points. If the process works, after a while the chains will be on top of each other, meaning that both are visiting the same part of the parametric space (the target distribution).

with $(\hat{\mu}_c, \hat{\sigma}^2_c)$ indicating the sample mean and variance for the n_{sims} simulations in the c-th of the n_{chains} used.

Heuristically, the ratio of $\left(\frac{n_{sims}-1}{n_{sims}}W + \frac{1}{n_{sims}}B\right)$ to W should converge to 1 as iterations increase, because, intuitively, this would indicate a situation where the variance within chains is approximately the same as the variance between chains. This in turn would suggest that the chains are subject to some healthy variation and they are both visiting the same portion of the parametric space.

For the example shown in Figure 2.13, we can compute the PSR using the following code.

```
# Here 'x' is a matrix containing 500 rows (simulations) and 2 columns (chains)
# We can show the first 4 rows of this matrix using the command
x |> head(4)
```

```
      Chain 1    Chain 2
[1,] 183.6060 -60.85966
[2,] 182.1367 -58.33558
[3,] 184.3697 -67.64598
[4,] 184.5805 -49.01882
```

```
# Now create a little function to compute the value of PSR
Rhat=function(x) {
  # Number of simulations (rows of x)
  nsims=nrow(x)
  # Number of chains (columns of x)
  nchains=ncol(x)
  # Vector of variances for the simulated values in each chain
  sigma2.hat=apply(x,2,var)
  # Vector of means for the simulated values in each chain
  mu.hat=apply(x,2,mean)
  # Computes W and B
```

```
  W=mean(sigma2.hat)
  B=nsims*var(mu.hat)
  # Now computes and returns the PSR
  ((((nsims-1)/nsims)*W+B/nsims)/W) |> sqrt()
}

# Now compute PSR for the whole 500 simulations
Rhat(x)
```

```
[1] 1.368965
```

```
# And compute PSR from simulation 250
Rhat(x[250:500,])
```

```
[1] 1.002365
```

We first create a little function that uses the simulated values (stored in the object `x`, of which we show the first few rows) to obtain the approximated value for PSR, exactly matching Equation 2.13. As is possible to see, when we use the whole set of 500 simulations for the two chains, the value of $\hat{R} = 1.368965 >> 1$, indicating lack of convergence. When we restrict the sample to the simulations after the 250-th iteration (as inspected in the traceplot of Figure 2.13), we get $\hat{R} = 1.002365$, which is now, consistently with the traceplot, closer to 1 and thus indicates convergence.

2.3.2.2 Autocorrelation

Because of how MCMC algorithms – and especially the Gibbs sampling – work, another issue to consider carefully when assessing the validity of a set of simulations to be used for MC estimation of a quantity of interest is the information load that it carries. The main reason for this is that, because of how they are obtained, successive MCMC iterations tend to be correlated. The s-th simulation for the q-th element of the parameter vector $\boldsymbol\theta = (\theta_1, \ldots, \theta_Q)$ is obtained from the full conditional distribution where $\boldsymbol\theta_{-q}$ are fixed to the value simulated last.

⚠ Information vs correlation

Here the main idea is that a sample of S simulated values may not actually contribute the same amount of information that the nominal sample size suggest. If we had S independent data points, then each would contribute 1 "information point" and thus the overall sample information load would be, intuitively, S. But because of correlation, it is likely that the information load is overall less than S.

Consider for instance a survey in which you want to collect information on the frequency of surnames. You may go around households and ask for the surname of the people living in a given one. Imagine that the first house you hit is a shared accommodation, where University students live. Because they are totally unrelated (i.e. statistically independent, as far as their surname is concerned), if you observe 4 data points (= people), you will probably get 4 separate responses, which means an overall "information load" of 4.

Imagine now that your next household is a traditional family home, where the 4 residents all share the same surname. In this case, while the number of data points is the same as before, the information load is simply 1 – because of the fact that all the

> residents are correlated, then every response contribute only 1 "information point", combined.

The consequence of the above issue is that if the MCMC sample is highly *autocorrelated* (i.e. successive iterations, even at higher lags, for instance every other l), then S data points will contribute a much lower "*effective sample size*" (ESS, see Lunn et al., 2013; Raftery and Lewis, 1992). This can be formally defined as

$$n_{eff} = \frac{n_{sims}}{1 + 2\sum_{l=1}^{\infty} \rho_l}, \tag{2.14}$$

where $\rho_l = \dfrac{\text{Cov}\left(\theta^{(t)}, \theta^{(t+l)}\right)}{\text{Var}(\theta)}$ is the autocorrelation between two simulations separated by a lag l.

We can provide an approximation to the ESS by computing

$$n_{eff} \approx n_{chains} n_{sims} \min\left[\frac{1}{B}\left(\frac{n_{sims}-1}{n_{sims}}W + \frac{B}{n_{sims}}\right), 1\right], \tag{2.15}$$

which is a measure of the equivalent number of independent observations to the correlated MCMC sample.

We can use Equation 2.15 and compute the ESS for both the whole sample in the object `x` (made by 500 iterations per chain) and the one restricted to the last 250 iterations and get values of $n_{eff} = 4.28$ and $n_{eff} = 230.47$, respectively. The sample "at convergence" has a much larger ESS, which is closer to the nominal sample size (250 iterations per chain, so 500 in total), although still lower, by effect of the intrinsic autocorrelation.

In addition to this analysis, we can use the following R code and the `bmhe` function `acfplot()` to visualise the amount of temporal correlation in the simulated values in Figure 2.14.

```
# Stacks the two chains into a vector of 500x2 iterations & plots AC function
c(x) |> bmhe::acfplot() +
  labs(title="Autocorrelation for all 1000 iterations")
# Stacks the two chains into a vector of 250x2 iterations & plots AC function
c(x[250:500,]) |> bmhe::acfplot() +
  labs(title="Autocorrelation for the last 500 iterations")
```

As is possible to see, when we select the whole sample of 500 iteration per chain (so 1000 in total), as in Figure 2.14a, the level of autocorrelation is large, even for large values of the lag: values $l = 1, \ldots, L$ along the x–axis indicate that we are considering the correlation between iterations that are l places apart. If things have worked, the level of autocorrelation should be reasonably small, even for small lags – this is clearly not the case in Figure 2.14a, when even at lag $l = 30$ correlation is around 0.75.

If we instead restrict the sample to the final 250 per chain (so 500 in total), things are much better – for the whole range of lags depicted in Figure 2.14b, the value of the correlation among iterations is much smaller and contained within a margin of Monte Carlo error (indicated by the horizontal dashed lines).

2.3.2.3 How many MCMC iterations should I use?

One of the critical questions in any MCMC procedure is about the size of the Markov chain sample to be used for the Monte Carlo estimation of the relevant quantities. As suggested

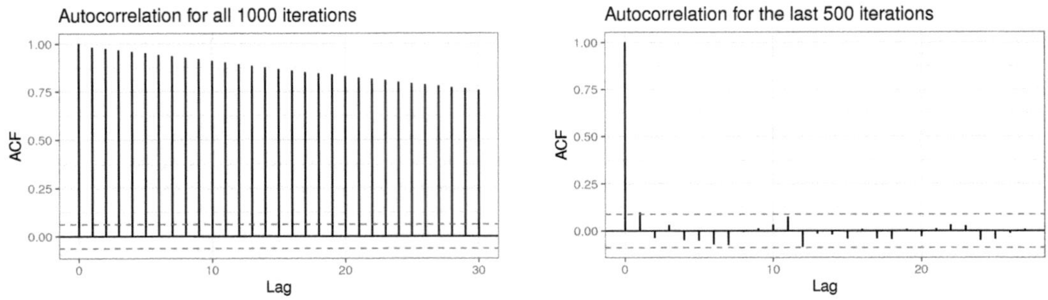

(a) $S = 1000$. (b) $S = 500$.

Figure 2.14: Autocorrelation functions for the simulated values of Figure 2.13. Panel (a) shows the while $S = 1000$ iterations, which display a large amount of autocorrelation, induced by the burn-in. Panel (b) only considers the simulations produced after convergence is reached (as visualised in Figure 2.13): in this case, autocorrelation is massively reduced.

above, ideally, we want n_{eff} to be as close as possible to the nominal sample size S, which indicates that the level of autocorrelation is minimal, thus leading to a MCMC sample that contains sufficient information. Raftery and Lewis (1995) suggest to get 95% posterior quantiles with true 94.5-95.5% coverage we typically need ESS > 4000.

On the other hand, almost invariably, the default choice is for $n_{sims} = 1000$ simulations. Historically, 1000 was a large enough, round-looking number, which would nicely balance the need for representativeness (which increases with the number of simulations) and the computational performance (which, in the 1990s was *much* less powerful than it is today, on a standard machine).

In very many applications, keeping 1000 simulations after convergence and using these to get the relevant estimates is probably sufficient – some of the examples we consider in the next chapters use exactly this strategy. But the choice of $n_{sims} = 1000$ after convergence should *not* be made dogmatically.

One important metrics to consider is the *Monte Carlo Standard Error* (MCSE), computed as the ratio of the standard deviation of the MCMC simulations to the effective sample size. So for a generic vector of S simulations $\left(\theta^{(1)}, \ldots, \theta^{(S)}\right)$, the MCSE is

$$\text{MCSE}(\theta) = \frac{\text{sd}\left(\theta^{(1)}, \ldots, \theta^{(S)}\right)}{\sqrt{n_{eff}}}$$

and it is a measure of how accurate the posterior mean is (Kruschke, 2015).

In the example shown above, we can compute the MCSE for the simulations stored in the object `x` by taking the standard deviation of the two chains stacked up as a vector and then dividing by $\sqrt{n_{eff}}$, which gives values of 24.343 and 0.34981, respectively.

Another helpful advice is to test the stability of the estimates (cfr. Figure 1.8), upon varying the length of the MCMC sample. This is generally helpful, because we may not have a good idea of how slow the process will be and thus we may start with a short run (to sort of "test the water"), then produce a longer sample and then may an even longer still. Comparing the resulting estimates may give us an indication of whether any marginal improvement is worth it – if the estimates do not vary very much, we are probably fine to stop.

2.3.2.4 Centring and thinning

When substantial autocorrelation is present, we have several options to try and mitigate it. Often, the best idea is to try and reparameterise the model – for instance, in a regression model

$$\begin{aligned} y_i &\sim \text{Normal}(\mu_i, \sigma) \\ \mu_i &= \alpha + \beta x_i, \end{aligned}$$

the posterior distributions for the two regression coefficients (α, β) tend to be highly correlated, which in turns slows down convergence. One easy and efficient way around it is to reparameterise the linear predictor as

$$\mu_i = \alpha^* + \beta^*(x_i - \bar{x}),$$

i.e. by considering the *centred* version of the covariate (see Section 2.4.7 of Baio, 2012). This changes the scale of the intercept α^*, but helps break the correlation among the coefficients, thus improving convergence.

An alternative to model reparameterisation is to use "brute force", i.e. run the model for a much longer time – there are theorems to ensure that if $S \to \infty$, convergence is guaranteed. Other than the computational effort, this has, possibly, some implications in terms of computer memory – if we run an MCMC process for, say, twenty parameters and for 1 000 000 iterations after a burn-in of 10 000 iterations, then we would be storing in the computer memory a very large object.

To limit this issue we can use *thinning* – this amounts to running the process for longer (which is what makes the actual difference), but only retaining one in every T simulations. The resulting sample that we save for the MC analysis is thus shorter than the actual number of simulations, which makes it more manageable. See the example discussed in Section 3.3 for more details.

Example 2.8. *Semi-conjugated model (continued): convergence.* As this model is semi-conjugated, convergence is not really an issue. However, to demonstrate this, we replicate the MCMC process shown in Example 2.7, using two different sets of starting points. We can do this using the following R code.

```
# Wrap up the MCMC code into a function; Takes the number of simulations
# as input, with default arbitrarily set at 1000
gibbs=function(nsim=1000) {
  for (i in 2:nsim) {
      sigma_n=sqrt(1/(1/sigma2_0 + n/sigma2[i-1]))
      mu_n=(mu_0/sigma2_0 + n*ybar/sigma2[i-1])*sigma_n^2
      mu[i]=rnorm(1,mu_n,sigma_n)

    alpha_n=alpha_0+n/2
    beta_n=beta_0 + sum((y-mu[i])^2)/2
    tau[i]=rgamma(1,alpha_n,beta_n)
    sigma2[i]=1/tau[i]
  }
  sigma=sqrt(sigma2)
  # Saves the output to a list
  list(mu=mu,sigma=sigma)
```

```
}

# Create a list object in which we will store the results
sims=list()

# First set of initial values
mu=tau=numeric()
sigma2=1/tau
mu[1]=rnorm(1,0,3)
tau[1]=runif(1,0,3)
sigma2[1]=1/tau[1]
# Run the MCMC algorithm and save the output in the first element of 'sims'
sims[[1]]=gibbs(5000)

# Then selects different initial values
mu=tau=numeric()
sigma2=1/tau
mu[1]=rnorm(1,10,3)
tau[1]=runif(1,5,10)
sigma2[1]=1/tau[1]
# Re-run the MCMC algorithm, saving the output in the second element of 'sims'
sims[[2]]=gibbs(5000)
```

Because the algorithm is quite cheap, computationally, we simulate $n_{sims} = 5000$ iterations in each chain, which we can use to assess convergence. For instance, we can use the function `Rhat()` defined above and apply it to a matrix with two columns (each a vector of simulations for either `mu` or `sigma` from the two MCMC chains), to compute $\hat{R}$.

```
# Uses the function Rhat() to compute the PSR for 'mu' and 'sigma'
Rhat(cbind(sims[[1]]$mu,sims[[2]]$mu))
```

```
[1] 0.9999104
```

```
Rhat(cbind(sims[[1]]$sigma,sims[[2]]$sigma))
```

```
[1] 0.9999196
```

For both variables, the value of $\hat{R}$ is extremely close to 1, indicating that convergence is achieved. This is also confirmed by the visual inspection of the two traceplots, shown in Figure 2.15. Again, as the model is semi-conjugated, even starting from very different initial values, the two chains converge immediately.

If we apply Equation 2.15 we can also compute $n_{eff} = 10\,000$ for both μ and σ. In this case, the combination of a large MCMC run and the fact that the model is semi-conjugated implies that for all parameters the ESS this coincides with the nominal sample size.

2.3.3 Hamiltonian Monte Carlo

Hamiltonian Monte Carlo (HMC – see Betancourt, 2018; Neal, 2011; Gelman et al., 2013; Kruschke, 2015) is another important MCMC algorithm, which has recently gained popularity. HMC is based on the physical concept of *Hamiltonian dynamics*, which can be used

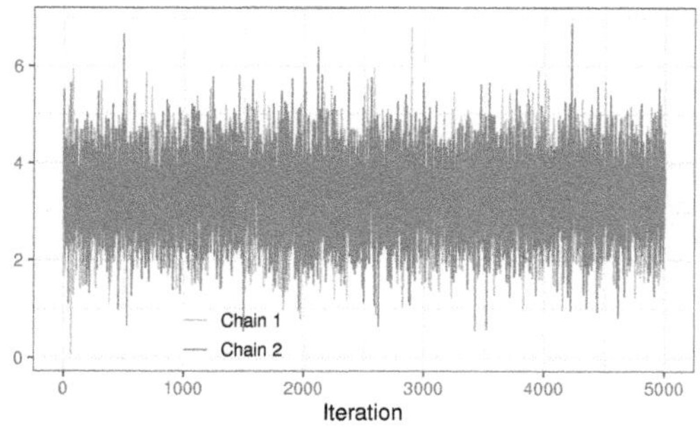

(a) $p(\mu \mid \boldsymbol{y})$.

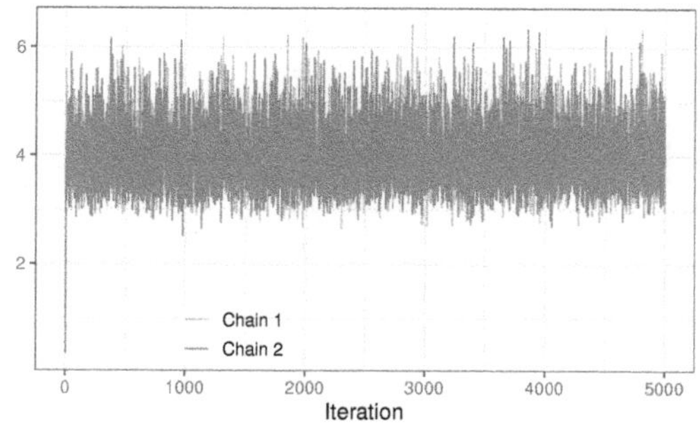

(b) $p(\sigma \mid \boldsymbol{y})$.

Figure 2.15: Traceplots for the simulations for $p(\mu \mid \boldsymbol{y})$ and $p(\sigma \mid \boldsymbol{y})$.

to model the idealised situation of a frictionless particle sliding over a surface of varying slope.

In a nutshell, HMC is an extension of simpler MCMC algorithms such as the Metropolis-Hastings, which are based on random walks through the parameter space, where successive moves are derived from a proposed symmetrical distribution (centred around the current parameter position) and accepted or rejected, depending on the relative density of the target (posterior) at the current parameter value.

The main innovation of HMC is that, to determine the next state of the parameters, it uses a proposal distribution that does not need to be symmetrical. In addition – and crucially – this proposal distribution changes depending on the current value of the model parameters. This makes the process highly adaptive and particularly efficient in cases where the number of parameters is very large.

Intuitively, we can think of HMC as a smart explorer navigating a rugged terrain whose height represents the (negative log-)density associated with different parameter values. The explorer uses information about the gradient of this density to guide its movement, allowing it to traverse the terrain more efficiently and sample from the distribution more effectively.

The classic analogy used to explain HCM is that of a marble travelling on a slope: the original position is generated randomly and the marble is given a random flick, to gain initial momentum. As shown in Figure 2.16, if the marble is in an area of low probability or, equivalently, high "potential energy" (i.e. the negative log-density), then it will tend to slide more quickly down the slope and will retain higher momentum before eventually stopping. If, on the other hand, it sits at the bottom of the valley (i.e. the area of highest density), the flick will have to be much stronger to make it climb over the hills.

The main idea is that, using complex Hamiltonian dynamics (based on differential equations) to approximate the physical movements of the marble, a single iteration of HMC involves letting the marble slide up and down the potential energy function for a set number of discrete times, at the end of which the new position is proposed. This is then subjected to a Metropolis-like acceptance step.

By using information about the gradient of the target distribution to propose more informed moves, HMC is able to explore the space more effectively and sample from the target distribution more efficiently. This is particularly true in high-dimensional spaces and for sampling from distributions with complex geometries or strong correlations, where traditional MCMC methods may struggle.

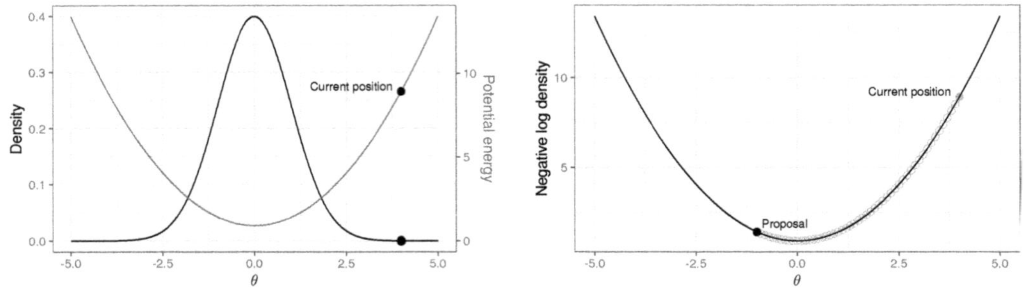

(a) (b)

Figure 2.16: A simplified schematic representation of HMC dynamics. Panel (a) shows the target density and the resulting 'potential energy', computed as the negative log-density. If the current value of the parameter
theta (the black dot) lies in an area of low probability under the target density, or, equivalently, an area of high potential under the negative log-density, then it is easier to slide down the steeper surface towards the area of higher density (i.e. lower potential). Panel (b) shows that when the 'particle' is flicked from its initial position, it starts to slide down the potential energy function. The trajectory observed over a set number of discrete times (obtained through Hamiltonian dynamics), starting from the current position, is described as the greyed-out area in panel (b). The arrival point, in black in panel (b) is the proposed move. Adapted from Kruschke (2015).

HMC vs Gibbs sampling

Generally speaking, HMC can be more computationally efficient than other MCMC schemes (including Gibbs sampling) because of the following features.

1. *Exploration of high-dimensional spaces.* HMC incorporates information about the geometry of the target distribution through Hamiltonian dynamics, allowing it to move more effectively through the space and explore distant regions in fewer steps. In contrast, Gibbs sampling updates each parameter individually, which can be less effective in high-dimensional spaces due to slow mixing.
2. *Adaptive proposals.* HMC can adaptively tune the proposal distribution during sampling by adjusting its defining features based on the local geometry of the target distribution. This adaptability can lead to more efficient exploration of complex distributions with varying scales and correlations. Gibbs sampling, on the other hand, generates samples based on the full conditionals for each parameter, which may not always be optimal for efficient exploration.
3. *Handling correlated variables.* HMC is better suited for sampling from distributions with strong correlations among the parameters. By using Hamiltonian dynamics to propose *joint* updates of the parameters, HMC can more effectively traverse the parameter space and capture dependencies between variables. In Gibbs sampling, updates are made independently for each parameter, which may result in slower convergence when dealing with correlated variables.

4. *Computational efficiency*. While HMC involves additional computational overhead due to the simulation of Hamiltonian dynamics and the need for gradient calculations, it can be more computationally efficient in high-dimensional settings compared to Gibbs sampling. This efficiency is especially pronounced when the target distribution exhibits complex geometric structures or strong correlations, as HMC can exploit this information to propose more effective moves in the parameter space.

In reality, in the majority of applications of Bayesian modelling to HTA problems (as presented in the rest of this book), there are only marginal gains in using the more complex HMC structure.

With the notable exceptions of highly structured hierarchical models (as those arising in the cases shown in Chapter 6 and more specifically in Chapter 11) and survival analysis (Chapter 8), Gibbs sampling is typically sufficient to fully and efficiently explore the target posterior distribution in which we are interested in the HTA context.

For this reason, we have presented here only a sketch of the main features of HMC – but refer the reader to, for example, Stan development team (2024), Kruschke (2015) or McElreath (2015) for more detailed and yet accessible descriptions.

2.4 Conclusions

This chapter has presented the process of Bayesian computation, with a view of combining background or contextual information (in the form of a prior distribution) with evidence from data, into a full posterior distribution. We have looked at ways in which we can define the prior distribution, aiming at not excerpting undue sensitivity on the final inference, but also allowing the inclusion of genuine information into the model.

We have also described in detail the basics of Markov Chain Monte Carlo algorithms (specifically the Gibbs sampling), which are used to make Bayesian inference. This process requires careful post-processing to ensure that the results are sensible and we have provided several diagnostic measures and a workflow to use in practice.

In the next chapter, we showcase specific software that can be used to make Bayesian inference. We consider `JAGS` as the software of choice throughout most of this book and we discuss in details the setup and machinery necessary to run Bayesian models.

3

Bayesian software

3.1 Introduction

As discussed in Section 2.3, if it is possible to sample from the full conditional distributions, suitable Markov Chain Monte Carlo algorithms (e.g. a Gibbs sampler) can be programmed in a relatively easy way. However, in most practical situations, the required conditional distributions are not analytically tractable and therefore it is necessary to approximate them (e.g. by means of algorithms such as Metropolis-Hastings or slice sampling) before a machinery such as the Gibbs sampling can be put in place.

In this chapter we look specifically at how Bayesian modelling can be performed using specialised software – we concentrate on popular Gibbs sampling programmes (such as the various flavours of BUGS). There are of course other possibilities and the review we provide below is far from exhaustive. On balance, however, for the vast majority of applications in health technology assessment, Gibbs sampling is probably sufficient; in addition, while not necessarily the most frequent tool for inference in this application area (yet...), BUGS-like models are reasonably popular with health economists (particularly in the case of evidence synthesis – see Chapter 6).

For this reason, we concentrate on them both in this chapter and for the vast majority of the rest of this book.

3.1.1 BUGS/JAGS

The most popular software that allows the semi-automation of MCMC procedures is probably BUGS – with this term we indicate the original incarnation (Spiegelhalter et al., 1996)[1], the MS Windows version WinBUGS (Spiegelhalter et al., 2002b) and its successor OpenBUGS (Lunn et al., 2009; Lunn et al., 2013), whose widespread use has arguably contributed to the establishment of applied Bayesian statistics, in the last thirty years.

The acronym BUGS stands for *Bayesian analysis Using Gibbs Sampling* and the process requires the user to specify a statistical model (e.g. a set of distributional and functional relationships among the quantities involved in the problem), for example such as the following code (we provide more details on the BUGS syntax in Example 3.1).

```
model {
  for (i in 1:N) {
     y[i] ~ dnorm(mu[i], tau)
     mu[i] <- alpha + beta*x[i]
  }
```

[1]The author is nerdly proud of sharing his birthday (only several years earlier...) with the day of the first ever public release of "classic BUGS", back in August 1996.

DOI: 10.1201/9781003771050-3

```
  tau ~ dgamma(0.1,0.1)
  sigma <- pow(tau,-0.5)
}
```

The BUGS code always starts with the keyword `model`, followed by "curly brackets" `{}` that enclose the model specification. The syntax maps very closely to the standard, "pen-and-paper" statistical notation, with the symbols `~` and `<-` indicating stochastic and logical relationship, respectively; for instance, the model described above can be written in statistical language as

$$\begin{aligned} y_i &\sim \text{Normal}(\mu_i, \sigma) \qquad \text{for } i = 1, \ldots, N \\ \mu_i &= \alpha + \beta x_i \\ \tau &\sim \text{Gamma}(0.01, 0.01) \\ \sigma &= \tau^{-0.5} \end{aligned}$$

– note that τ is the *precision* (= inverse variance), which is used in BUGS to index the Normal distribution, alongside the mean.

Note 7: Precision vs standard deviation

The fact that BUGS defines the Normal distribution in terms of the precision is pretty much a historical accident. In a Normal model, the precision is useful because it is possible to derive a conjugate prior (see Section 2.2.2 and Example 2.7) and thus when designing BUGS in the early days of the "Gibbs sampling revolution" (see Section 2.3), the coders took advantage of this specific parameterisation, which could be vital in speeding up the computation.

The notation has since stuck and even later versions of BUGS have continued to use this parameterisation. Other Bayesian software (e.g. `Stan` – see Section 3.1.2) have favoured a more natural parameterisation for a Normal distribution (i.e. in terms of mean and standard deviation), which is sometimes easier to deal with.

BUGS has a built-in *parser*, which inspects the set of declarations and translates them into a DAG (see Section 1.1), exploiting as much as possible the underlying conditional independence relationships. These generally make the computation simpler and faster, because only a small portion of the whole model needs to be considered at any given time (Lunn et al., 2013).

The DAG resulting from the code above is shown in Figure 3.1, where nodes are represented in ovals; single arrows indicate probabilistic relationships, while double-edged arrows indicate logical relationships, e.g. the node `sigma` depends logically on the node `tau` through the relationship `sigma <- pow(tau,-0.5)`, which maps onto the mathematical relationship $\sigma = \tau^{-0.5}$. The "plate" (i.e. the rectangles) enclosing the nodes `y[i]`, `x[i]` and `mu[i]` indicate that their values and underlying relationships hold `for (i in 1:N)`, i.e. for the N observations.

By and large, BUGS allows models of (almost) arbitrary complexity. The software includes an "expert system", which determines an appropriate MCMC scheme to be used in the simulation procedure. When possible, BUGS exploits conjugacy (see Section 2.2.2) to speed

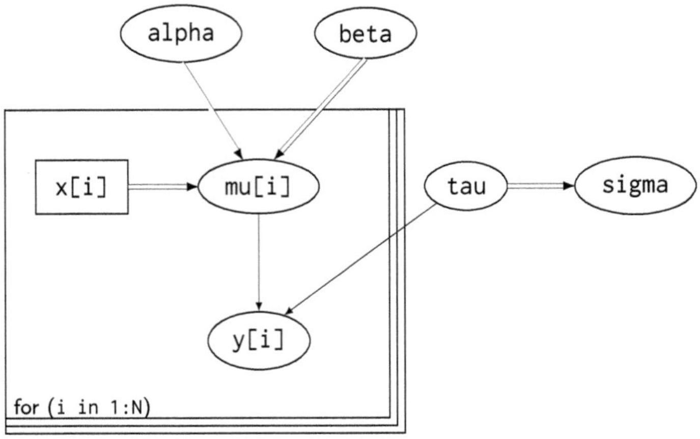

Figure 3.1: The DAG constructed by BUGS starting from the linear regression model assumptions passed by the user. Ovals indicate modelled variables, while rectangles indicate observed, but unmodelled data. Single-edged arrows indicate probabilistic dependence, while double-edged arrows indicate logical relationships. The “plates” surrounding the variables indexed by `[i]` indicate that the structure of relationships and data are for N overall units.

up the process; when this is not possible, alternative algorithms are used to obtain the required MCMC estimation.

As mentioned above, there are three main versions of BUGS. The first one (called WinBUGS), which can be downloaded at https://www.mrc-bsu.cam.ac.uk/software is an established and stable, stand-alone version of the software. While still available (the latest and last version is 1.4, dating back to August 2007), WinBUGS is not further developed.

The second (OpenBUGS, also available at https://www.mrc-bsu.cam.ac.uk/software) is an open-source version of the software. At the time of writing this book, the latest release of OpenBUGS is 3.2.2 and it has been designed to be at least as efficient and reliable as WinBUGS over a wide range of test applications.

Finally, the most recent version is called MultiBUGS (Goudie et al., 2020), downloadable from https://www.multibugs.org, which automatically parallelises the MCMC algorithm to speed up computation. The syntax for the three versions of BUGS is essentially identical and the same code should work on either.

Another very relevant and popular “dialect” of the BUGS language is JAGS (*Just Another Gibbs Sampler* – Plummer, 2010; Kruschke, 2015), which can be downloaded from the website https://mcmc-jags.sourceforge.io. While WinBUGS and OpenBUGS are written in Component Pascal[2], JAGS is written in C++, which effectively makes it platform-independent. Because every operating system has a C++ compiler and standard library, JAGS can be run natively under MS Windows, Unix/Linux or Mac. Similar to BUGS, JAGS can be interfaced with R by means of suitable libraries.

[2]This is a relatively obscure language implemented in a particularly low-level environment, known as *Black Box Component Builder*, with compiler available only for MS Windows (although the latest release of OpenBUGS does run under Linux and, using a virtual machine, under Mac too).

For this reason[3], JAGS is the preferred tool for Bayesian inference in this book.

3.1.2 Other Bayesian software

Following the introduction of BUGS, much research has also been devoted to developing more software specifically designed for Bayesian analysis. More recently, new MCMC methods have been developed in the form of Hamiltonian (or Hybrid) Monte Carlo (HMC, Duane et al., 1987) – see also Section 2.3.3. Hoffman and Gelman (2013) and Betancourt (2018) have implemented a very clever algorithm that is at the heart of Stan (https://mc-stan.org/), another Bayesian sampler programmed in C++ that can be used very efficiently, particularly for hierarchical models (Gelman et al., 2013). The package rstan interfaces the C++ original code from R, which has contributed to the increasing popularity of this mode of inference. Kruschke (2015) and McElreath (2015) provide extensive examples of implementation of Bayesian models using R and rstan.

Another very interesting development is Integrated Nested Laplace Approximation (INLA, Rue et al., 2009; Blangiardo et al., 2013; Blangiardo and Cameletti, 2015; Wang et al., 2018; Gómez-Rubio, 2020). INLA (implemented in the package R-INLA, downloadable at http://www.r-inla.org/) is a very fast approximate Bayesian inference method; for a relatively wide class of models, INLA can be used to compute the marginal posterior distribution of the parameters without using MCMC, which usually produces a substantial decrease in the computational time. In the context of this book and HTA in general, both Stan and R-INLA can be used in survival modelling (Chapter 8), while Stan is the core engine for Bayesian modelling of indirect treatment comparisons (Chapter 11).

As suggested above, a common characteristic of all these programmes is the possibility to interface each of these with statistical software, e.g. with R. This means that the whole process of Bayesian analysis can be run using R to pre-process the data (e.g. by loading a dataset and creating relative variables), run the Bayesian analysis (e.g. MCMC, HMC or INLA) using BUGS, JAGS, Stan or INLA in the background and then use R to post-process the resulting posterior distribution, for example to assess convergence, plot histograms or compute functions of the parameters. This simplifies and help standardise the whole process of Bayesian analysis.

In a slightly different, but related way, NIMBLE (https://r-nimble.org/, NIMBLE Development Team, 2016) and greta (https://greta-stats.org/) are R packages that can be used to perform MCMC inference directly from R; instead of leaving the simulation from the posterior distributions to a specific software, NIMBLE works by letting the user specify the model in a BUGS-like syntax and then uses C++ to compile and run the required algorithms. greta builds statistical models interactively in R, and then sample from them by different types of MCMC algorithms, including HMC. Finally, Python (https://www.python.org/) and Julia (https://julialang.org/) are very popular with "data scientists" and have specific modules for Bayesian inference.

Pragmatically, what software is used for Bayesian modelling is not really *that* relevant, provided the user is able to understand the actual modelling specification and what the underlying inferential algorithm is actually doing. As mentioned above, however, we feel that BUGS-like programmes are probably still the most cost-effective for applications in HTA.

[3] Upon joining UCL in 2005, the then IT manager told me: "I'll install Linux on your machine. You will probably hate it for a while, but then you will never look back". I have not looked back.

3.2 Running JAGS from R

Historically, BUGS was built to run as stand-alone, with a specific graphic user interface. Pretty soon, however, this has been effectively superseded by several packages, macros or add-on that would allow to interface it with "proper" statistical software, such as R, Matlab, Stata or SAS.

The main reason for this is that in essence, BUGS is not a statistical language; rather it is a set of instructions that are used to figure out the most efficient way of producing simulations from a target probability distribution. As such, pre-processing, data wrangling, graphing and reporting facilities are extremely limited in BUGS. Interfacing with statistical software overcomes this limitation – and this has further contributed to the success and wide use of BUGS.

We thus need a suitable library to interface R with the MCMC software of choice. For JAGS, we use R2jags (Su and Yajima, 2010), which is based on rjags (Plummer, 2023), while for BUGS it is possible to use packages such as R2WinBUGS (Sturtz et al., 2005) or R2OpenBUGS (Sturtz et al., 2019). These packages allow the user to perform the analysis from within R by running BUGS/JAGS in the background and they can be installed as usual.

```
install.packages("R2jags")
install.packages("R2OpenBUGS")
```

Note that we do not require both BUGS and JAGS (and thus the respective R packages) – we can choose the one we prefer (which may depend on the operating system and/or other considerations) and just have that installed on the machine. Again, in the examples in the next chapters, we will use primarily JAGS.

In general, the process works as follows:

1. Use R to pre-process the relevant data; this may entail loading a dataset from a spreadsheet or external file, creating new variables, by aggregating or modify existing ones, etc.
2. Code the statistical model to be run (typically in an external text file) and use suitable commands to launch either JAGS or BUGS in background.
3. Once the MCMC run is finished, the simulations become available in the R session where the user is able to post-process them to complete the Bayesian analysis, for instance to produce tables and graphs.

Example 3.1. *Drug (continued): conjugate analysis calling* JAGS *from* R. Consider again the situation described in Example 2.3, where we have managed to perform a small pilot study in which we have observed $y = 15$ in $n = 20$ individuals to whom we have given the back-pain relief drug. We can replicate the analysis using JAGS, but we also expand the scenario shown in Example 1.5. In that case, we propagated the uncertainty in the prior distribution and produced MC samples from the prior predictive distribution.

In the current case, we have already gone beyond that stage, because we have observed y – thus we can update the uncertainty in θ to the posterior $p(\theta \mid y)$ and then use that to propagate the revised level of knowledge and compute, by means of simulations, the *posterior* predictive distribution

$$p(y^* \mid y) = \int p(y^* \mid \theta)p(\theta \mid y)d\theta \tag{3.1}$$

(compare this with Equation 1.7).

In other words, we may want to assess what we could reasonably expect if we were able to observe, in the future, a further sample (say of m new observations): how many y^* would we reasonably observe, given the current evidence?

We need to map the modelling assumptions in the BUGS language. Fortunately, this is fairly straightforward as most of the syntax is relatively similar to how we would describe the model in "pen and paper". For the current example, the model code is something like the following.

```
model {
   theta     ~ dbeta(a,b)                 # prior distribution
   y         ~ dbin(theta,m)              # sampling distribution
   y.pred    ~ dbin(theta,n)              # predictive distribution
   P.crit   <- step(y.pred - ncrit + 0.5) # =1 if y.pred >= ncrit
                                          # =0    otherwise
}
```

In the code above, `y` and `y.pred` share the same distributional assumption.

In DAG terms, we could represent this situation as in Figure 3.2: panel (a) shows the alleged data-generating process. The two observ*able* variables y and y^* are assumed to be generated by a common mechanism, depending on a parameter θ, for which we are willing to describe our current uncertainty using a distribution $p(\theta)$ and suitable observed constants (hence represented in grey squares), n and m – technically, y and y^* are said to be *exchangeable* (see Section 6.2.4). Random, yet unobserv*ed*, or simply unobserv*able* variables are depicted in white circles.

Panel (b) in Figure 3.2 shows the update process. When data y are observed (indicated by the fact that the node y is now represented in a grey circle), then the information travels "against the arrows" of the DGP, to update first the uncertainty on the unobserv*able* parameter θ into the posterior $p(\theta \mid y)$. This in turn is used to update the uncertainty in yet unobserv*ed*, but potentially observ*able* y^*

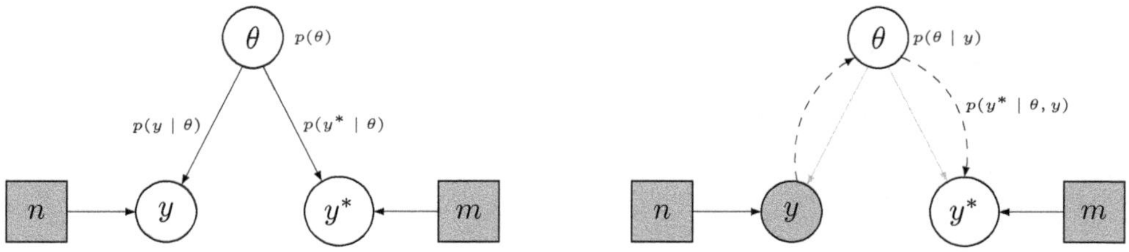

(a) The data-generating process. (b) The update process.

Figure 3.2: The data-generating process and the updating from observed data to posterior and predictive distributions in terms of a DAG.

step() function and assignments

Note the use of the `step()` function, which acts as a logical operator: if its argument is `TRUE`, then the function returns `1`, while it returns a `0` otherwise. The `JAGS` manual (Plummer, 2010, sec. 9.1) provides a list of available logical and mathematical functions. Examples include `log()`, `logit()` or `equals()` and `ifelse()`.

Also, note that in `JAGS/BUGS`, unlike `R`, assignments are made using the `<-` operator – we cannot use `=` instead. Finally, **stochastic** relationships are given using the `~` operator (read: "is associated with a XX distribution")

There are several ways to pass the model code to `JAGS`; the easiest is to save the code above onto a text file, say `drug-MCMC.txt`. Other alternatives are possible, which may be more efficient, in some cases, when integrating the `JAGS` analysis into an `R` script – we return to this in Note 8 below.

The second piece of key information that we need to pass onto `JAGS` is the list of data. We can do so with the following `R` code.

```
# Creates the list of data
data=list(
  a = 9.2, b = 13.8, # prior parameters
  y = 15,             # number of successes
  m = 20,             # number of trials
  n = 40,             # future number of trials
  ncrit = 25          # critical value of future successes
)
```

This is a "list" (we shall see a lot more of this). It is generally a good idea to keep the code general and then pass values that can be changed separately, rather than "hard-coding" them in the model code.

Finally, we can provide a list of "initial values". In a `JAGS/BUGS` file, all variables that are associated with a probabilistic statement (i.e. a "~" symbol after the variable name) **and** are *not* observed need to be initialised so that `BUGS` can run the Gibbs sampler. In this particular case, although `y` is defined as a random variable, because it is also observed, then there is no uncertainty about its value and so we should not initialise it. Conversely, although `y.pred` has exactly the same nature as `y`, because it is not observed, then we need to initialise it[4]. We can either pass specific values for those variables, or leave to `JAGS` the job of specifying them (more on this later).

Running the model

We are now ready to call `JAGS` in the background and perform the MCMC analysis

```
# First load the 'R2jags' package
library(R2jags)

# Then calls the function 'jags' to call 'JAGS' in the background
# and perform the MCMC analysis
```

[4]In fact, we may get away with not initialising `y.pred` too, because it is a deterministic function of other random nodes (`theta`, in this case) and thus, by initialising `theta`, we provide enough information for `JAGS` to initialise `y.pred` too.

```
model=jags(
  data=data,
  parameters.to.save=c("y.pred","theta","P.crit"),
  inits=NULL,
  model.file="PATH_TO_THE_MODEL_CODE_FILE",
  n.chains=2,
  n.iter=6000,
  n.burnin=1000,
  n.thin=1,
  DIC=TRUE
)
```

– note that we can run the model using BUGS instead, by simply modifying the command `library(R2jags)` to `library(R2OpenBUGS)` and then `model=jags(...)` to `model=bugs(...)`.

Once the package `R2jags` is loaded, we can use the function `jags()`, which takes several inputs – the following are the most important, but others are discussed in later examples and chapters.

- `data=data`: instructs JAGS to look for data in the object `data` (defined as a list, above);
- `parameters.to.save`: these are a vector of strings including names of the variables defined in the model code and that we want JAGS to monitor (i.e. to store values simulated from their relevant distributions);
- `inits`: we use this option to specify the initial values from which JAGS should start the MCMC process. In this case we set it to NULL, which means that JAGS will take care of this steps;
- `model.file`: here we specify the path to the (external) file in which we have saved the model code. If the file is *not* in the current directory, we should specify the full path to it (but see also Note 8 below);
- `n.chains`: this specifies the number of chains to be run by JAGS (in this case, 2);
- `n.iter`: the number of iterations of the Gibbs sampler that we want JAGS to run;
- `n.burnin`: the number of iterations that we want JAGS to discard. This is typically a very important part of the process as, in general, it may take some time for the Gibbs sampler to converge to the target (posterior) distributions in its exploration of the parametric space. In this particular case, because the underlying model is conjugated (and thus we do not really need to do MCMC), we could even set `n.burnin` to 0, knowing that convergence is immediate. In more general cases, we should ensure that this stage of the process is run for long enough before we can trust the simulations to be drawn from the actual target posterior (see Section 2.3.2);
- `n.thin`: the thinning of the chains. It instructs JAGS to only store one every `n.thin` iterations (again, see Section 2.3.2 for details). By default, JAGS does apply some thinning (see Section 3.3), but here we set it to 1;
- `DIC`: if set to TRUE (and in the presence of observed data), instructs JAGS to store the "Deviance Information Criterion", a measure that can be used to assess model fit (we return to this in Section 5.3.1).

Note 8: Model code as an R function

As mentioned above, sometimes it is more efficient to code the model assumptions directly into the R script we are using to run the whole analysis. We can do this by creating an R function in which we store the JAGS code, as we have done to save it to the .txt file. For example, we can create the object model.code as in the following code

```
model.code=function(){
   theta ~ dbeta(a,b)                      # prior distribution
   y ~ dbin(theta,m)                       # sampling distribution
   y.pred ~ dbin(theta,n)                  # predictive distribution
   P.crit <- step(y.pred - ncrit + 0.5) # =1 if y.pred >= ncrit,
}
```

and then call the function jags() specifying that the option model.file is set to the object model.code

```
model=jags(
  data=data,parameters.to.save=c("y.pred","theta","P.crit"),
  inits=NULL,n.chains=2,n.iter=6000,n.burnin=1000,DIC=TRUE,n.thin=1,
  # This specifies the model code as the function 'model.code'
  model.file=model.code
)
```

— technically, this calls in the background the function write.model() from the R2WinBUGS package, which is automatically loaded when R2jags is (see Note 21 in Example 7.3).

Obviously, the naming convention is entirely up to the user – there is no requirement to call the model code model.code and we can choose any name we prefer, as long as we are consistent and refer to the correct variable/path in the call to jags().

In this case, the model is so simple that this operation is almost immediate and R regains control of the session very quickly.

Post-processing of the model output

The JAGS output is the object model, which can be post-processed using specific functions from R2jags (as well as other packages) – see also Section 3.3 for some more details. For example, we can summarise the simulations using the print() method (here we also use the option digit=3 to specify the number of significant digits to show in the summary table).

```
print(model,digit=3)
```

```
Inference for Bugs model at "drug-MCMC.txt",
 2 chains, each with 6000 iterations (first 1000 discarded)
 n.sims = 10000 iterations saved. Running time = 0.045 secs
         mu.vect sd.vect   2.5%    25%    50%    75%  97.5% Rhat n.eff
P.crit     0.327   0.469  0.000  0.000  0.000  1.000  1.000 1.001 10000
theta      0.563   0.075  0.415  0.512  0.564  0.615  0.706 1.001 10000
y.pred    22.511   4.306 14.000 20.000 23.000 25.000 31.000 1.001 10000
deviance   6.640   2.400  3.397  4.828  6.189  7.963 12.463 1.001 10000

For each parameter, n.eff is a crude measure of effective sample size,
and Rhat is the potential scale reduction factor (at convergence, Rhat=1).

DIC info (using the rule: pV = var(deviance)/2)
pV = 2.9 and DIC = 9.5
```

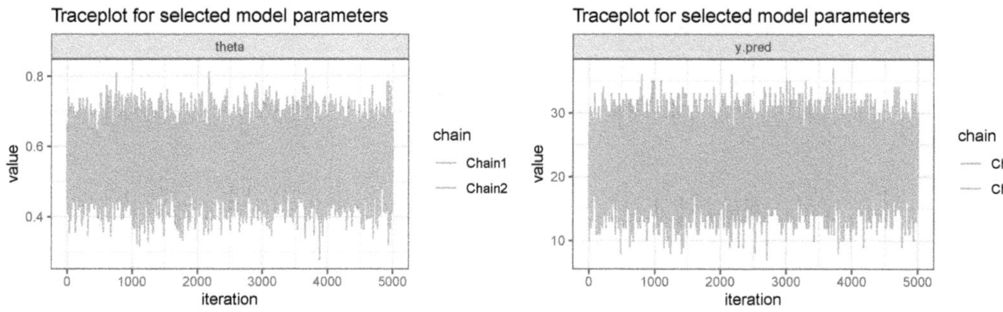

(a) Traceplot for θ. (b) Traceplot for y_{pred}.

Figure 3.3: Traceplots of selected variables in the model.

```
DIC is an estimate of expected predictive error (lower deviance is better).
```

The summary statistics indicate that, given current evidence, we revise our uncertainty about the true success rate of the drug from a distribution centred on 0.4 and with most of the mass in [0.2; 0.6] to another centred around 0.563 and with most of the probability mass included in [0.415; 0.706]. As for `y.pred` and `P.crit` we can see that the expected number of successes in the next phase of the trial is around 23 and the probability of exceeding the critical threshold (25) is 32.68%.

The output `model` is a very structured object, which contains several other variables and information. These can be accessed and processed, for instance to produce traceplots to assess convergence[5] We can use the specialised function `traceplot()` from the package `bmhe`, to show the traceplots for selected nodes (among those we have monitored).

```
bmhe::traceplot(model,"theta")
bmhe::traceplot(model,"y.pred")
```

In both cases, already at iteration 1 of the MCMC the two chains that we have run in parallel are on top of each other (we can barely see the lighter lines under the darker ones) and evidently visiting the same portion of the parametric space. This is also confirmed by looking at the more formal convergence statistics: $\hat{R}$ (`Rhat`) and the effective sample size n_{eff} (`n.eff`), presented in the last two columns of the summary table shown above (see Section 2.3.2). The former has a value of 1 for all the nodes, well below the rule-of-thumb cutoff of 1.1 – again, given the fact that the model is conjugate, this is not surprising. The model does not present problems in terms of autocorrelation as the effective sample size (giving a measure of how many equivalent independent simulations from the posterior distribution are associated with the possibly dependent vector of MCMC draws) is identical to the nominal sample size (i.e. the number of iterations stored for the MCMC analysis). Figure 3.4 shows the autocorrelation plot for the monitored nodes, using the `bmhe` function `acfplot()`.

```
bmhe::acfplot(model,parameter=c("theta","y.pred"),col="red")
```

The way in which we need to interpret Figure 3.4 is to look at the level of autocorrelation across different lags. These indicate how much correlation exists across consecutive, lagged simulations in the MCMC procedure. It is expected that consecutive iterations be relatively

[5]Again, *in this case* we do not have to worry about this because of conjugacy (see Section 2.2.2), but we use this example to make the point.

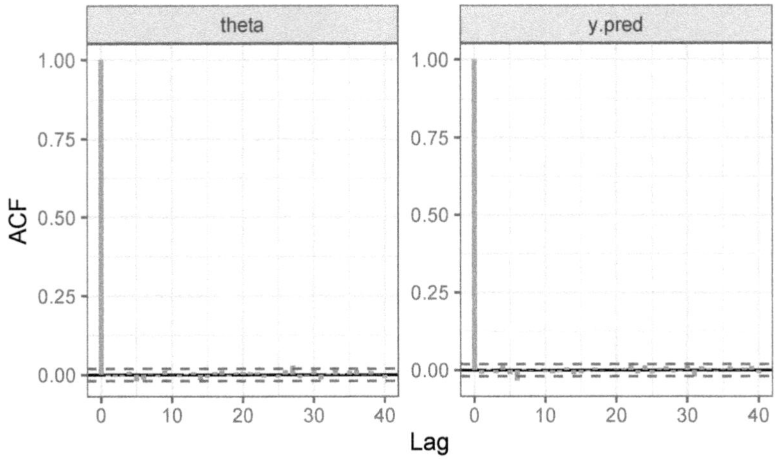

Figure 3.4: Autocorrelation plot for θ and y_{pred}.

correlated (because of how the Gibbs sampling is constructed, the s−th simulated value for the q−th parameter $\theta_q^{(s)}$ depends on the distribution at the $(s-1)$−th run for all the other parameters). But it is also expected that this level of correlation should fade away as we consider simulations that are further apart. So if the autocorrelation graph looks like the ones in Figure 3.4, we can say that actually the simulations are close to a series of independent values because the autocorrelation is very low, in fact at low lags as well.

The formal statistics for convergence ($\hat{R}$ and n_{eff}) can be visualised using the bmhe specialised function `diagplot()`, as in the following code.

```
bmhe::diagplot(model,what="Rhat")
bmhe::diagplot(model,what="n.eff")
```

Numerically, when the effective sample size is "close enough" to the nominal sample size (i.e. the number of iterations we use to draw the inference), then autocorrelation is not a problem. In this case, we have considered 2 chains, each with 5000 iterations (so a total of 10 000). The value of `n.eff` is 10 000 for `y.pred`, 10 000 for `theta` and 10 000 for `P.crit`.

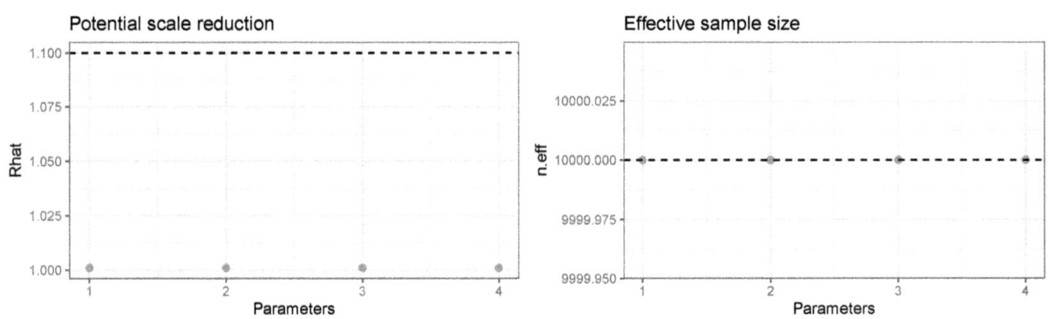

(a) The potential scale reduction (Gelman-Rubin statistics) $\hat{R}$.

(b) The effective sample size n_{eff}.

Figure 3.5: Formal convergence diagnostics.

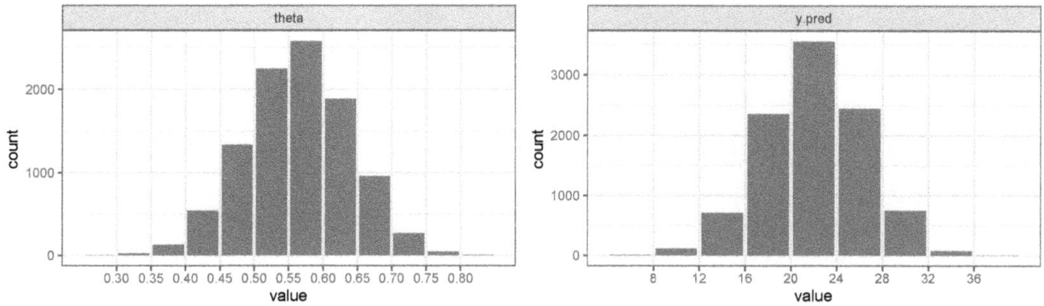

(a) θ.

(b) y_{pred}.

Figure 3.6: Posterior densities for the nodes monitored.

The ratios of effective to nominal sample size are then 1, 1 and 1, respectively, which clearly indicate no issues.

We can also use `bmhe` to visualise the various posterior densities. We choose to do so using the option `plot=bar`, which shows histograms, but the default `plot=density` would produce smoothed density estimation for the distributions of interest.

```
bmhe::posteriorplot(model,plot="bar",parameter="theta")
bmhe::posteriorplot(model,plot="bar",parameter="y.pred")
```

Note that while the graphs look very similar for (the posterior of) `theta` and (the predictive distribution for) `y.pred`, the nature of the variables is fundamentally different (cfr. Example 2.1). The former is about the model parameter θ, which represents a probability and it is thus constrained in the range [0-1], Conversely, y_{pred} represents the number of successes out of a sample size $n = 40$ and is thus a very different quantity – and in addition, θ is continuous and y_{pred} is discrete!

3.3 Differences between BUGS and JAGS

While a piece of code written in BUGS has almost 100% compatibility with JAGS, there are still some built-in differences between the two; more importantly there are some key distinctions between the R packages used to run the MCMC models, R2OpenBUGS and R2jags.

If we look at the R help for the two main functions[6] `R2OpenBUGS::bugs()` and `R2jags::jags()`, we can see that quite a few of the default values are not actually aligned, which explains why we may get different numbers when running one or the other – that is with a *vanilla* version, that does not control for all the underlying options.

```
# Default inputs for the `R2OpenBUGS::bugs()` function
R2OpenBUGS::bugs(
  data, inits, parameters.to.save, n.iter, model.file="model.txt",
```

[6]To highlight that the functions come from different packages, we use the `pkg::func()` notation – see the discussion in Note 4 in Section 1.2.4.

```
  n.chains=3, n.burnin=floor(n.iter / 2), n.thin=1, saveExec=FALSE,
  restart=FALSE, debug=FALSE, DIC=TRUE, digits=5, codaPkg=FALSE,
  OpenBUGS.pgm=NULL, working.directory=NULL, clearWD=FALSE, useWINE=FALSE,
  WINE=NULL, newWINE=TRUE, WINEPATH=NULL, bugs.seed=1, summary.only=FALSE,
  save.history=(.Platform$OS.type == "windows" | useWINE==TRUE),
  over.relax = FALSE
)

# Default inputs for the `R2jags::jags()` function
R2jags::jags(
  data, inits, parameters.to.save, model.file="model.bug", n.chains=3,
  n.iter=2000, n.burnin=floor(n.iter/2),
  n.thin=max(1, floor((n.iter - n.burnin) / 1000)), DIC=TRUE,
  working.directory=NULL, jags.seed = 123, refresh = n.iter/50,
  progress.bar = "text", digits=5,
  RNGname = c(
    "Wichmann-Hill", "Marsaglia-Multicarry", "Super-Duper", "Mersenne-Twister"
  ), jags.module = c("glm","dic"), quiet = FALSE
)
```

More specifically, let us see what happens when we actually run them both on the same data without thinking too much. We do this using the "eight schools" example presented in the `R` help for both `R2OpenBUGS::bugs()` and `R2jags::jags()` and originally discussed in Sturtz et al. (2005).

```
# An example model file is given in:
model.file=system.file(
  package="R2OpenBUGS", "model", "schools.txt"
)
# Can visualise the model uncommenting the following command
# file.show(model.file)

# Some example data (see ?schools for details):
data(schools)

# Makes relevant variables
J=nrow(schools)
y=schools$estimate
sigma.y=schools$sd

# Puts the data in a list
data=list ("J", "y", "sigma.y")

# Functions to generate initial values
inits=function(){
    list(theta=rnorm(J, 0, 100),
         mu.theta=rnorm(1, 0, 100),
         sigma.theta=runif(1, 0, 100)
    )
}
```

```
# Defines the model parameters
parameters=c("theta", "mu.theta", "sigma.theta")

# Runs the model using a vanilla BUGS
mbugs=bugs(
  data, inits, parameters, model.file,n.chains=3, n.iter=5000
)

# Runs the model using a vanilla JAGS
mjags=jags(
  data, inits, parameters, model.file,n.chains=3, n.iter=5000
)
```

The first slightly annoying quirk is that if we inspect the two objects `mbugs` and `mjags` we can see that they have a different structure.

```
names(mbugs)
```

```
 [1] "n.chains"         "n.iter"          "n.burnin"        "n.thin"
 [5] "n.keep"           "n.sims"          "sims.array"      "sims.list"
 [9] "sims.matrix"      "summary"         "mean"            "sd"
[13] "median"           "root.short"      "long.short"      "dimension.short"
[17] "indexes.short"    "last.values"     "isDIC"           "DICbyR"
[21] "pD"               "DIC"             "model.file"
```

```
names(mjags)
```

```
[1] "model"                "BUGSoutput"           "parameters.to.save" "model.file"
[5] "n.iter"               "DIC"
```

`R2jags` is perhaps more organised and creates a nested object `BUGSoutput`, in which it stores all the, well... `BUGS` output. `R2OpenBUGS`, on the other hand, stores all the main output directly in the object (in this case, named `mbugs`). We can use the `$` notation to access the elements of the nested object `mjags$BUGSoutput`; thus, for instance, we can visualise the first few simulated values using the following `R` code

```
mjags$BUGSoutput$sims.matrix |> head() |> round(4)
```

```
     deviance mu.theta sigma.theta theta[1] theta[2] theta[3] theta[4] theta[5]
[1,]  63.1957   3.4785     14.2200  26.2666 -16.7075  -9.2396  11.9437   2.4603
[2,]  60.1780   5.0820      2.8610   0.4945   6.6275   1.4543   6.6836   4.9866
[3,]  59.1257  11.6818      9.6859  19.9707   3.7033  -1.6391   5.4203  17.2153
[4,]  59.6005   7.7004      0.6455   8.1408   7.0607   7.2135   5.8920   7.8793
[5,]  57.7529   3.8825      9.1391  12.7300   8.0826   4.1697  -0.7808   8.4334
[6,]  60.2013   4.8843      0.6047   4.7616   5.5125   6.1149   4.9416   5.3324
     theta[6] theta[7] theta[8]
[1,]   3.8333  11.0219  -8.8492
[2,]   6.4765   8.2986   4.2943
[3,]  -0.3253  17.0090   6.8228
[4,]   8.1308   6.8901   7.4641
[5,]  -1.1303  14.1492  12.4989
[6,]   5.3788   4.5440   5.2419
```

while we could simply write `mbugs$sims.matrix |> head()` if we were post-processing a R2OpenBUGS object. All in all, we can get access to the same information from both packages – it is just in different places and we need to know where to look. Note that the package bmhe, which we use throughout this book somehow mitigates this by using specialised functions that *do know where to look* and pick up the relevant information, whether the object to be processed is obtained through R2jags or R2OpenBUGS.

Another important difference is perhaps even more subtle. In both cases, we are using n.iter= 5000 (that is the number of total iterations per chain) with n.chains=3 (the default number of parallel chains). In both cases, by default (i.e. unless we say something explicitly different), n.burnin=n.iter/2 and so we have a total of (n.iter-n.burnin) × n.chains= $(5000 - 2500) \times 3 = 7500$ iterations. That is the length of the MCMC process.

However, by default, BUGS assumes n.thin=1 (see Section 2.3.2.4), which means that it retains all the 7500 iterations for the MCMC analysis (that is actually stored in the variable n.sims), as we can see from the table below.

```
print(mbugs,digits=3)
```

```
Inference for Bugs model at "schools.txt",
Current: 3 chains, each with 5000 iterations (first 2500 discarded)
Cumulative: n.sims = 7500 iterations saved
               mean    sd     2.5%    25%    50%    75%  97.5%  Rhat n.eff
theta[1]     11.185 8.892  -2.787  5.500  9.806 15.663 32.897 1.006   400
theta[2]      7.481 6.504  -4.901  3.363  7.368 11.480 20.810 1.006   380
theta[3]      5.800 8.013 -12.037  1.330  6.370 10.520 20.950 1.003  1000
theta[4]      7.106 6.741  -6.251  3.049  7.133 11.182 20.980 1.005   580
theta[5]      4.908 6.339  -8.841  0.958  5.510  9.134 16.380 1.004   620
theta[6]      5.798 6.787  -9.097  1.754  6.126 10.120 18.356 1.005   490
theta[7]     10.376 7.224  -2.110  5.615  9.710 14.582 26.280 1.008   280
theta[8]      8.092 8.010  -7.132  3.365  7.770 12.440 25.675 1.006   390
mu.theta      7.619 5.439  -2.693  4.123  7.606 11.000 18.630 1.008   290
sigma.theta   6.681 5.877   0.241  2.273  5.283  9.403 21.862 1.004   560
deviance     60.533 2.279  57.005 59.170 60.060 61.560 66.230 1.002  1700

For each parameter, n.eff is a crude measure of effective sample size,
and Rhat is the potential scale reduction factor (at convergence, Rhat=1).

DIC info (using the rule, pD = Dbar-Dhat)
pD = 2.879 and DIC = 63.410
DIC is an estimate of expected predictive error (lower deviance is better).
```

Conversely, JAGS uses by default `n.thin=max(1, floor((n.iter - n.burnin)/1000))`, which in this case is `max(1, floor((5000 - 2500)/1000)) = 2`. In other words, of the 7500 iterations that are considered, JAGS retains only one every 2, which means the overall value for n.sims is actually half as that produced, **by default** by BUGS[7].

```
print(mjags,digits=3)
```

```
Inference for Bugs model at "schools.txt",
 3 chains, each with 5000 iterations (first 2500 discarded), n.thin = 2
```

[7] `floor()` is an R function that takes a single numeric argument x and returns a numeric vector containing the largest integers not greater than the corresponding elements of x. Thus `floor(2.5)` = 2.

```
 n.sims = 3750 iterations saved. Running time = 0.071 secs
            mu.vect sd.vect    2.5%    25%    50%    75%  97.5%  Rhat n.eff
mu.theta      7.846   5.106  -1.758  4.758  7.725 10.804 18.247 1.002  3800
sigma.theta   6.975   5.524   0.131  2.908  5.892  9.674 20.873 1.022   230
theta[1]     11.808   8.956  -1.977  6.059 10.181 15.909 34.503 1.001  3800
theta[2]      7.638   6.423  -5.300  3.704  7.419 11.387 21.196 1.001  3800
theta[3]      5.950   7.855 -11.879  1.667  6.330 10.431 21.241 1.004  2500
theta[4]      7.453   6.659  -6.156  3.381  7.186 11.428 21.263 1.001  3800
theta[5]      5.109   6.251  -8.358  1.493  5.626  9.063 16.594 1.004  1000
theta[6]      5.800   7.036  -9.660  1.704  6.174  9.900 19.810 1.005   670
theta[7]     10.750   7.083  -1.275  6.084  9.928 14.827 26.562 1.003  3500
theta[8]      8.488   7.870  -6.659  3.751  8.100 12.784 25.586 1.001  3800
deviance     60.378   2.266  56.851 59.039 59.930 61.456 65.924 1.008   780

For each parameter, n.eff is a crude measure of effective sample size,
and Rhat is the potential scale reduction factor (at convergence, Rhat=1).

DIC info (using the rule: pV = var(deviance)/2)
pV = 2.6 and DIC = 62.9
DIC is an estimate of expected predictive error (lower deviance is better).
```

As a result, the efficiency of the two processes is also different – in the case above, note the values of n_{eff}, which are generally higher (with a smaller nominal sample size) for JAGS than they are for BUGS, again due to the impact of thinning, which reduces the autocorrelation in the former in comparison to the latter.

Effective vs nominal sample size and autocorrelation

The summary table for the JAGS model indicates that for some nodes the effective sample size (`n.eff`) is even bigger than the nominal MC sample size (`n.sims`), for instance for the node `mu.theta`. This apparent quirk is due to the fact that n_{eff} is a function of the underlying autocorrelation in the simulations (see Equation 2.14). When this autocorrelation is negative, the effective sample size gets artificially inflated to values larger than the theoretical upper bound, indicated by the MC sample size. This artefact is also common to Stan, which can return $n_{eff} > n_{sims}$ for parameters whose posterior is close to a Normal and have little dependency on other parameters (Stan development team, 2024).

More specifically, this means that what is an **apparently** identical process may in fact be much slower in BUGS, simply because of how it handles the thinning. In BUGS, if we specify `n.iter`=10 000 and `n.thin`=20, then BUGS will run the MCMC process for $10\,000 \times 20 = 200\,000$ iterations so that it can in fact retain one every 20 – that is 10 000 overall. In JAGS, conversely, this would be handled by running the actual number of iterations requested (`n.iter`=10 000); then, because of the thinning, only 1 in 20 will be retained and so we would end up with only 10 000/20=500 iterations saved.

When initial values are not specified by the user, the two programmes also have slightly different ways of generating them. BUGS generates initial values by forward sampling from the prior distribution for each parameter. Thus, when using very vague priors, it is possible that, by random chance, one of the chains for a given parameter is initialised from a point that is very far from the target area of the posterior distribution, which may slow down convergence. JAGS on the other hand sets all initial values from the "middle" (either the mean or the mode, depending on the distribution) of the prior. On occasions, this may be a safer approach – but ultimately, it is always helpful to at least try a model run with user-specified initial values.

Finally, another important distinction is in the default random seed[8]: `BUGS` sets its seed to `1`, while `JAGS` sets its to `123`. Generally speaking, none of these differences matter greatly, once the model has converged and run for long enough. A larger `n.sims` would generally imply a smaller MC error and more precision (and, crucially, a better characterisation of the whole posterior distribution – not just the mean and central part). Even in the case above, for most parameters, the individual statistics are fairly aligned and using one set of estimates instead of the others does not make a huge difference...

3.4 Defining non-standard distributions in BUGS/JAGS

Both `BUGS` and `JAGS` have a number of built-in distributions, which cover a vast number of applied cases. There are however circumstances in which we may need to use a formulation that is not available, either for the sampling or the prior distribution.

For example, imagine that we want to model a variable $y \sim p(y \mid \theta)$, where $p(y \mid \theta)$ is the required non-standard distribution, indexed by a parameter θ. The main idea is to use the "zero-trick" (Lunn et al., 2013, sect. 9.5), i.e. to create some fake observation, $w = 0$, which is modelled as $w \sim \text{Poisson}(\phi)$.

Because we "pretend" that w is observed to be 0, then its contribution to the overall likelihood is $\exp(-\phi)$, as is possible to see from Equation 1.1. If we set $\phi = -\log \mathcal{L}(\theta \mid w, y)$ and model y using a very flat, non-informative prior, then we retrieve the correct overall contribution to the likelihood and effectively model $p(y \mid \theta) \propto \exp(-\phi) = \mathcal{L}(\theta \mid w, y)$ – cfr. the discussion in Section 2.2.1.

Notice that we may or may not observe y (which, in fact, may have the role of a model parameter, when we are trying to define a non-standard prior and thus may not be at all observable, as we show in Example 3.2); if we have no observation on y, we can still construct a likelihood based on the "observation" of w.

Example 3.2. *Zero-trick to code a PC prior for Binomial parameter.* The PC prior in Equation 2.11 has a highly non-standard format and thus it is not implemented as a built-in distribution to directly use in `BUGS/JAGS` code. However, if we give θ a Beta(1, 1) prior (which effectively does not contribute anything to the posterior – see again Section 2.2.1) and set $\phi = -\log \mathcal{L}(\theta \mid w) = -\log p(\theta)$, where $p(\theta)$ is defined in Equation 2.11, then we will imply the correct likelihood contribution and therefore we will have effectively modelled $\theta \sim \text{PC prior}(\lambda, \theta_0)$.

We can do so in the `JAGS` code below.

```
model_pc_bern=function(){
  # "Pseudo-observation", w=0
  w ~ dpois(phi)
```

[8]See `??seed` in an `R` terminal for some information about how `R` treats (pseudo-)random number generation.

```
  # Defines the likelihood from the PC prior
  d <- pow(
    2*theta*log(theta/theta0)+2*(1-theta)*log((1-theta)/(1-theta0)), 0.5
  )
  deriv <- abs((log(theta)-log(1-theta)-log(theta0)+log(1-theta0))/d)
  # Models phi as a function of the likelihood for theta
  phi <- -log(lambda*exp(-lambda*d)*deriv) + C

  # "Non-informative" prior for theta, to combine with the likelihood
  # contribution from phi and effectively imply that theta ~ PC prior
  theta ~ dbeta(1,1)
  # Possible data - if not observed, sampling from the prior only
  y ~ dbin(theta,10)
}

# Runs the model in JAGS with no data for y to check what the prior looks like
test=R2jags::jags(
  data=list(y=NA,w=0,C=10000,lambda=1,theta0=0.5),parameters.to.save=c("theta"),
  model.file=model_pc_bern,n.chains=2,n.thin=4,n.iter=100000,DIC=FALSE,
  inits=list(list(theta=0.1), list(theta=0.9))
)
```

Notice that here we add a large constant $C = 10\,000$ to the expression for ϕ, to ensure that it is positive (as is required, since ϕ is the mean of a Poisson distribution and hence constrained in $\mathbb{R}^+$) – this is just a scaling factor.

The results can be summarised by using the `print()` method. In this case, convergence is reached satisfactorily although, in general, the "zero-trick" method can be prone to poor mixing of the chains.

```
# Summary results
print(test,digits=3)
```

```
Inference for Bugs model at "/tmp/Rtmpot5hec/modelf0aae5072cd58.txt",
 2 chains, each with 100000 iterations (first 50000 discarded), n.thin = 4
 n.sims = 25000 iterations saved. Running time = 0.238 secs
      mu.vect sd.vect  2.5%   25%   50%   75% 97.5%  Rhat n.eff
theta   0.503    0.27 0.026 0.293 0.502 0.715 0.976 1.001 25000

For each parameter, n.eff is a crude measure of effective sample size,
and Rhat is the potential scale reduction factor (at convergence, Rhat=1).
```

```
# MC estimate for Pr(theta>0.75)
sum(test$BUGSoutput$sims.list$theta>0.75)/test$BUGSoutput$n.sims
```

```
[1] 0.21656
```

We can see that the empirical estimate or $\Pr(\theta > 0.75)$ agrees with the numerical integration we performed in Example 2.6 ($\approx$ 0.22) and the resulting prior distribution depicted in Figure 3.7 is also similar to the analytic form presented in Figure 2.10.

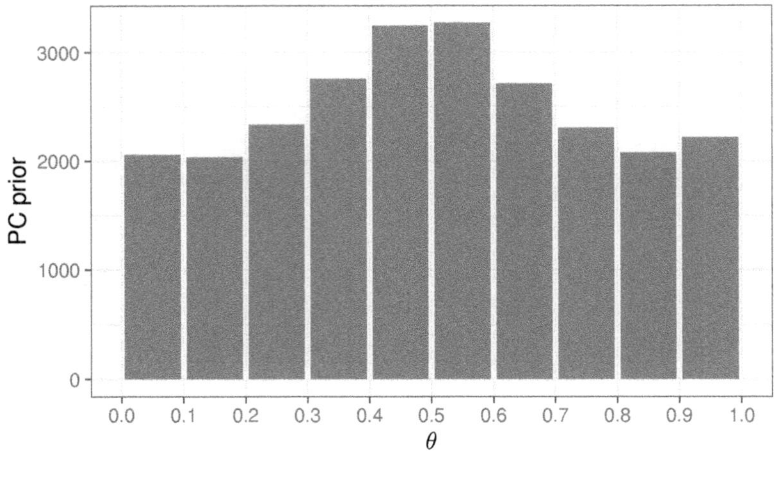

Figure 3.7: The implied PC prior for the parameter θ, obtained using the "zero-trick". This is aligned with the analytic form described in Equation 2.11.

In the vast majority of applications of Bayesian modelling to HTA, the practitioner would not be required to define their own specific probability distribution (either to model sampling variability for observable data y or epistemic uncertainty for parameters θ). If that becomes a necessity, perhaps more "modern" software (usually classified as "probabilistic languages"), e.g. `Stan` or `Nimble` may be more appropriate and efficient.

For instance, in `Stan` there is no need to use the zero-trick to adjust the likelihood; instead, it is possible to define a customised distribution in a `functions` block (see Section 8.3.5 for a specific example and more details on coding `Stan` models). This would generally work in a more efficient and generalisable way.

Custom-defined distributions in `JAGS`

In fact, a bit like `Stan`, `JAGS` also allows to build new distributions and add them to the catalogue of "modules" that are available in the default installation.

In order to do so, the user must be able to implement a new `C++` class, including suitable functions to calculate the log-density, draw random samples and return "typical" values (to be used at initialisation). This is then built into a module containing this class, which in turns makes available the new distribution in a `JAGS` code, by simply using something like the following.

```
model {
  ...
  y ~ dmybrandnewdistribution(theta1,theta2,theta2)
}
```

While, in theory, opening up `JAGS` to any custom-made distribution, this does require obvious mathematical expertise as well as familiarity with coding in `C++`, as discussed in the tutorial by Wabersich and Vandekerckhove (2014).

As an example, the PC prior for the Binomial parameter described above is implemented as an extra `JAGS` module at `https://github.com/giabaio/bmhta-examples`.

3.5 Conclusions

This chapter has given a brief introduction to all-purpose Bayesian software, presenting a list of the most popular and focusing specifically on JAGS and BUGS. These are both based on Gibbs sampling and have already been used relatively extensively in the Health Technology Literature and thus we have selected them (and specifically JAGS) as the main alternative, for the purpose of modelling discussed in this book.

We have given a general introduction to the main setup (which is fairly common for both JAGS and BUGS) and have looked at how it is possible to interface the Bayesian software with R, the language of choice for statistical modelling – other are of course possible (including ones that are very popular in fields such as Data Science, e.g. Python). We have also discussed the general workflow of Bayesian analysis based on running a model in JAGS.

In the next chapter, we will concentrate on a general introduction to the field of Health Technology Assessment (HTA), particularly from a Bayesian perspective. We will present the basic decision problem and the various metrics used to perform the economic evaluation of healthcare interventions and then prepare the setting for later chapters, in which we will go over various statistical modelling specifically for HTA.

4

Introduction to health technology assessment

4.1 Introduction

In this chapter we provide a brief introduction to the principles of *health economic evaluation*. While we acknowledge that this is a very broad label that can be used to indicate a number of quantitative techniques aimed at analysing data generated in the healthcare context, we consider specifically the situation of health technology assessment (HTA), in which the objective is to determine the *value-for-money* associated with a given intervention, in comparison to at least another one.

More specifically, to put it with Luce et al. (2010):

> *Health technology assessment (HTA) is a method of evidence synthesis that considers evidence regarding clinical effectiveness, safety, cost-effectiveness and, when broadly applied, includes social, ethical, and legal aspects of the use of health technologies. The precise balance of these inputs depends on the purpose of each individual HTA. A major use of HTAs is in informing reimbursement and coverage decisions, in which case HTAs should include benefit-harm assessment and economic evaluation.*

"Health economics"[1] is a relatively young discipline, which has come to the fore in the late 1970s. In particular, since the establishment of the *National Institute for Clinical Excellence* (later renamed as National Institute for Health and Care Excellence, but commonly still indicated as NICE) by the UK Government in 1997, HTA has firmly become a fundamental part of decision-making in a large number of jurisdictions. NICE has since gained prominence as the global powerhouse for HTA and has been instrumental in developing most of the underlying theoretical underpinning, as well as guidance for practitioners.

Today, the principles of HTA guide healthcare decisions in many countries and agencies such as *Canada's Drug Agency* (CDA, originally known as the *Canadian Agency for Drugs and Technologies in Health*, CADTH), the *Zorginstituut Nederland* (ZiN; the Dutch agency), the *Tandvårds- och läkemedelsförmånsverket* (TLV; the Swedish agency), the *Scottish Medicine Consortium* (SMC) or the *All Wales Medicines Strategy Group* (AWMSG), to name only a few, who, similarly to NICE in England, are responsible for providing national guidance and advice to improve health and social care. This focuses specifically on advising governments on whether particular healthcare interventions (most notably, pharmaceuticals) should be paid for by the healthcare provider, typically through taxation.

[1] On occasions when he wants to be particularly annoying (even more than usual), the author would argue that the naming is to some extent a "historical accident" – health economics has been invented by economists and certainly is grounded in economic theory. But by necessity this process does involve many other key components (among which, arguably, Statistics is a cornerstone).

DOI: 10.1201/9781003771050-4

In this chapter, we give some basic definition and notation that is then used throughout the following ones; in particular, we consider the overall structure that is generally associated with HTA.

4.2 Cost-effectiveness analysis

Throughout this book, we almost interchangeably refer to the process of using data to produce an economic evaluation of healthcare interventions as HTA, or *health economic evaluation*, or *cost-effectiveness analysis* (CEA). Technically speaking, this is an abuse of the terminology, because, in economic terms, there is a marked distinction between different types of economic analysis (e.g. cost-*effectiveness* vs cost-*utility* analysis) and, from the purely economic point of view, conflating these terms is perhaps bad practice – readers should be aware of the nuances in these terms and we refer them to the classic textbooks by Briggs et al. (2006) and Drummond et al. (2015).

Despite this, we also acknowledge that, by and large, the basic process and methodologies applied have several points in common, as we highlight in the following. For this reason, we resist the urge of detailing all the theoretical distinctions in the various economic evaluation methods and provide a unified presentation instead.

Note 9: Basic notation for HTA Modelling

Generally speaking, throughout this book we indicate observed or observable variables using Roman letters, e.g. y or x, typically to indicate a main outcome or some covariate. In the HTA context, the main outcome typically represents effects e and costs c (suitably defined, as in the sections below). One of the most important covariate is usually the treatment arm, or the intervention applied to a given group or population. We index this using $t = 1, \ldots, T$.

When we have individual-level data (as in Chapter 5), we index them using $i = 1, \ldots, N$. If the data have a longitudinal nature (e.g. repeated measures over time), we use $j = 0, \ldots, J$ to index the time points at which measurements are taken (as in Table 5.1 and Section 8.5.2), or to describe the time horizon of our analysis (see Chapter 9). In the case of aggregated level data (e.g. Chapter 6), we generally indicate the units of observation as $s = 1, \ldots, S$ (for each "study").

Occasionally, we slightly abuse this basic notation and change the meaning of a variable or index (e.g. when indicating time to a particular event as t, in Chapter 8). When this is not obvious, we highlight the change specifically.

In particular, in our view, the process of a cost-effectiveness analysis in HTA can be described by a graph such as the one shown in Figure 4.1, which consists of four interconnected building blocks.

The main building block is represented by the "Statistical model", which uses observed data $\boldsymbol{y}$ to obtain estimates of a set of population parameters, say $\boldsymbol{\theta}$. Generally speaking, the observed outcome is in fact a bivariate quantity, which we generally indicate as (e, c), although the actual nature of the data (and therefore of the model) may vary: for instance, in Chapter 5, we present the case in which individual-level data are available (e.g. alongside

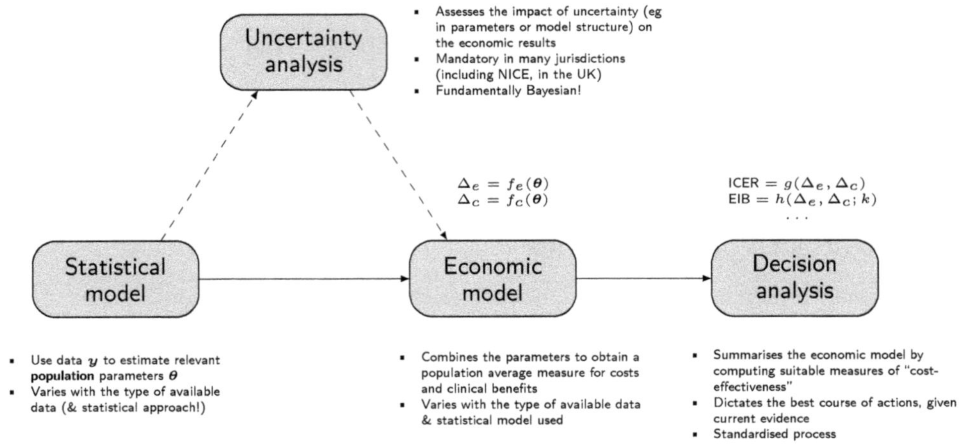

Figure 4.1: A graphical representation of the decision making process. Adapted from Baio et al. (2025a).

a clinical trial), while in Chapter 6 we consider the case in which summary statistics are available, e.g. from a literature review.

As suggested in Note 9 above, we assume that T alternatives are under consideration; typically, $t = 1, 2, \ldots, T-1$ are the interventions currently implemented, i.e. the "standard of care" or "status quo", while $t = T$ is the new therapeutic option being investigated. For simplicity of exposition, we can consider the case where $T = 2$, but this is not strictly necessary and, in fact, it is recommended that a full economic evaluation does consider all the relevant options.

The output of the statistical model feeds into a second building block, termed the "Economic model" in Figure 4.1, which is used to derive suitable economic quantities for each intervention, that are used to summarise the performance of the competing interventions. More specifically, in an economic context, we are interested in the *differential* performance of a given intervention against a comparator (typically $t = 1$). This is generically indicated by the quantities

$$\Delta_e = f_e(\boldsymbol\theta) \qquad \text{and} \qquad \Delta_c = f_c(\boldsymbol\theta),$$

for suitable functions $f_e(\cdot)$ and $f_c(\cdot)$. For instance, when performing an economic evaluation alongside a clinical trial, we may obtain the relevant economic summaries directly from the Statistical model – in that case, $f_e(\cdot)$ and $f_c(\cdot)$ are the identity functions (see Chapter 5). In more complex situations, however, the output of the Statistical model may be estimates for a set of relevant parameters that need to be processed using highly non-linear and often complex functions to map them back to the scale of the population average benefits and costs (as in Chapters 6 and 7).

Note 10: Quality-Adjusted Life Years

Typically, experimental clinical studies set their primary outcome at some hard measure of relative effectiveness: examples include physical measurements (e.g. blood pressure), the incidence of a specific clinical outcome (e.g. cardiovascular failure), or the time until a clinically meaningful event occurs (e.g. time to death). These are obviously relevant and, depending on the specific intervention under study, they allow the clinicians to quantify the actual benefits associated with it.

From a wider decision-making perspective, however, these sorts of outcomes are not necessarily ideal. Firstly, the economic evaluation must be performed to optimise the allocation of resources to the provision of healthcare across the whole range of diseases that are relevant for the target population. Thus, it becomes complex to compare the economic performance of a highly specialised cancer drug (whose main outcome is reduction in cancer mortality) against an innovative form of physiotherapy to relieve from back pain – note that the actual cost-effectiveness analysis would not necessarily compare these two very different interventions against each other, but, eventually, a choice must be made in how to allocate the finite resources and thus it may be rationale to prioritise one over the other as more appropriate to maximise health across the entire target population.

Secondly, hard clinical outcomes may fail to account for both the *quantity* and the *quality* of life for a given individual under a particular intervention. This is of course a very relevant aspect, although it may be hard to fully capture. To try and do so, we generally define the measure of "clinical benefit" based on *health related quality of life* (HRQL) data. These are utility-based scores to value health. Notable examples include the EQ-5D (The EuroQol Group, 1990) and the SF-36 (Ware and Sherbourne, 1992) instruments. Typically, these are obtained through specific questionnaires administered to individuals to map the underlying health state, possibly over time.

Using these tools, we can assign a utility score to each specific health state and then compute the overall *Quality-Adjusted Life Years* (QALYs, Loomes and McKenzie, 1989). Figure 4.2 shows this process graphically, highlighting how the QALYs can be considered as the "area under the curve" identified by the HRQL values (on the y–axis) over a range of measurements (time, on the x–axis).

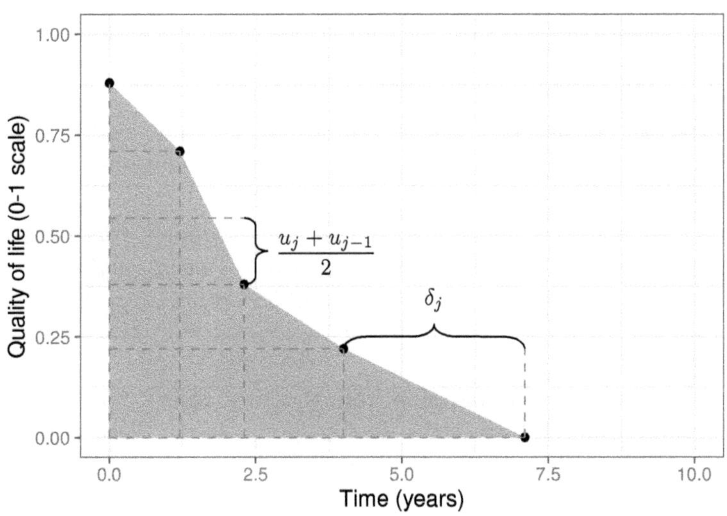

Figure 4.2: A graphical representation of the concept of Quality-Adjusted Life Year, as "area under the curve".

Here, the dots represent the value of the utility measured for an individual and generically indicated as u_j, at given measurement time points $j = 0, \ldots, J$ – in this fictional case, we assume that at beginning of observation (time $j = 0$) the measured utility is 0.88. At the next measurement (time $j = 1.2$), the utility decreases to 0.71 and so on, until it hits 0 at time $j = 7.1$ (end of follow-up).

The quantity δ_j indicates the length of interval between two successive measurements. The trapezoids shown in Figure 4.2 encode the assumption that quality of life as measured by the utility score decreases linearly between two consecutive measurements. The overall QALYs are effectively computed as the area under each trapezoid and summed over all of them, to obtain an aggregated measure for the HRQL component

$$\text{QALYs} = \sum_{j=1}^{J} \frac{(u_j + u_{j-1})}{2} \delta_j \tag{4.1}$$

– we consider more specifically a worked example for the computation of QALYs starting from individual-level data on HRQL in Chapter 5.

Another useful way to interpret QALYs is by mapping the actual time alive onto an equivalent amount in "perfect health". In the example above, the individual is alive for 7.1 years during the observation period, but applying Equation 4.1 this is computed to be equivalent to 2.40 years in perfect health.

The main advantage of using QALYs as a standardised measure of clinical benefit, is that they facilitate resource allocation decisions. In addition, through the incorporation of utility values, they allow to reflect the subjective experiences and preferences of individuals regarding their health states.

On the other hand, several ethical objections have been raised against QALYs: the main one is that they implicitly quantify the monetary value of a human life, which is often seen as problematic, in particular because health states are generally evaluated on a scale 0 (= death) to 1 (= perfect health), while allowing for health states that are "worse than death" and are therefore given a negative utility. This is considered unethical and increasingly advised against (Schneider, 2022).

Neumann and Cohen (2018) review other potential advantages and pitfalls of QALYs, including the fact that they tend to prioritise common conditions over rare diseases, but conclude that

> *Without QALYs, health systems would still have difficult trade-offs. Decision makers would still confront and make difficult choices about paying for the health care that people need and desire. But they would lack a practical instrument to aid in the process.*

Irrespective of how we obtain the mapping from the "Statistical model" to the "Economic model", the quantities (Δ_e, Δ_c) are then used to perform the "Decision analysis", which is aimed at selecting the alternative that offers the largest "value", both in terms of benefits and costs. There are various suitable metrics that can be defined as functions of the differential benefits and costs, (Δ_e, Δ_c), to conduct the decision analysis.

For example, historically, a common summary of the decision-making process has been represented by the *Incremental Cost-Effectiveness Ratio* (ICER)

$$\begin{aligned}\text{ICER} &= \frac{\text{Population average cost differential}}{\text{Population average effectiveness differential}} \\ &= \frac{\text{E}[c_2] - \text{E}[c_1]}{\text{E}[e_2] - \text{E}[e_1]} = \frac{\text{E}[\Delta_c]}{\text{E}[\Delta_e]},\end{aligned} \tag{4.2}$$

which quantifies the "cost-per-outcome", or, in other words, the monetary cost that the healthcare provider needs to bear in order to increase the population average benefits by one unit. Here, we generically indicate with $\text{E}[e_t]$ and $\text{E}[c_t]$ the intervention-specific population average measures of benefits and costs, respectively.

Given current evidence and *assuming that the modelling assumptions are reasonable*, the ICER can be used to guide the decision-making process, i.e. to determine whether to switch to the new intervention $t = 2$ or stick with the status quo $t = 1$. In particular, when comparing two interventions, if ICER < 0, then one of two situations occurs:

- $\text{E}[\Delta_e] > 0$ and $\text{E}[\Delta_c] < 0$; in this case, the new intervention is associated with higher benefits and generates savings, in comparison to the status quo. Thus, $t = 2$ *dominates* $t = 1$ and, *given current evidence*, it should be selected as the most cost-effective alternative;
- $\text{E}[\Delta_e] < 0$ and $\text{E}[\Delta_c] > 0$; in the opposite situation, the new intervention is more expensive and decreases the population benefits. In this case, $t = 2$ is *dominated* by $t = 1$ and, *given current evidence*, it should be rejected, with the status quo maintained as the most cost-effective alternative.

Similarly, when ICER > 0, there are two possibilities:

- If both $\text{E}[\Delta_e], \text{E}[\Delta_c] < 0$, then the new intervention generates monetary savings, but it does so by producing fewer health benefits.
- If both $\text{E}[\Delta_e], \text{E}[\Delta_c] > 0$, then the new interventions improves health, but at an increased cost.

In both these situations, it is more complicated to make a decision based on the value of the ICER, as it is unclear up to what point we can accept an increase in costs to produce more benefits or a decrease in benefits to generate savings that we can re-invest in other interventions.

As a more specific example, consider the comparisons between a reference intervention, say A, and four different comparators: B, C, D and E. These are shown in Figure 4.3, which presents the "cost-effectiveness plane" (Black, 1990), where the $x-$ and $y-$axes describe, respectively, the population effectiveness and cost differentials (we return to this in the discussion of Figure 4.5). In this case, E dominates A, because the corresponding ICER falls in the North-Western quadrant, indicating that A produces, on average, lower benefits and increased costs. On the other hand, A dominates B, C and D because it produces more benefits while saving costs (with all three corresponding ICERs in the South-Eastern quadrant). The greyed areas in Figure 4.3 (the North-Eastern and the South-Western quadrants) indicate the parts of the cost-effectiveness plane in which the decision is undetermined, just by looking at the ICER.

An additional inconsistency of the analysis based on the ICER is that it is not an ordered statistic: in this simple example, we can look at the ICERs and the actual cost and benefit differentials to see that A fares best against D (highest increase in benefits and highest decrease in costs), then against C and finally against B; yet, the ICERs do not respect this ordering, since $\text{ICER}_{\text{AB}} = -1$, $\text{ICER}_{\text{AC}} = -1/2$ and $\text{ICER}_{\text{AD}} = -1$. Moreover, the sign

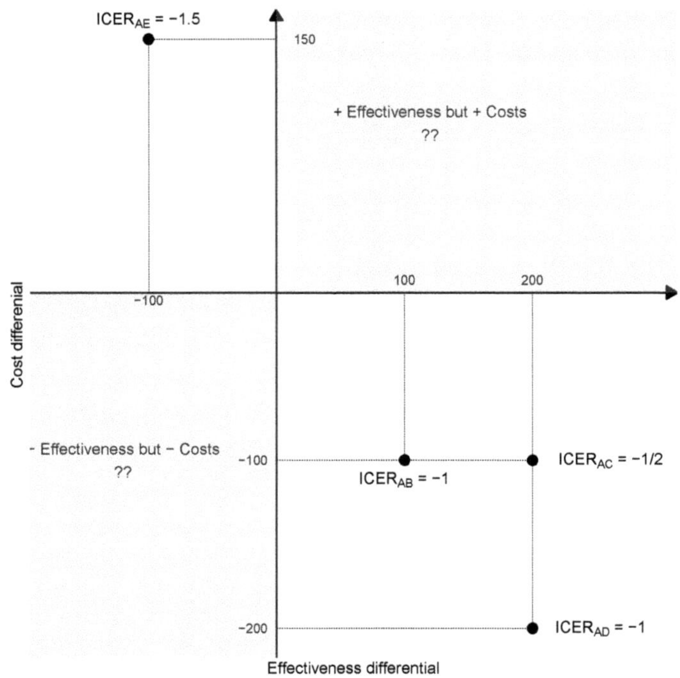

Figure 4.3: A graphical representation of the cost-effectiveness plane for different pairwise comparisons, highlighting the inconsistencies of the analysis based purely on the ICERs.

of the ICER is the same for all the comparisons, even though A is dominated by E and dominates the other interventions.

To overcome these limitations of using the ICER as the basic criterion for decision-making, we can use a fully decision-theoretic approach. This is based on defining a utility function to associate with each intervention t and then determine the most cost-effective alternative as the one maximising the expected utility. In HTA, the standardised choice is for the *monetary net benefit* (MNB)

$$nb_t = ke_t - c_t \tag{4.3}$$

where k is a "willingness to pay" deterministic parameter, used to place the benefits and costs on the same monetary scale – in other words, k determines the cost-per-outcome.

Pros and cons of the monetary net benefit

As suggested above, there is no reason why other utility functions should not be considered in place of the the monetary net benefit, in HTA. Nonetheless, this is effectively an unchallenged choice, basically because of its ease of interpretation (at least at face value) and because of its linearity in (e, c), which means that the computations are simplified – the expected utility is computed with respect to a bivariate quantity, but thanks to linearity the two components can be separated out.

There are some underlying complexities in the use of the MNB: firstly, it assumes that we are willing and able to rescale health benefits in monetary terms. We generally do and accept that we can put a monetary value to, effectively, a human life. This is of course not free from controversy (see for example Donaldson et al., 1997; Friedman, 2021).

In addition, from a more mathematical perspective, we can also prove that the MNB assumes risk-neutrality on the part of the decision-maker, i.e. in other words that k is all that is needed to put costs and benefits on equal footing – this is most often not the case in real applications, where decision-makers tend to be risk-averse. Baio (2012, sec 3.7.1) discusses the expansion of the utility function to include a risk-aversion parameter (Raiffa, 1968).

For each intervention, we can compute the expected net benefit

$$\mathcal{NB}_t = \mathrm{E}\left[nb_t\right],$$

The intervention associated with the highest expected net benefit $\mathcal{NB}^* = \max_t \mathcal{NB}_t$ is then selected as the most cost-effective.

In the simple case of only two interventions being compared, we can make decisions based on the *Expected Incremental Benefit*

$$\begin{aligned}\text{EIB} &= \mathcal{NB}_2 - \mathcal{NB}_1 \\ &= \mathrm{E}\left[ke_2 - c_2\right] - \mathrm{E}\left[ke_1 - c_1\right] \\ &= k\,\mathrm{E}\left[e_2 - e_1\right] - \mathrm{E}\left[c_2 - c_1\right] \\ &= k\,\mathrm{E}\left[\Delta_e\right] - \mathrm{E}\left[\Delta_c\right]. \end{aligned} \tag{4.4}$$

Using this metric, $t = 2$ is deemed to be cost-effective if EIB > 0, in which case its expected utility is higher than that of the comparator. Because the value of k is explicitly considered in the definition of the EIB, there is no confusion over the decision rule. Interestingly, this is equivalent to the case in which $k >$ ICER if $\mathrm{E}\left[\Delta_e\right] > 0$ or $k <$ ICER if $\mathrm{E}\left[\Delta_e\right] < 0$, as can be seen by simply re-arranging Equation 4.4.

i How they made the threshold

Historically, NICE have usually considered that interventions associated with an ICER between £20 000 and £30 000 represent good value for money for the healthcare provider – given the discussion above, this implies a threshold of $k \in$ £[20 000; 30 000]. However, the range of values for the willingness to pay selected by NICE has a long and complicated history.

As mentioned in McCabe et al. (2008), NICE's official methods guides did not refer to a fixed threshold; nonetheless, Rawlins and Culyer (2004) reported that NICE had up to that point basically always accepted interventions with ICER $<$ £20 000 and hardly ever recommended those with ICER $>$ £30 000.

Much to marked disappointment among some members of the original NICE panel, that range has become received wisdom and has often been taken at face value, leading to some heated debates – see for example Claxton et al. (2000) and, more recently, Barnsley et al. (2013) and Claxton et al. (2015), who suggest lower optimal values for k. Sampson et al. (2022) present an econometric analysis of the cost-effectiveness threshold as determined by the supply-side.

Very recently (and with a view for full implementation starting from April 2026), the threshold suggested for use by NICE has been increased to £25 000 and £35 000 (NICE,

2025). This has been justified with the possibility of approving medicines that deliver significant health improvements but might have previously been declined purely on cost-effectiveness grounds, although critics have argued that increases in the price paid by the healthcare provider by raising the threshold is not guaranteed to bring additional benefits for the whole population (notably among others, Claxton and Sculpher, 2025).

The cost-effectiveness threshold around the world

It is difficult to keep a close record of official values for the "cost-per-QALY" sanctioned in different jurisdictions. This is because not all have formal HTA processes and agencies and even when they do, they may decide to apply more or less rather general rules, sometimes subject to specific exceptions (e.g. in the case of interventions for high-impact disease areas or end-of-life care).

In some cases, the national threshold is, at least informally, set at some equivalent to that suggested by NICE – for instance, while there is no formally pre-specified cost-effectiveness threshold, in Italy interventions are typically evaluated against an informal benchmark of €25 000 to €40 000 per QALY (Russo et al., 2023), which occasionally raises up to €50 000.

Some recent examples of international estimates include Vallejo-Torres et al. (2018), who suggest a range of €22 000 to €25 000 per QALY, in Spain, while separate work by van Baal et al. (2019) and Stadhouders et al. (2019) estimate a cost-per-QALY ranging from €41 000 to €71 600, in the Netherlands. Siverskog and Henriksson (2019) place the threshold at SEK 370 000 (approximately equivalent to €39 000 in 2019 currency) for Sweden, while Vanness et al. (2021) estimate a cost-per-QALY of $104 000, in the US. Finally, Edney et al. (2018) give an estimate of AUD 21 000 to AUD 38 000 for Australia and Ochalek et al. (2020) estimate a range of RMB 28 000 to RMB 52 000 for China.

4.3 Uncertainty analysis

The straight path from the "Statistical model" to the "Decision analysis" in Figure 4.1 represents the decision-making process *given current evidence* and conditionally on the assumptions made in the statistical analysis. This, however, does not fully account for the inherent uncertainty in the estimates for the model parameters, which in turn determine the economic summaries and therefore have a potentially substantial impact on the uncertainty in the decision-making process. For example, this may be because the relevant data may be obtained from a relatively small clinical trial, possibly with a follow-up that is not long enough to capture potential side effects.

More importantly, the decision is generally not binary, because we could always consider a third option: what if we are not confident in making a decision just yet, because the data are not definitive and thus there remains too much uncertainty? In that case, the optimal decision is in fact to postpone it until we can obtain more data to reduce the current uncertainty and thus be able to make a better one (we return more formally to this point in Chapter 12).

Consequently, the uncertainty underlying decisions over the adoption, implementation or reimbursement of new interventions must also be assessed thoroughly and, crucially, its

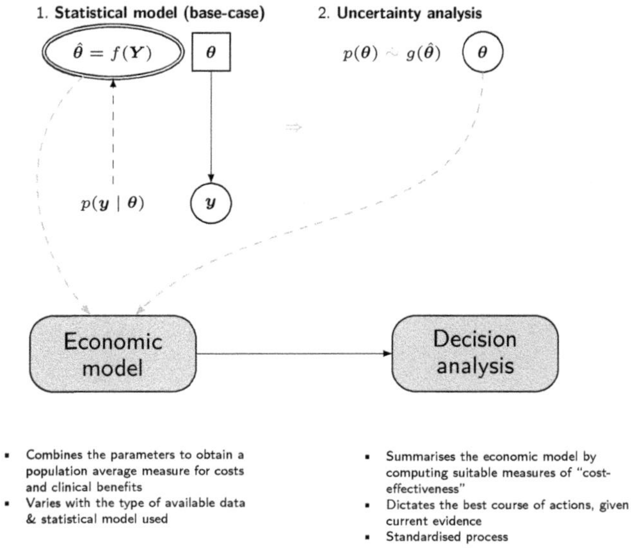

Figure 4.4: "Standard", frequentist perspective (termed "two stage" in Spiegelhalter et al., 2004).

impact on the decision-making must be formally included in the assessment. For this reason, it is generally mandatory to "take a detour" from the straight path from "Statistical model" to "Decision analysis" through the "Uncertainty analysis" building block, as shown in Figure 4.1 – this process is often referred to as "Probabilistic Sensitivity Analysis" (PSA), in the HTA literature.

4.3.1 "Standard", frequentist approach to uncertainty analysis

From a frequentist perspective (which has been historically used when HTA was formalised as a discipline, in the late 1970s), while in principle the only relevant source of uncertainty is represented by the sampling variability associated with the observed data, the cost-effectiveness analysis tends to be performed as a two-stage process (Spiegelhalter et al., 2004), as shown graphically in Figure 4.4.

First, the statistical analysis is used to obtain an estimate for the "base-case" analysis, for instance using the point estimate described by the maximum likelihood estimator for the parameters of interest. This value is fed to the "Economic model" to obtain suitable measures of population benefit and costs, with which we can then perform the decision analysis, for instance to construct the ICER or the expected net benefit. In this case, all the expectations are computed with respect to the sampling variability associated with the observed data.

Then, separately, in order to account for the uncertainty in the parameter estimates, we use Monte Carlo or bootstrap simulations to construct a pseudo-distribution $g(\hat{\boldsymbol\theta})$ – see again Figure 4.4, where we use the symbol $\dot{\sim}$ to indicate that the distribution $p(\theta)$ can*not* model epistemic uncertainty on the parameters, as there is no such thing for a frequentist/maximum likelihood approach. Conversely, $g(\hat{\boldsymbol\theta})$ is a function of the data and the only variability is generated by the sampling process, in line with the frequentist/maximum likelihood philosophy (see also Baio, 2025 for more details on the distinction between Bayesian and non-Bayesian inference).

Table 4.1: A tabular representation of the concept of uncertainty analysis. Each row in the table represents a simulation from the distribution for the model parameters. At each simulation, we can perform the decision analysis *as if this were the realised value of the parameters*. The intervention with the highest *row-wise* utility is marked in italics, while the highest overall ($t = 2$, in this case) is typeset in bold

	Parameter simulations				Expected utility		
Sims	θ_1	θ_2	...	θ_Q	$\text{NB}_1(\boldsymbol{\theta})$	$\text{NB}_2(\boldsymbol{\theta})$	$\text{IB}(\boldsymbol{\theta})$
1	0.58	0.38	...	0.42	*77480*	67795	-9685
2	0.51	0.02	...	0.08	87165	*106535*	19370
3	0.61	0.14	...	0.06	*58110*	38740	-19370
4	0.2	0.73	...	0.73	77480	*87165*	9685
...	...	...	...	...	...	...	...
1000	0.03	0.2	...	0.56	48425	*87165*	38740
				Average:	$\mathcal{NB}_1 = 72365.35$	$\mathcal{NB}_2 = \mathbf{77403.49}$	$\text{EIB} = 5038.14$

To give an example, a parameter θ may indicate a proportion and we may consider $g(\hat{\theta}) = \text{Beta}(a, b)$ to first map the range of values supported by the 95% confidence interval around the point estimate $\hat{\theta}$ (a process similar to the one described in Example 1.4, in Section 1.2.4 and then in Section 1.2.6) and then to forward-sample a large number of possible values, to capture the underlying uncertainty in the parameter estimates. These simulated values are passed onto the Economic model and the analysis is repeated all the way to the Decision analysis, in order to construct a pseudo-distribution of the entire decision-making.

We can think of this process using a tabular format, as shown in Table 4.1. Here, we report in each row the simulations from the posterior distribution: we assume that the model is characterised by Q parameters $\theta_1, \ldots, \theta_Q$ – some models will only have a relatively limited number of parameters, but more complex ones (e.g. in network meta-analysis, see Chapter 7) may include a very large number.

If we treat each row separately and pretend that the simulated values for the parameters are the "true" ones, then we can compute the "known-distribution" expected utilities

$$\text{NB}_t(\boldsymbol{\theta}) = \text{E}\left[nb_t \mid \boldsymbol{\theta}\right]$$

and, assuming $T = 2$, the "known-distribution" incremental benefit

$$\text{IB}(\boldsymbol{\theta}) = \text{NB}_2(\boldsymbol{\theta}) - \text{NB}_1(\boldsymbol{\theta}).$$

With these, we can check which intervention is associated with the highest value.

For instance, in simulation 1 in Table 4.1, the status quo $t = 1$ is associated with a known-distribution expected utility $\text{NB}_1(\boldsymbol{\theta}) = 77\,480$. In this case, this is larger than the resulting value for $t = 2$, $\text{NB}_2(\boldsymbol{\theta}) = 67\,795$. Consequently, if we were able to resolve the uncertainty in the parameter to the values simulated at this iteration, we would select $t = 1$ as the most cost-effective treatment (for this reason, the value for $\text{NB}_1(\boldsymbol{\theta})$ is typeset in italics, in the first row of Table 4.1).

In other words, if the future turned out to be as characterised by the parameters profile in iteration 1, then $t = 1$ would be the most cost-effective intervention – this is also consistent with the fact that, in the first row of Table 4.1, the incremental benefit $\text{IB}(\boldsymbol{\theta}) < 0$, indicating that $t = 2$ would produce a lower expected utility.

Of course, this is only one simulations and in order to characterise fully the underlying parametric uncertainty, we need to consider the whole lot – say 1000 simulations as in Table 4.1, effectively deriving a full distribution of decisions.

We can summarise the process overall (i.e. given current evidence and assumptions) by taking the averages over the distribution of $\boldsymbol{\theta}$ for the two known-distribution expected utilities

$$\mathcal{NB}_t = \text{E}\left[\text{NB}_t(\boldsymbol{\theta})\right],$$

and selecting as optimal the intervention associated with the highest value

$$\mathcal{NB}^* = \max_t \mathcal{NB}_t, \tag{4.5}$$

or, in the case of $T = 2$, equivalently by computing

$$\text{EIB} = \text{E}\left[\text{IB}(\boldsymbol{\theta})\right]$$

and comparing it with 0.

In the case of Table 4.1, $\mathcal{NB}_1 = 72\,365.35 < \mathcal{NB}_2 = 77\,403.49$ and thus it would $t = 2$ to in fact represent the most cost-effective alternative, overall – this is why the value for $\mathcal{NB}_2$ is typeset in bold and, for the same reason, why $\text{EIB} > 0$, in Table 4.1.

Note 11: Tell me you're a Bayesian without telling me you're a Bayesian...

The uncertainty analysis described above sounds suspiciously similar to a full Bayesian approach, in which we formally express uncertainty in the model parameters using a probability distribution. Technically speaking, the two are quite not the same – in the standard, frequentist approach to cost-effectiveness analysis, there is no such thing as a full joint distribution for the model parameters. The Monte Carlo pseudo-distribution is used to try and account for the fact that the evidence base is naturally not definitive and this will have an impact on the confidence with which we can make a decision.

Another way of describing the full process of economic evaluation and uncertainty analysis is graphically using the cost-effectiveness plane (previously introduced in Figure 4.3), as shown in Figure 4.5.

Figure 4.5a shows the ICER (the dot, obtained in correspondence of the averages for Δ_e and Δ_c). In line with the discussion above, the new intervention dominates the status quo in the south-eastern quadrant and is dominated in the north-western quadrant of the cost-effectiveness plane. In the south-western and the north-eastern quadrant, the decision based purely on the ICER is not immediate.

Figure 4.5b shows the full economic evaluation obtained by "exploding" the point estimate (the ICER) through the pseudo-distribution of the model parameters. This describes the uncertainty associated with the base-case decision.

Figures 4.5c and 4.5d show the decision-making process based on including a willingness to pay threshold, k. The two graph also show the "sustainability area" (Baio, 2012), i.e. the

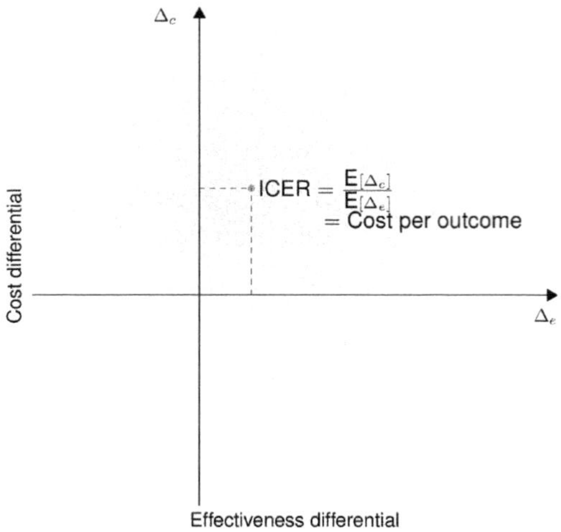

(a) Base-case analysis.

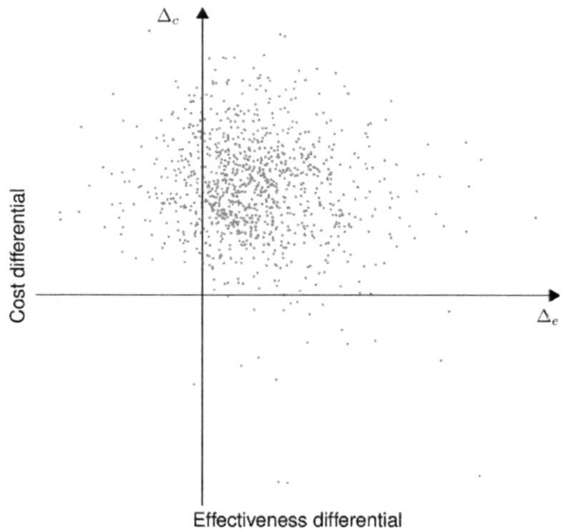

(b) Uncertainty analysis.

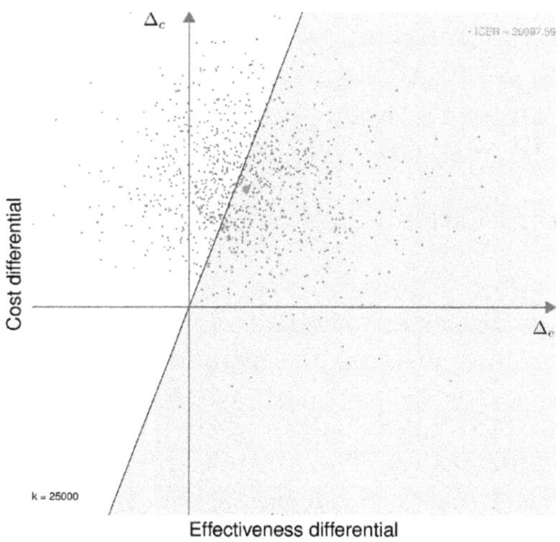

(c) ICER lying inside the sustainability area.

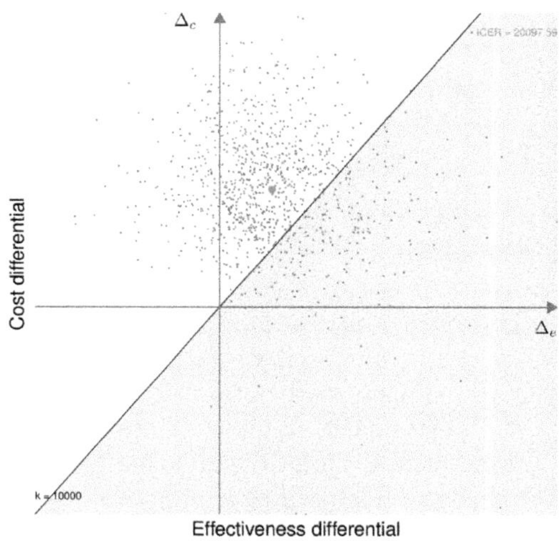

(d) ICER lying outside the sustainability area.

Figure 4.5: The cost-effectiveness plane. In the base-case scenario, we consider the ICER, as derived by the ratio of the point estimate for the cost and benefit population average differential. The PSA is based on constructing a pseudo-distribution of possible values to characterise the underlying uncertainty in the model parameters.

part of the cost-effectiveness plane which lies below the line $\Delta_c = k\Delta_e$. In Figure 4.5c, the ICER lies in the grey area (in this case for a value of $k = 25\,000$ monetary units), where $t = 2$ is an acceptable choice because the additional benefit is achieved at a smaller unit cost than the selected value of k (or, in other words, ICER $< k$). Conversely, if a different willingness-to-pay threshold had been selected, e.g. $k = 10\,000$ monetary units, as in Figure 4.5d, then $t = 2$ would be unacceptable. Similar considerations would apply if the ICER was in the south-western quadrant of the cost-effectiveness plane inside or outside the sustainability area.

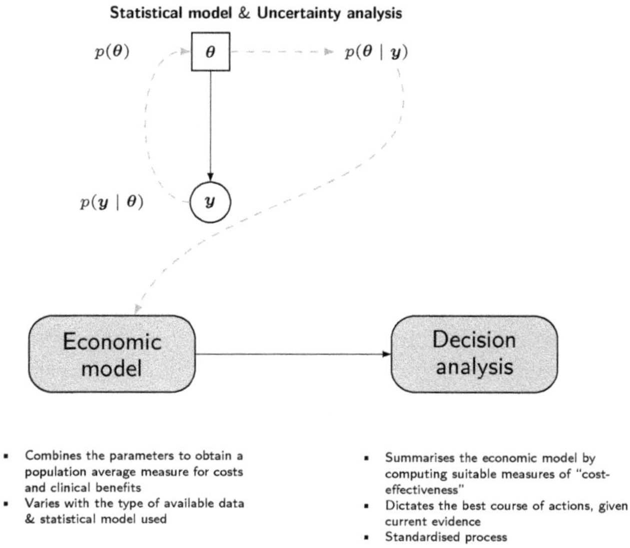

Figure 4.6: Bayesian, "integrated" approach to HTA.

Generally speaking, the proportion of points in the sustainability area gives an indicative measure of the uncertainty underlying the decision-making process – the more "possible futures" end up in the sustainability area, the more confident we can be about the decision made under current evidence (e.g. as described by the ICER).

4.3.2 Bayesian approach to cost-effectiveness analysis

In many ways, the process of uncertainty analysis is much more natural from a Bayesian perspective, in which everything happens "in one go", as shown in Figure 4.6: the prior and the sampling distribution are combined and, once the posterior distribution $p(\boldsymbol{\theta} \mid \boldsymbol{y})$ is obtained, then we can use for example MCMC simulations to characterise its uncertainty and feed each simulation directly to the "Economic model" and then the "Decision analysis" block, effectively creating a full distribution of decision-making processes as the basic model output. In other words, Figure 4.5b is the direct result of the Bayesian decision-making process – the order is somehow "flipped around" in comparison to the frequentist counterpart.

The only difference with a "normal" Bayesian analysis, where the estimates for the quantities of interest are obtained by marginalising out all the sources of uncertainty (sampling variability and epistemic uncertainty), is that in the process of PSA we want to examine the impact of the parameter uncertainty on the decision-making.

In order to do so, we effectively consider the induced full distribution of decisions to quantify how much the uncertainty in the model parameters affect the final cost-effectiveness assessment, though the conditional quantities $\text{NB}_t(\boldsymbol{\theta})$ and $\text{IB}(\boldsymbol{\theta})$. The tabular description of the process shown in Table 4.1 remains the same – but in a Bayesian context, the simulations for the Q model parameters come directly from the joint posterior distribution $p(\boldsymbol{\theta} \mid \boldsymbol{y})$ and, more importantly, they are the core output of the statistical analysis.

The best decision based on current evidence is obtained by averaging out all the uncertainty (e.g. by considering $\mathcal{NB}_t = \text{E}\left[\text{NB}_t(\boldsymbol{\theta})\right]$), but we can also assess how much uncertainty there is around that overall best decision, in terms of the posterior distribution of the model parameters. This quantifies the impact of parameter uncertainty on the decision-making process.

It's good to be Bayesian (in HTA)

The Bayesian and frequentist approaches may look very similar at face value, in this context – but there are fundamental differences.

- Firstly, while it is in principle possible to construct a multivariate version of the Monte Carlo psuedo-distribution $g(\hat{\boldsymbol{\theta}})$ from which to simulate values for the PSA, this process would involve increasing complexity and, in practice, most often the simulations are drawn independently for the Q model parameters. Conversely, the Bayesian analysis returns as the primary outcome a full joint posterior distribution for all the model parameters. For simplicity, we may assume prior independence among some of the Q parameters, but, by effect of the observed data, the posterior will capture any correlation present among the parameter.
- Related to the first point, in models characterised by a very simple structure, running a MCMC analysis may increase the computational cost by a large factor, at least relatively speaking (we return to this point, for instance, in Note 26 in Section 8.3.4). However, when the model becomes more and more complex and we start adding relevant structure (including composite sources of evidence, as we show in Chapter 6 and Chapter 7), building a frequentist version also involves notable computation, e.g. to maximise a highly dimensional likelihood function. In that case, the MCMC process is likely to become a more cost-effective tool, also in terms of running time and certainly in allowing more flexibility in the modelling framework.
- From a philosophical point of view, a Bayesian approach seems to apply naturally to the problem of decision-making: the evidence upon which we must base our decision is naturally subject to uncertainty (that is the very reason why we consider PSA) and if we are willing to model this (very possibly epistemic) source of uncertainty using a probability distribution, then we are able to formally propagate this across all the decision-making process – this is effectively what we want from PSA!

4.3.3 Summarising uncertainty analysis

Very often, uncertainty analysis is summarised using the concept of *Cost-Effectiveness Acceptability Curve* (CEAC, Van Hout et al., 1994). This is computed as

$$\text{CEAC} = \Pr(\text{IB}(\boldsymbol{\theta}) > 0)$$

– technically, from a Bayesian point of view, this is a posterior probability given the observed data and thus, perhaps, a more formal notation would be $\Pr(\text{IB}(\boldsymbol{\theta}) > 0 \mid \boldsymbol{y})$. The value of the CEAC depends specifically on the willingness-to-pay parameter, k; basically, for each choice of k in a usually discrete grid of values, e.g. $k = (0, 100, 200, 300, \ldots, 10\,000)$, we can compute the proportion of PSA simulations that fall in the sustainability area – see Figures 4.5c and 4.5d.

Figure 4.7 shows the CEAC computed for the example shown schematically in Table 4.1. Here, we consider a grid of k values from 0 to 50 000 monetary units, with increments of 100. For each of these values, we plot the resulting proportion of PSA simulations for which $\text{IB}(\boldsymbol{\theta}) > 0$ – these computations happen automatically when using the `R` package `BCEA` (Baio et al., 2025a). We present more details throughout the next chapters and specifically in Example 5.6.

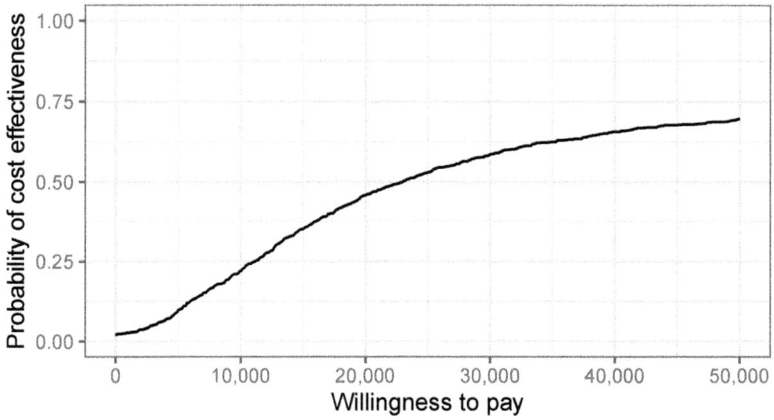

Figure 4.7: The Cost-Effectiveness Acceptability Curve derived in the case of Table 4.1, considering all the 1000 simulations from the uncertainty analysis.

Generally speaking, for a given willingness-to-pay threshold, we would like the CEAC to have "large enough" values, to indicate that decision uncertainty is negligible – typical thresholds are often somewhat artificially put at around 80%. In addition, in general, the CEAC alone cannot be used to determine the optimal intervention, for a given value of the willingness-to-pay: by definition, the CEAC only quantifies the probability that the intervention under consideration ($t = 2$, in this case) is optimal, for any particular value of k (Fenwick et al., 2001).

When the number of interventions $T > 2$, we can still process each pairwise comparison, e.g. set $t = 1, 2, 3$ as the comparators and $t = 4$ as the main intervention, for which we want to assess the cost-effectiveness and then produce $(T-1)$ CEACs, describing the probability that $t = 4$ is the most-cost-effective intervention against either of the other options.

Figure 4.8a shows this graph over a grid of values for k in $[0; 1000]$. As is possible to see, in this case, for all pairwise comparisons, the CEAC is increasing and, by the end of the range in the x–axis, it exceeds 0.5 against all the alternative intervention, in fact reaching larger values (close to 0.8 for the comparison against $t = 2$ and close to 1 for the comparison against $t = 1$).

In addition, we may also want to assess the overall performance of the alternatives. Figure 4.8b shows the absolute probability that each of the $T = 4$ interventions is the one associated with the highest net benefit, for each value of k in the grid $[0; 1000]$ – these probabilities are computed as the proportion of PSA simulations in which $t = \arg\max_t \mathcal{NB}_t$.

In this case, the probability that $t = 1$ is optimal is very large for very small values of k, only to tail off very rapidly towards 0. $t = 4$ becomes the intervention associated with the highest chance of being the most cost-effective at around 200 monetary units along the x–axis, but there is a short interval in which $t = 2$ is the optimal intervention.

We can consolidate these findings into the *Cost-Effectiveness Acceptability Frontier* (CEAF, Fenwick et al., 2001). This is shown in Figure 4.8c and Baio et al. (2025a) detail how to obtain the resulting graphical output using the R package BCEA. The CEAF is computed for each given value of the threshold k as the probability of cost-effectiveness for the optimal intervention (i.e. the one associated with the highest expected utility, in correspondence of

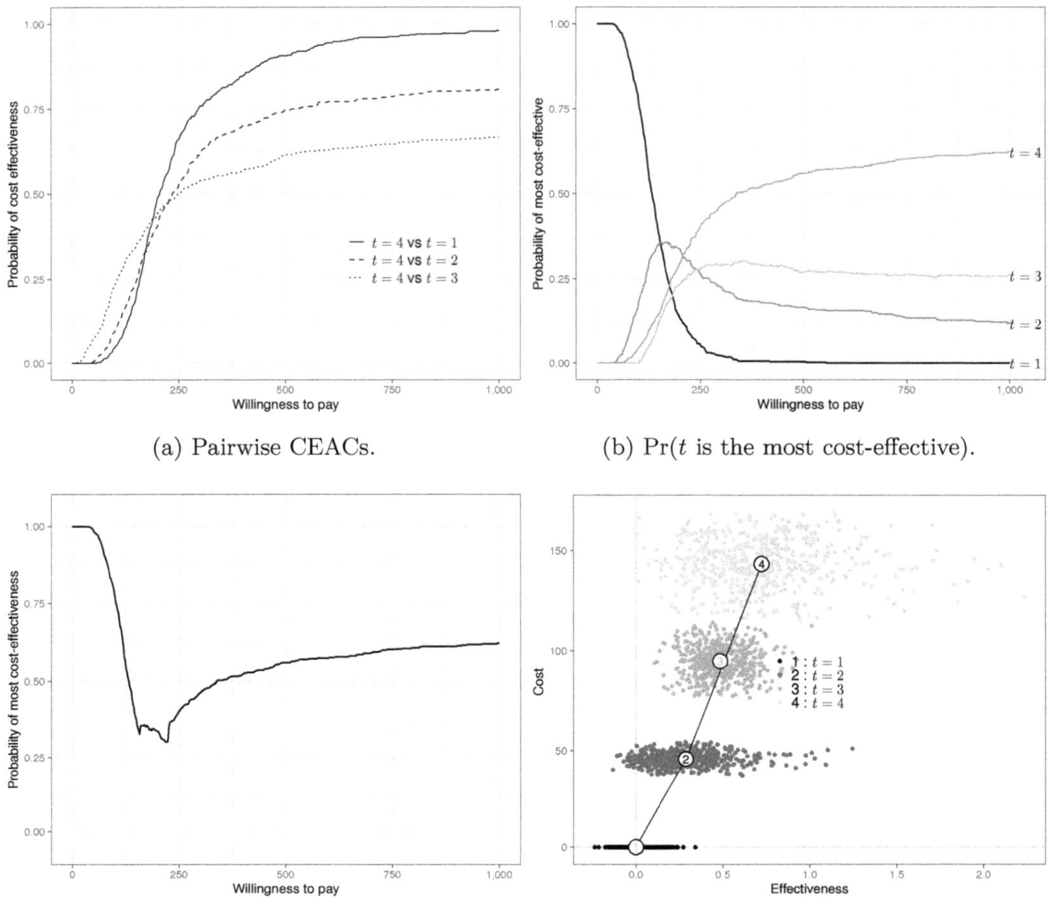

(a) Pairwise CEACs.

(b) Pr(t is the most cost-effective).

(c) Cost-effectiveness acceptability frontier.

(d) Cost-effectiveness efficiency frontier.

Figure 4.8: Uncertainty analysis in the case of multiple comparators.

that value of k). This analysis reveals "switch points" where the best strategy changes. In this case the piecewise curve shown in Figure 4.8c is the combination of the three parts in which $t = 1$, then $t = 2$ and then $t = 4$ are the optimal interventions.

Figure 4.8d shows also the *Cost-Effectiveness Efficiency Frontier* (CEEF, Fenwick et al., 2001). This is a graphical representation that illustrates the most efficient interventions in terms of cost versus health outcomes (benefits). More specifically, it shows the trade-off between cost and effectiveness for various health technologies or interventions.

In the graph, each intervention is plotted as a point based on its average cost and health outcome – in Figure 4.8d, these are the numbered circles and we also display the underlying uncertainty around this average estimate in terms of the PSA simulations. In this case, we scale the axes so that $t = 1$ sits in the point $(0, 0)$, by using the option `start.from.origins=TRUE` in the `BCEA` function `ceef.plot()`.

The efficiency frontier is formed by connecting the points of interventions that provide the best possible trade-off between cost and effectiveness. Interventions on the frontier are considered efficient because no other intervention offers greater effectiveness for the same or lower cost. In contrast, interventions below the efficiency frontier are generally less cost-effective; they require more resources for less health benefit. The slope of the line connecting different points on the efficiency frontier is equivalent to the ICER.

For example, in Figure 4.8d interventions $t = 1$, $t = 2$ and $t = 4$ are directly connected by the frontier. This is consistent with the analysis of Figures 4.8b and 4.8c, in which we have identified them as the optimal intervention for different choices of k. Conversely, $t = 3$ is *just* inside the frontier, i.e. it does not lie on the segment connecting $t = 2$ and $t = 4$: it sits slightly to its left, to indicate that there is no value of k in correspondence of which $t = 3$ is the most cost-effective intervention.

Note 12: Limitations of the CEACs

A major limitation of CEACs is that they do not account for the actual consequences of the underlying decision uncertainty. For example, consider the following, admittedly rather silly example:

1. Intervention $t = 2$ is deemed to be more cost-effective than a comparator $t = 1$, given current evidence and CEAC $= \Pr(t = 2 \text{ is cost-effective} \mid \text{current data}) = 0.51$. In this case, the uncertainty in the model inputs generates substantial uncertainty in the decision. However, imagine that, if we "get it wrong" and in fact given more evidence we would be able to determine that $t = 1$ is more cost-effective, we would need to bear: *a)* an increase in population average costs of 3 monetary units; and *b)* a decrease in population average effectiveness of 0.000001 benefits.
2. Intervention $t = 2$ is again deemed to be more cost-effective than a comparator $t = 1$, given current evidence, this time with CEAC $= \Pr(t = 2 \text{ is cost-effective} \mid \text{current data}) = 0.999$. However, in this case, if we get it wrong and more information would tell us that the opposite is true, we would face consequences of *a)* an increase in population average costs of 100 million monetary units; and *b)* a decrease in population average effectiveness of 100 million benefits.

In case 1., although the uncertainty is substantial, there really is no point in agonising over it and perhaps delaying making a decision until more evidence becomes available, because the pay-offs are effectively negligible. In case 2., conversely, although the uncertainty is minimal, the consequences in the rare event where we make the wrong decision are dire and therefore we may want to consider postponing a firm commitment to the new intervention, until we can remove, or at least reduce the possibility of making it. We return to these considerations in Chapter 12, in which we discuss the analysis of the value of information.

4.3.4 Structural uncertainty

All the discussion above has been based on the premise that the main sources of variation in the decision-making process are given by the sampling distribution that characterises the observed data and the uncertainty associated with the model parameters (with the caveats of Note 11 above, in terms of the frequentist approach). In other words, as mentioned throughout the chapter, the decision is made *given current evidence and the model assumptions*.

However, there is often a strong sense that in fact we cannot be entirely confident in the "structural assumptions" underpinning our model. Critical examples include the assessment of how the down-stream decision-making process would change if we used a given sampling distribution instead of a potential alternative one (see specifically the analyses in Chapter 5 and the discussion in Chapter 8), or whether we should use 'fixed' or 'random' effects, to build up a Network Meta-Analysis (see Sections 6 and 7).

One obvious solution is to run different version of the overall model and then perform some sort of "scenario sensitivity analysis" by reporting the results of the decision analysis for each different modelling choice. This may be a reasonable idea, but it has the considerable downside that each scenario is considered separately and we still need to find a way to rank them, possibly in terms of how well the underlying modelling assumption align with the observed data – we return to this point in Sections 5.3 and 6.2.6.

Baio (2012, sec. 3.6) presents a possible framework for structural uncertainty based on a form of model averaging, where separate distributional assumptions are tested and then the various models are combined in a sort of weighted average, where the weights are proportional to measures of model fit. This type of analysis can be implemented for the health economic evaluation using the `BCEA` function `struc.psa()` – see also Baio et al. (2025a, sec. 4.4). We return to this point in Section 5.3.5, Example 5.6 and, briefly, in Note 19 in Example 6.6.

4.4 Conclusions

This chapter has described a general introduction to the statistical foundations underpinning the general problem of health technology assessment; in particular, we have discussed the fundamental nature as a decision problem, as well as the importance of the assessment of the impact of uncertainty in the model inputs onto the final decision-making process.

This is closely related to the Bayesian framework of the problem, in which this uncertainty is handled naturally as a *prima-facie* feature of the modelling structure. We have also shown the general measures of analysis, which will be used in the rest of the book to quantify the "value for money" associated with various interventions.

In the next chapter, we begin the exploration of the most important modelling framework for HTA, starting from the case of individual-level data, typically relevant for economic evaluation alongside clinical trials.

Part II

Statistical modelling in HTA

5

Cost-effectiveness analysis with individual-level data

5.1 Introduction

Ideally, when comparing the economic performance of a set of alternative interventions, we would have access to full data on individuals, which inform about a range of variables. Obviously, we need a measure of some pre-specified clinical outcome, depending on the specific intervention applied to a given individual; in addition, important information include the use of healthcare resources (e.g. GP visit, hospital, drugs, etc.), which we can use to compute the corresponding cost for the healthcare provider. Finally, in order to be able to provide a balanced assessment of the "value-for-money" for a given intervention, we generally prefer to measure "effectiveness" through specific *Health-Related Quality of Life* data (HRQL, see Section 4.2).

Generally speaking, this framework is not limited to any single study design and can accommodate data arising from randomised studies, observational cohorts or routine data sources. The central aim is to exploit the granularity of patient-level observations to appropriately characterise heterogeneity, handle missingness (see Chapter 10) adjust for prognostic factors (see Chapter 11 for more discussion on this), as well as propagate uncertainty in the relevant model inputs, when estimating incremental costs, effects and cost-effectiveness measures over the relevant analytic horizon (as discussed in Chapter 4).

When such data are collected alongside clinical studies (not necessarily, but very often in the context of randomised trials), individual-level modelling also supports an immediate or short-term economic assessment grounded in the observed follow-up. Here, the economic analysis is aligned with the clinical analysis, sharing the same unit of observation while focusing on costs and health outcomes rather than treatment efficacy alone. This contrasts with wider decision-analytic modelling, which is often, though not necessarily, built on aggregated level evidence and designed to extrapolate beyond the available data, synthesise multiple sources and project long-term consequences for decision making at the population level – we return to these ideas in Chapters 6, 7 and 9, in particular.

Table 5.1 shows a simplified version of a possible dataset containing relevant individual-level data (ILD), which we may want to use to perform economic evaluation, typically alongside the clinical study.

Here, we assume that the data have a *longitudinal* nature, where we observe time-varying variables over a number of times – this is indicated by the use of the indices $0, \ldots, J$ to indicate that there are J measurements after the baseline time $j = 0$. The variables y_{ij} indicate the main clinical outcome, for example the survival time (see Chapter 8), event indicator (e.g. occurrence of cardiovascular disease), the number of events, or some continuous measurement (e.g. blood pressure), for each individual $i = 1, \ldots, N$ and time points $j = 0, \ldots, J$. Similarly, we may be able to record a set of HRQL data (see Note 10 in Section 4.2) – we indicate these as u_{ij}.

DOI: 10.1201/9781003771050-5

Table 5.1: A typical individual-level dataset. Each row characterises an individual (ID), for whom we observe a treatment indicator, a set of demographic variables (e.g. age and sex). We also typically observe a set of clinical measurements $\boldsymbol{y} = (y_0, y_1, \ldots, y_J)$ for a number J of time points after the baseline $j = 0$. The economic data consist of the health-related quality of life measurements $\boldsymbol{u} = (u_0, u_1, \ldots, u_J)$ and the cost data $\boldsymbol{c} = (c_0, c_1, \ldots, c_J)$. These may or may not be repeated over time, although, typically, there are at least two measurements (baseline and end of follow-up)

		Demographics			Clinical outcomes			HRQL data			Cost data		
ID	Trt	Sex	Age	...	y_0	...	y_J	u_0	...	u_J	c_0	...	c_J
1	1	M	23	...	y_{10}	...	y_{1J}	0.32	...	0.44	103	...	80
2	1	M	23	...	y_{20}	...	y_{2J}	0.12	...	0.38	1204	...	877
3	2	F	19	...	y_{30}	...	y_{3J}	0.49	...	0.88	16	...	22
...	...	...	...	...	...	...	...	...	...	...	...	...	...

As for the cost data c_{ij}, these typically consider the use of specific healthcare resources (e.g. the cost of the relevant drugs, hospital visits or GP appointments). In practice, we may access the actual number of occurrences for each at any given time point measurement and apply a cost multiplier – for instance, the unit cost for a specific dose of a drug, or the tariff associated with a set duration for a stay in hospital under a given condition.

While it is possible (and in fact, desirable) to fully exploit the underlying longitudinal nature of the data, often measurements are aggregated into cross-sectional summaries and for each individual we end up considering the pair (e_i, c_i), defined as

$$e_i = \sum_{j=1}^{J} \frac{(u_{ij} + u_{ij-1})}{2} \delta_j, \tag{5.1}$$

where $\delta_j = \left[\frac{\text{Time}_j - \text{Time}_{j-1}}{\text{Unit of time}} \right]$ is the duration of the interval between two consecutive measurements and

$$c_i = \sum_{j=0}^{J} c_{ij}.$$

Discounting

One key feature of many healthcare interventions is that costs and clinical outcomes may typically occur at very different times, with respect to the point at which the intervention is implemented, for a given population.

An example is given by vaccination programmes, such as that against Human Papilloma Virus (HPV), implemented in several jurisdictions. Infection with HPV is transmitted through sexual intercourse and it is one of the key drivers of serious illnesses, notably cervical cancers. Current HPV population vaccination programmes are available for boys and girls as young as 12 (e.g. in the UK or Italy); however, while the cost of vaccination is born by the healthcare provider *now*, the real benefits will not materialise for a long time – for instance, cervical cancer rates tend to peak in the 30-35 year old age group.

Often, we thus find ourselves in a situation where the time horizon associated with the implementation of a given intervention is long-term, but we need to somehow "rebalance" the timing at which costs and benefits arrive – and, generally speaking, society tends to value benefits that arrive closer to the present time more than those that will be achievable in the (possibly very distant) future.

Discounting can be used to account for the differential timing of costs and benefits, by reducing the value of costs and effects that occur in the future. This is particularly relevant for economic evaluation spanning over a time horizon > 1 time unit (e.g. year) – Markov models (see Chapter 9) and Value of Information (see Chapter 12) are a specific example of this and thus discounting is a key issue when using them.

The general principle is to define a *discount rate*, d, in order to ensure that costs sustained and benefits gained closer to now have more weight. With that, we can then compute the Present Value as

$$\text{PV}_i^e = \sum_{j=0}^{J} \frac{u_{ij}}{(1+d)^j} \quad \text{and} \quad \text{PV}_i^c = \sum_{j=0}^{J} \frac{c_{ij}}{(1+d)^j}. \tag{5.2}$$

NICE suggests using $d = 3.5\%$ for costs and outcomes (NICE, 2016), although sometimes different or differential values are accepted. Despite the choice of the set discount rate being historically subject to some criticism (O'Mahony and Paulden, 2014), the value suggested by NICE tends to be used almost universally, across jurisdictions.

Discounting has the effect of weighting down future costs and benefits, whose face value becomes increasingly lower than the present value, as further times are considered.

Example 5.1. *10TT (adapted and expanded from Keng et al., 2025).* The 10 Top Tips trial (10TT, Beeken et al., 2017) is a two-arm, individually randomised, controlled trial of a weight-loss intervention for obese adults attending general practices in the UK. In the original study, a total of 537 participants were randomised to receive either the 10TT intervention or the standard of care from their general practices. The intervention was designed to behavioural change in forming good habits through self-help materials including a leaflet with ten simple weight-control tips and a log-book to record progress.

We use here a synthetic version of the original data, where the variables presented in Table 5.2 (which shows the first few rows of the resulting dataset) have been simulated to mimic the 10TT study. In particular, in this chapter we consider the "complete-case analysis", i.e. we discard the records subject to some form of missingness (see Chapter 10 for more discussion). This leaves the available sample size at 167.

We can use the following `R` code to manipulate the original data and compute the QALYs (see again Note 10 in Section 4.2), given the HRQL measurements at the various time points in the follow-up of the study, essentially applying Equation 5.1.

First, we create a function `disc()`, which applies a default 3.5% discount rate to the HRQL measurements at the various time points. The inputs to the function are `x`, the outcome to discount; `year`, representing the time variable (at which the discounting occurs); and `disc_rate`, the value selected for the discount rate (default at 0.035 = 3.5%).

```
# Defines a simple function to do the discounting.
disc=function(x, year, disc_rate = 0.035) {
```

Table 5.2: The first few rows of the 10TT dataset

		Demographics[a,b]				HRQL data[c]						
ID	Trt	Sex	Age	BMI	GP	u_0	u_3	u_6	u_{12}	u_{18}	u_{24}	c[d]
2	1	F	66	1	21	0.088	0.85	0.69	0.088	0.69	0.59	4230
3	1	M	57	1	5	0.796	0.8	0.8	0.62	0.8	1	1585
4	1	M	49	2	5	0.725	0.73	0.8	0.848	0.8	0.29	331
12	1	M	64	2	14	0.85	0.85	1	1	0.85	0.73	1034
13	1	M	66	1	9	0.848	0.85	0.85	1	0.85	0.73	1321
21	1	M	64	1	3	0.848	1	1	1	0.85	1	521

[a] BMI=Categorised body mass index
[b] GP=Number of GP visits
[c] QoL measurements at baseline, 3, 6, 12, 18 and 24 months
[d] Total costs

```
  x / ((1 + disc_rate)^(year - 1))
}
```

Then we first transform the original dataset (named `ttt` for "ten-top-tips", in the code below) from "wide" to "long" format (one in which each row contains a time measurement and thus individuals are replicated as many times as there are measurements), using the `tidyverse` function `pivot_longer()` – see also the discussion in Example 7.2.

In the next part of the code, we group by individual and first create the variables `du` and `delta` (same as in Equation 5.1), to represent the sum of two consecutive HRQL measurements and the duration of time across them. We do this using the `dplyr` function `lag()`, which determines the previous value in a vector.

With that, we compute the "area under the curve" value (see Figure 4.2) and then the full QALYs for each individual in the dataset. This last operation is performed using the `dplyr` function `summarise()`, where we divide the original value of the area under the curve by 12 (as it is defined in months, but we want to obtain the relative value in years).

```
# Temporary computation of QoL + QALY with discounting by using long format
df_qol=ttt |>
  ## select columns of interest
  select(id, arm, contains("qol")) |>
  ## convert dataframe from wide to long format
  pivot_longer(
    contains("qol"), names_to = "month", names_prefix = "qol_",
    names_transform = list(month = as.integer), values_to = "qol"
  ) |>
  # convert month to follow-up year; set baseline to be in year 1
  mutate(year = pmax(1, ceiling(month/12))) |>
  ## apply discounting
  mutate(qol_disc = disc(qol, year)) |>
  # group by individual
  group_by(id) |> mutate(
```

```
  # time duration between measurements
    delta=month-dplyr::lag(month,default = 0),
  # sum of utilities between two consecutive time points
    du=qol_disc+dplyr::lag(qol_disc,default = 0),
  # area under the curve (AUC)
    auc=du*delta/2
  ) |>
  # compute the QALYs (in years so divide by 12!), as sum of the AUC
  # for all time points
  summarise(qaly=sum(auc)/12) |> ungroup()
```

The final command merges the computed QALYs from the temporary dataset `df_qol` back into the original dataset `ttt`, which now contains an extra column with the resulting values.

```
# Merges the overall QALYs to the main dataset
ttt=ttt |> left_join(df_qol,by=c("id"="id")) |>
  mutate(
    Trt=arm+1,arm=factor(arm),
    arm=case_when(arm=="0"~"Control",TRUE~"Treatment")
  )
```

Figure 5.1 shows the histograms for the distributions of the discounted QALYs and the total costs, grouped by treatment arm. As is possible to see, the QALYs are highly skewed to the left; this is sensible, because we have a time horizon of 2 years and given the underlying disease is not life-threatening, it is reasonable to imagine that most individuals would be in a state of good health, with quite a few even in "perfect health", resulting in very high QALYs over the two year range.

5.2 Modelling ILD in HTA

5.2.1 Normal/Normal independent model

The "standard" and most basic statistical modelling (often implicitly) assumes normality and linearity and models *independently* individual benefits/HRQLs and total costs by controlling for the treatment arm Trt_i and the *centred* baseline values, e.g. $u^*_i = (u_i - \bar{u})$ and $c^*_i = (c_i - \bar{c})$

$$e_i = \alpha_0 + \alpha_1 \text{Trt}_i + \alpha_2 u^*_{0i} + \varepsilon_{ei}\,[+\ldots], \qquad \varepsilon_{ei} \sim \text{Normal}(0, \sigma_e) \tag{5.3}$$

$$c_i = \beta_0 + \beta_1 \text{Trt}_i + \beta_2 c^*_{0i} + \varepsilon_{ci}\,[+\ldots], \qquad \varepsilon_{ci} \sim \text{Normal}(0, \sigma_c), \tag{5.4}$$

where the notation $[+\ldots]$ indicates that we may want to include additional covariates in the model, for instance some demographic measurements on the individuals.

Statistics vs econometrics

Equations 5.3 and 5.4 describe two linear regression models where the observable variable is expressed in terms of a 'fixed' component (the linear predictor) and some

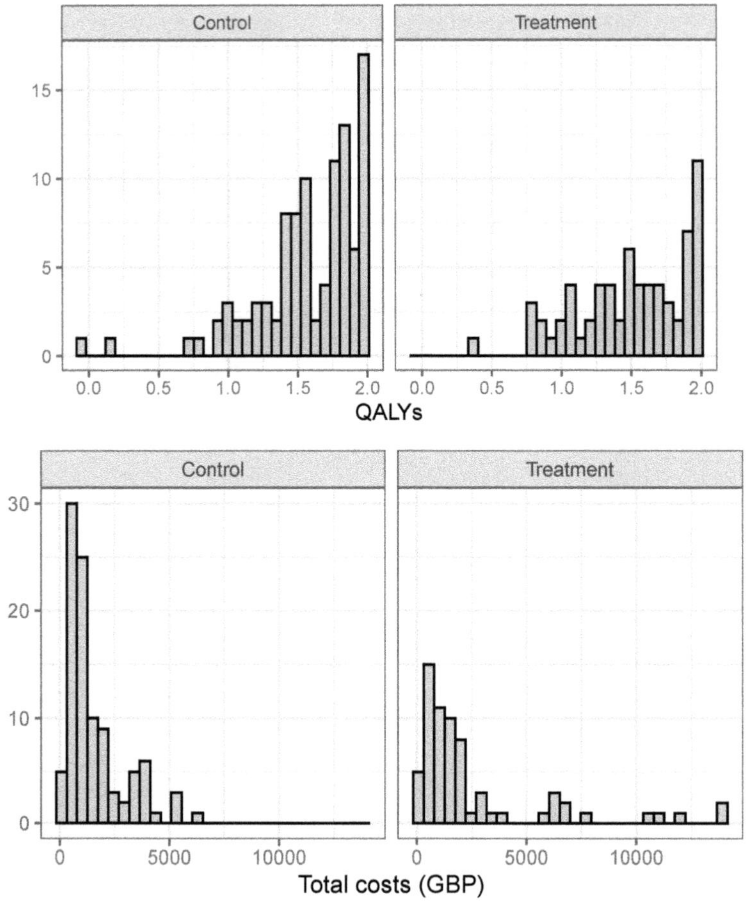

Figure 5.1: Empirical distribution for QALYs and total costs in the two treatment arms of the 10TT.

random noise (the error terms ε_{ei} and ε_{ci}), in a form that is perhaps more familiar in Econometrics than it is in Statistics.

If you prefer to speak Statistics than Econometrics[1], a more common description of this model is probably to consider

$$\begin{aligned} e_i &\sim \text{Normal}(\phi_{ei}, \sigma_e) \\ \phi_{ei} &= \alpha_0 + \alpha_1 \text{Trt}_i + \alpha_2 u^*_{0i} \, [+ \ldots] \end{aligned}$$

(of course, this extends obviously to c_i).

The two models are identical as they encode the same assumptions, in slightly different semantic ways.

Even with underlying randomised data, it is usually a good idea to control for the baseline values of utility and costs. The reason for this is that, most often, randomisation is performed with respect to the main clinical outcome y, rather than to the economic ones (e, c) and thus

[1]Unsurprisingly, the author does prefer to speak Statistics.

it is still possible that the baseline measurements for (e, c) may be unbalanced among the different treatment or intervention arms. Using a centred version of these covariates typically simplifies the interpretation of the results (and we come back to this in Section 5.2.2).

The models in Equations 5.3 and 5.4 can produce directly an estimate of the population average effectiveness and cost differentials – under these specifications, they are directly $\Delta_e = \alpha_1$ and $\Delta_c = \beta_1$. In a fully frequentist/maximum likelihood analysis, we can use basic functions such as `lm()`, in `R` to obtain the estimates for the model parameters and then quantify the impact of uncertainty in model parameters on the decision making process using resampling methods, such as the bootstrap.

Example 5.2. *10TT (continued): Normal/Normal independent model.* We start by modelling the 10TT data using the specification in Equations 5.3 and 5.4.

For each of the $i = 1, \ldots, N = 167$ observations we model $e_i \sim \text{Normal}(\phi_{ei}, \sigma_{et})$, where $t = 1, 2$ are the two intervention arm ($t = 1$ indicates the standard of care, while $t = 2$ is the active intervention – note here that we assume a treatment-specific variance). The linear predictor is defined as

$$\phi_{ei} = \alpha_0 + \alpha_1(\text{Trt}_i - 1) + \alpha_2(u_{0i} - \bar{u}_0)$$

– note that because for each individual we code in the data the treatment indicator as $\text{Trt}_i = 1, 2$, we use the rescaled version $(\text{Trt}_i - 1)$, so that when $\text{Trt}_i = 1$ (the control intervention), then the term disappears from the linear regression model and thus α_1 indicates the effect of the active intervention. In line with Equation 5.3, we control for the scaled (centred) version of the baseline HRQL, $u^*_{0i} = (u_{0i} - \bar{u}_0)$, whose effect is measured by the coefficient α_2. Consequently, we can define the population average effects as

$$\mu_{et} = \alpha_0 + \alpha_1(t - 1),$$

for $t = 1, 2$, so that, in the control arm $(t = 1)$, the effect of the treatment disappears.

As for the costs, we model $c_i \sim \text{Normal}(\phi_{ci}, \sigma_{ct})$ and, in a similar way to what we have done for the effects, the linear predictor as

$$\phi_{ci} = \beta_0 + \beta_1(\text{Trt}_i - 1).$$

Here, β_0 is the value of the linear predictor ϕ_{ci} when the treatment arm is $\text{Trt}_i = 1$ (i.e. the standard of care). Thus, we estimate of the population average costs as

$$\mu_{ct} = \beta_0 + \beta_1(t - 1),$$

for $t = 1, 2$. Because we only have data on the total costs over the course of the study, unlike for the effects, here we do not control for the background level.

⚠ Individual (conditional) vs population (marginal) averages

In the modelling presented above, we consider two forms of averages: the first ones are the linear predictors ϕ_{ei} and ϕ_{ci}; because they are defined as functions of the covariates, which are measured for each individual in the sample, these represent the *individual* (or conditional) average benefits and costs.

Conversely, the parameters μ_{et} and μ_{ct}, do not depend on the index i, because they are constructed by averaging ϕ_{ei} and ϕ_{ci} over the entire range of individual profiles (i.e. combination of values for the covariates), thus identifying the *population* (marginal) average benefit and costs. These are the object of the economic evaluation and thus the main parameter of our analysis (we return to this point later in Section 5.2.2 and Example 5.4, as well as in Chapter 11).

Finally, we define the prior distributions. For the regression coefficients we use minimally informative Normal priors

$$\alpha_0, \alpha_1, \alpha_2, \beta_0, \beta_1 \stackrel{iid}{\sim} \text{Normal}(\text{mean} = 0, \text{sd} = 100)$$

(this means of course a precision of $100^{-2} = 0.0001$). Note that we could probably do much better than this – given the scale of the observed data, it is unlikely that α_0 and α_1 have such a large range. However, given we have a reasonably large sample size, this very vague prior will probably not impact on the convergence of the model (see the results below).

As for β_0 and β_1, in fact we need to pay a little more attention: as shown in Figure 5.1, the range of the costs is quite large: [71.34; 13 899.28], overall. For this reason, a "lazy" prior centred on 0 may fail to accommodate the full range in the data and thus place some unduly mass away from where the posterior should actually be, by effect of the observed data.

One way around this would be to use more sensible priors – after all, β_0 indicates the average cost for the control, so we can expect it to be well away from 0 (and certainly to be positive). Alternatively and perhaps more easily, we can rescale the observed costs, e.g. by dividing them by £1000. This makes the assumption that $\beta_0, \beta_1 \stackrel{iid}{\sim} \text{Normal}(\text{mean} = 0, \text{sd} = 100)$ much more sensible and allows the posterior to explore a wide enough range. Of course, when taking this approach, we need to rescale up (by a factor of £1000) the estimates for the population average costs (see also the discussion in Note 14, below).

For the standard deviations for the observed costs and effects, we consider a PC prior (see Section 2.2.3 and Example 2.5 in particular). Given knowledge of the scale of the two outcomes, we assume that $\Pr(\sigma_{et} > 0.8) \approx 0.01$, leading to an Exponential distribution with rate $-\frac{\log(0.01)}{0.8} \approx 5.75$; and, on the scale of £1000, $\Pr(\sigma_{ct} > 2) \approx 0.5$, which implies an Exponential distribution with rate $-\frac{\log(0.5)}{2} \approx 0.35$.

Figure 5.2 shows these prior distributions. As is possible to see, the regression coefficients are widely spread and the data standard deviations have decreasingly small mass for higher values. In all cases, we do not rule out *a priori* the possibility that the evidence would change these distributions to different shapes.

The full modelling assumptions under a Bayesian framework can be written into suitable `JAGS` code. We do so by creating an `R` function (as in Note 8 in Example 3.1).

```
# Normal/Normal independent model - JAGS code
nn_indep=function(){
  for (i in 1:N) {
    # Model for the effects
    e[i] ~ dnorm(phi.e[i], tau.e[Trt[i]])
    phi.e[i] <- alpha0 + alpha1*(Trt[i]-1) + alpha2*u0star[i]
    # Model for the costs
    c[i] ~ dnorm(phi.c[i], tau.c[Trt[i]])
    phi.c[i] <- beta0 + beta1*(Trt[i]-1)
  }
```

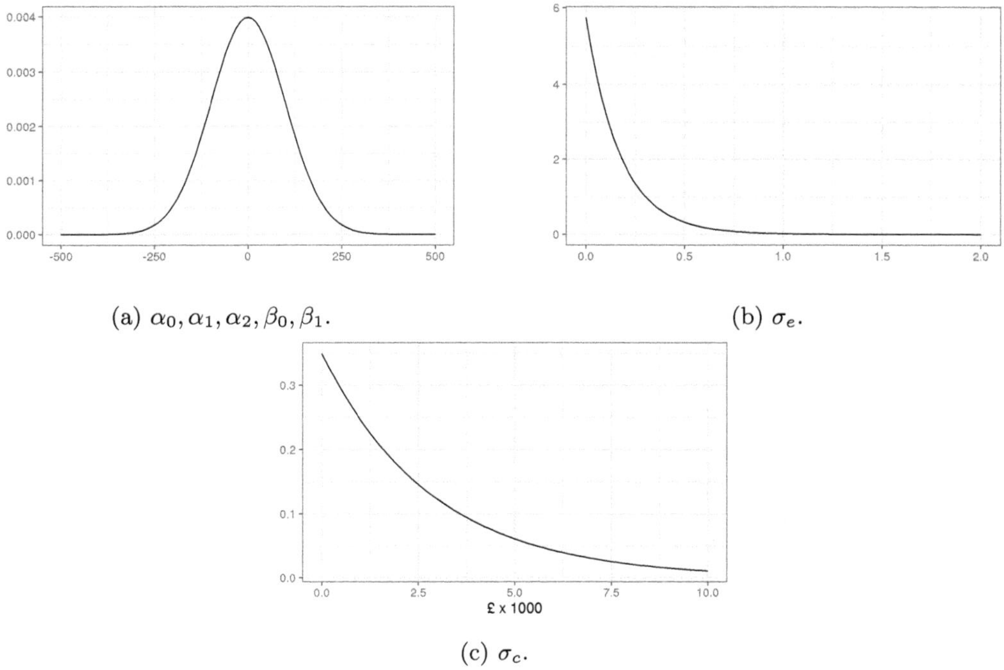

Figure 5.2: The prior distributions for the parameters of the 10TT model. For β_0, β_1 and σ_c, the x–axis is scaled to £1000, given that the original data are given as $c_i/1000$.

```
  # Rescales the main economic parameters
  for (t in 1:2) {
    mu.e[t] <- alpha0 + alpha1*(t-1)
    # (NB costs need to be scaled up by 1000)
    mu.c[t] <- 1000*(beta0 + beta1*(t-1))
  }
  # Minimally informative priors on the regression coefficients
  alpha0 ~ dnorm(0,0.0001)
  alpha1 ~ dnorm(0,0.0001)
  alpha2 ~ dnorm(0,0.0001)
  beta0 ~ dnorm(0,0.0001)
  beta1 ~ dnorm(0,0.0001)
  for (t in 1:2) {
  # PC-prior on the sd with Pr(sigma_e>0.8) \approx 0.01
    sigma.e[t] ~ dexp(5.75)
    tau.e[t] <- pow(sigma.e[t],-2)
  # PC-prior on the sd with Pr(sigma_c>2) \approx 0.5
    sigma.c[t] ~ dexp(0.35)
    tau.c[t] <- pow(sigma.c[t],-2)
  }
}
```

Vectorising the linear predictor

Unlike BUGS (but similarly to other related software, such as Stan – see Section 8.3.5), JAGS allows *vectorisation.* This means that, instead of having to specify fully the linear predictor in a regression model, by adding all the relevant covariates, we could more economically use matrix algebra and code up the general relationship $\mu = \boldsymbol{X}\boldsymbol{\beta}$, where

$$\boldsymbol{X} = \begin{pmatrix} 1 & X_{11} & X_{12} & \cdots & X_{1C} \\ 1 & X_{21} & X_{22} & \cdots & X_{2C} \\ \vdots & \vdots & \vdots & \ddots & \vdots \\ 1 & X_{n1} & X_{n2} & \cdots & X_{nC} \end{pmatrix}$$

is a matrix with n rows and $K = (C+1)$ columns (a vector of ones and then the C "active" covariates), while $\boldsymbol{\beta} = (\beta_0, \beta_1, \ldots, \beta_C)$ is the vector of regression coefficients, including the intercept β_0.

Back to the Normal/Normal independence model discussed above, we could use something like the following code to construct the covariates matrix and define the overall number of them to a variable K and then modify the JAGS code to vectorise the linear predictor.

```
# Pre-processing to make the matrix of covariates
X=cbind(
  rep(1,N),     # vector of 1s (intercept)
  Trt-1,        # first covariate (Treatment arm)
  u0star        # second covariate (centred baseline utility)
)
# Define number of covariates (including intercept)
K=ncol(X)

# JAGS model
nn_indep=function(){
  for (i in 1:N) {
    # Model for the effects
    e[i] ~ dnorm(phi.e[i], tau.e[Trt[i]])
    # Vectorised linear predictor using the operator %*%, which
    # computes alpha_1*X[i,1] + alpha_2*X[i,2] + ... + alpha_K*X[i,K]
    phi.e[i] <- X[i,]%*%alpha
    ...
  }
  # Prior on the K coefficients (including intercept)
  for (k in 1:K) {
    alpha[k] ~ dnorm(0,0.0001)
  }
  ...
}
```

Vectorisation means that we would not have to modify the JAGS code if we decided to include an extra covariate, or exclude an existing one – we would simply pass a different matrix X in the data list and compute a different value for K, depending on the number of its columns.

This format allows us to be more economic with setting up the priors for the regression coefficients, which we can do in a loop – and note that we do not have any restriction on assigning to each the exact same prior distribution: for example, we could index the Normal distribution for `alpha[k]` as a function of a specific mean `mu.alpha[k]` and precision `tau.alpha[k]`, say, which would be passed on as data.

As discussed in Note 7 in Section 3.1.1, recall that `BUGS/JAGS` index the Normal distribution in terms of the precision, which we define as $\tau_{et} = \sigma_{et}^{-2}$, to encode the assumption that each treatment arm has a specific measure of variance. Note also that we use the observed treatment indicator t to construct the index to assign to the precision. This is consistent with the prior distributions definition – the block

```
for (t in 1:2) {
   sigma.e[t] ~ dexp(5.75)
   tau.e[t] <- pow(sigma.e[t],-2)
   ...
```

specifies a separate prior for each treatment arm on the standard deviation scale and then maps it on the precision scale, which is required for `BUGS/JAGS` to run the model.

We now run the model using `JAGS` and `R2jags`, with the following `R` commands. Once the model has completed the run, we can visualise the summary statistics using the `print()` method for the resulting `JAGS` object.

```
# Defines the data list
data=list(e=e,c=c,Trt=Trt,u0star=u0star,N=N)

# Initialises the object 'model' as a list to store all the results
model=list()

# Runs JAGS in the background
library(R2jags)
# Stores the BUGS output as an element named 'nn_indep' in the object 'model'
model$nn_indep=jags(
  data=data,
  parameters.to.save=c(
    "mu.e","mu.c","alpha0","alpha1","alpha2","beta0","beta1","sigma.e","sigma.c"
  ),
  inits=NULL,n.chains=2,n.iter=5000,n.burnin=3000,n.thin=1,DIC=TRUE,
  # This specifies the model code as the function nn_indep()
  model.file=nn_indep
)

# Shows the summary statistics from the posterior distributions.
print(model$nn_indep,digits=3,interval=c(0.025,0.5,0.975))
```

```
Inference for Bugs model at "/tmp/RtmpERtvsp/modeld78bd757721ee.txt",
 2 chains, each with 5000 iterations (first 3000 discarded)
 n.sims = 4000 iterations saved. Running time = 0.54 secs
            mu.vect sd.vect    2.5%     50%   97.5%  Rhat n.eff
alpha0        1.552   0.021   1.510   1.552   1.593 1.001  4000
alpha1       -0.007   0.039  -0.082  -0.007   0.068 1.002  1600
```

```
alpha2          1.280   0.073    1.138    1.279    1.423 1.001  4000
beta0           1.557   0.134    1.286    1.559    1.817 1.001  4000
beta1           1.082   0.432    0.224    1.092    1.914 1.001  4000
mu.c[1]      1556.947 133.875 1285.589 1558.759 1817.013 1.001  4000
mu.c[2]      2639.237 409.117 1837.599 2642.336 3441.981 1.001  4000
mu.e[1]         1.552   0.021    1.510    1.552    1.593 1.001  4000
mu.e[2]         1.545   0.033    1.480    1.545    1.609 1.002  1400
sigma.c[1]      1.358   0.098    1.181    1.354    1.571 1.001  4000
sigma.c[2]      3.333   0.295    2.820    3.307    3.982 1.003   710
sigma.e[1]      0.208   0.015    0.181    0.207    0.242 1.009   330
sigma.e[2]      0.268   0.024    0.226    0.266    0.318 1.002  1500
deviance      676.766   4.273  670.356  676.146  686.641 1.001  4000

For each parameter, n.eff is a crude measure of effective sample size,
and Rhat is the potential scale reduction factor (at convergence, Rhat=1).

DIC info (using the rule: pV = var(deviance)/2)
pV = 9.1 and DIC = 685.9
DIC is an estimate of expected predictive error (lower deviance is better).
```

The weird path for the model file (in this case `/tmp/RtmpERtvsp/modeld78bd757721ee.txt`) depends on the fact that we are coding up the model as a function. `JAGS` will write data and model files onto a temporary folder (`/tmp/RtmpERtvsp`, in this case).

As is possible to see from the summary statistics, convergence seems to be reached for all the model parameters and, according to the ESS (see Section 2.3.2.2) is reasonably large for almost all the parameters, indicating that there are no crucial issues with autocorrelation. We can use `bmhe` and other packages to produce other diagnostics visualisations and summaries, as in Section 2.3.2.

The intervention seems to produce slightly lower QALYs than the standard of care (on average, 1.545 against 1.552). These differences do not seem substantial, though, with much of the underlying distributions crossing each other. The difference in population average costs seem to be more marked, with average values of £2639.24 against £1556.95. As mentioned above, these relative differences are equivalent to the observed posterior values for the regression parameters α_1 and β_1.

The posterior summaries for the parameters σ_{et} and σ_{ct} indicate that the evidence from the data perhaps is stronger than implied in the prior, with the former shrunk towards smaller values and the latter pushed to higher ones. Then again, the PC priors are able to not force too much information and can be modified if a strong signal is observed in the data.

The first important issue with the basic structure described above is that it fails to account for the potential correlation between costs and clinical benefits. In general, this may materialise as a positive correlation, since effective treatments are innovative and result from intensive and lengthy research and are thus associated with higher unit costs. However, it may also arise as negative correlation, because more effective treatments may end up reducing total care pathway costs e.g. by reducing hospitalisations, side effects, etc.

Either way, modelling costs and benefits separately and (more or less implicitly) assuming independent error terms in the regression models in Equations 5.3 and 5.4 simply fails to allow for the possibility of correlation, potentially leading to biased estimates.

In a frequentist/maximum likelihood setting, one possible way around this limitation is to use so-called "seemingly unrelated regression" (SUR) models, originally proposed by Zellner (1962). SUR models essentially imply a correlation structure between the error terms $(\varepsilon_{ei}, \varepsilon_{ci})$ – this is effectively the same model as in Equations 5.3 and 5.4, but with the added assumption that

$$\begin{pmatrix} \varepsilon_{ei} \\ \varepsilon_{ci} \end{pmatrix} \sim \text{Normal}\left(\begin{pmatrix} 0 \\ 0 \end{pmatrix}, \begin{pmatrix} \sigma_e^2 & \rho\sigma_e\sigma_c \\ & \sigma_c^2 \end{pmatrix} \right).$$

Earlier advice on statistical modelling for HTA did consider this – see for instance Willan and Briggs (2006).

A second potential issue is that joint or marginal normality is generally not a realistic assumption. This is because costs are usually skewed and certainly bounded in $[0; \infty)$, while benefits may be bounded in an interval $[a; b]$, for some problem-specific constants, e.g. when representing QALYs – see Figure 5.1.

One obvious solution to this would be to use suitable transformations, for instance to model $\log c_i$ to make the Normal sampling distribution more plausible; while this is reasonably easy to do, care is needed when back transforming to the natural scale – see also Section 5.2.3 and recall that the objectives of the economic evaluation are the population *average* (mean) cost and benefits, because it is them we need to feed to the decision analysis (see Chapter 4). We return to this problem in Example 5.4 and in Section 5.2.3.

5.2.2 Marginal/conditional factorisation model

To overcome the issues highlighted above, we can take a set of countermeasures, which allow us to build models capable of producing estimates of the population average cost and benefit accounting for potential correlation as well as for the underlying nature of the observed data. This is of course an important objective – but it does mean using a much more structured modelling framework, as we explain below.

The main objective is to consider as target for our inference the *joint* probability distribution $p(e, c \mid \boldsymbol{\theta})$, for some vector of model parameters $\boldsymbol{\theta}$. A useful strategy that allows us to move away from the normality assumption without too many complications makes use of the fundamental properties of probability, under which we can always factorise a joint distribution into the product of a (univariate) marginal and a (univariate) conditional:

$$p(e, c) = p(e)p(c \mid e) = p(c)p(e \mid c) \tag{5.5}$$

– note that we temporarily drop the dependence to the model parameters, for simplicity. We label this modelling strategy as "marginal/conditional factorisation" (MCF) model.

From a purely probabilistic point of view, the two different factorisations are equivalent and represent fully the target joint distribution. Pragmatically, we may have some underlying causal construct, whereby, for instance, it is more appropriate to think of a DGP in which the effects have an impact on the costs (and thus we may favour the first factorisation in Equation 5.5).

Figure 5.3 shows a graphical representation of this structured modelling framework – indeed, we assume that the joint is factorised as $p(e, c \mid \boldsymbol{\theta}) = p(e \mid \boldsymbol{\theta}_e)p(c \mid e, \boldsymbol{\theta}_c)$, for some specific subset of parameters $\boldsymbol{\theta} = (\boldsymbol{\theta}_e, \boldsymbol{\theta}_c)$. The dashed box indicates the marginal model for the benefits $e_i \sim p(e \mid \phi_{ei}, \boldsymbol{\xi}_e)$. Here, $\boldsymbol{\theta}_e = (\phi_{ei}, \boldsymbol{\xi}_e)$; ϕ_{ei} is a *location* parameter indicating a measure of central tendency for the underlying distribution, while $\boldsymbol{\xi}_e$ is a set of *ancillary*

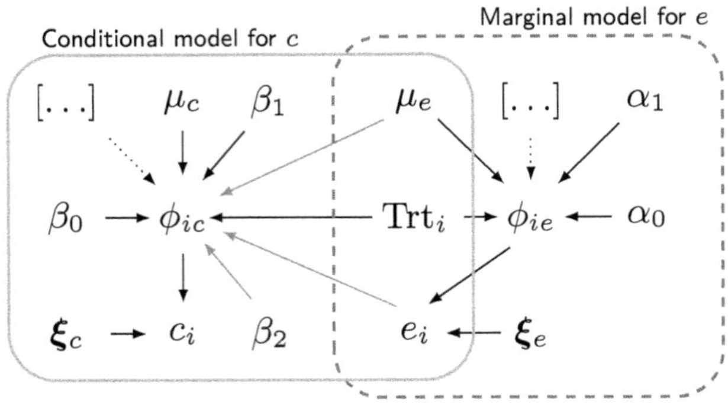

Figure 5.3: A DAG representation of the marginal/conditional factorisation model for effects and costs (aligned with the formulation in Equations 5.6 and 5.7).

parameters, which may indicate a measure of shape, or variance – these may or may not be present, depending on the form of the distribution $p(\cdot)$ that we choose. We can model the location parameter using some generalised linear regression

$$g_e(\phi_{ei}) = \alpha_0 + \alpha_1 \text{Trt}_i \, [+\ldots]. \tag{5.6}$$

The solid box in Figure 5.3 shows the conditional model for the cost, given the effects. We describe $c_i \sim p_c(c \mid e, \phi_{ci}, \boldsymbol\xi_c)$, where, again, ϕ_{ci} is a location and $\boldsymbol\xi_c$ is a vector of ancillary parameters. We include the dependence between costs and effects through the location parameter, which is again modelled using a generalised linear regression

$$g_c(\phi_{ci}) = \beta_0 + \beta_1 \text{Trt}_i + \beta_2 \, (e_i - \mu_e) \; [+\ldots], \tag{5.7}$$

where this time we definitely have one (centred) covariate, i.e. the observed individual benefits, scaled by the estimated population average (which we get from the previous module).

In Equation 5.7, the coefficient β_2 quantifies the level of correlation between e and c – in the simplest case of a Normal/Normal model (which we describe in more details in Example 5.3), we can prove analytically the relationship

$$\beta_2 = \rho \frac{\sigma_c}{\sigma_e} \qquad \Rightarrow \qquad \rho = \beta_2 \frac{\sigma_e}{\sigma_c}, \tag{5.8}$$

where $\rho \in (-1, 1)$ is the *linear* correlation coefficient between costs and benefits (see Example 5.3).

It is very much possible that the evidence in the data suggests that, in fact, there is no substantial correlation among the two outcomes and thus the estimate for its value would be close to 0 – in a frequentist setup, this would be "non-significantly different from 0". On the other hand, the model does allow for the possibility that the two outcomes are indeed correlated and if the evidence supported this assumption, then β_2 would be estimated with a value away from 0.

In addition, the modelling structure encoded in Figure 5.3 do make the simplifying assumption that the correlation between costs and benefits only happens through the location parameter. However, this is by no means a requirement and it would be possible to add even further structure and build another generalised linear regression component in which $\boldsymbol\xi_c$ does depend probabilistically on e_i. We make a similar remark in the context of survival modelling, in Section 8.3.3.

If no further covariates are included in the two generalised linear regressions of Equations 5.6 and 5.7, we compute $\mu_{et} = g_e^{-1}(\alpha_0 + \alpha_1(t-1))$ and $\mu_{ct} = g_c^{-1}(\beta_0 + \beta_1(t-1))$ – i.e. setting $(e_i - \mu_e) = 0$ to obtain the average cost in correspondence of the average benefits profile.

If we do consider additional covariates in Equations 5.6 and/or 5.7, we can still use the rescaled intercepts to estimate the population average benefits and costs. However, in this case, the two models target directly two *conditional* estimates, given the "profile" of covariates and so a little care is needed.

For example, consider the case

$$g_e(\phi_{ei}) = \alpha_0 + \alpha_1 \text{Trt}_i + \alpha_2(u_{0i} - \bar{u}_0) + \alpha_3 \text{Sex}_i,$$

where $(u_{0i} - \bar{u}_0)$ is the centred baseline HRQL continuous measurement and Sex_i is a discrete variable taking values $(0,1)$ for males and females, respectively. Under this specification, $g_e^{-1}(\alpha_0 + \alpha_1(t-1))$ = population average benefits for a male with average baseline HRQL measurement, while $g_e^{-1}(\alpha_0 + \alpha_1(t-1) + \alpha_3)$ = population average benefits for a female with average baseline HRQL measurement. We can approximate the *marginal* population average benefit as

$$\mu_{et} \approx p_M g_e^{-1}(\alpha_0 + \alpha_1(t-1)) + p_F g_e^{-1}(\alpha_0 + \alpha_1(t-1) + \alpha_3), \tag{5.9}$$

where p_M and p_F are the frequencies with which males and females are observed in the population of interest. Note that marginalisation of continuous covariates is automatic with centring (because it makes sense to determine the "average" profile, with respect to these covariates). Conversely, for discrete covariates we need to effectively compute a weighted average over their levels – we return to the distinction between marginal and conditional estimates in Example 11.2 in Section 11.3.1.

To be or not to be... (Bayesian)?

While there is nothing inherently Bayesian about the modelling framework described in Figure 5.3, there are several advantages to using a Bayesian approach.

1. As the model becomes more and more realistic and its structure more and more complex, to account for skeweness and correlation, the computational advantages of using maximum likelihood estimations become increasingly smaller. This is because writing and optimising the likelihood function becomes more complex analytically and even numerically and might require the use of simulation althorithms. A Bayesian approach, conversely, can scale up with minimal changes – whether we consider the simple Normal-Normal model or more convoluted distributional assumptions, MCMC methods effectively require almost no modification. The computation may be more expensive, but the marginal computational cost is in fact diminishing.
2. As mentioned above, it is very possible that realistic models be based on highly non-linear transformations; from a Bayesian perspective, this does not pose a substantial problem, because once we obtain simulations from the posterior distribution for α_0 and β_0, it is possible to simply rescale them to obtain samples from the posterior distribution of μ_e and μ_c. This in turn allows us to fully characterise and propagate the uncertainty in the fundamental economic parameters to the rest of the decision analysis with essentially no extra computational cost. A frequentist/maximum likelihood

approach would resort to resampling methods, such as the bootstrap to effectively produce an *approximation* to the joint posterior distribution for all the model parameters $\boldsymbol{\theta}$ and any function thereof.

3. Prior information can help stabilise inference (especially with sparse data, as shown in Example 1.2). Most often, we do have contextual information to mitigate limited evidence from the data and stabilise the evidence – for instance, we may be confident in thinking that odds ratio for drug-related treatment effects are rarely very large (say, larger than 1.5 or 2 — see Note 17 in Example 6.3); similarly, when looking at time-to-event data, we know for instance that cancer patients are unlikely to outlive the general population and thus we may "anchor" estimates for sick individuals using population life tables. Using a Bayesian approach allows us to use this contextual information in a principled way.

Example 5.3. *10TT (continued): Normal/Normal MCF model.* The simplest version of the modelling framework of Figure 5.3, which is equivalent to a standard implementation of the SUR model, is:

$$\begin{aligned} e_i &\sim \text{Normal}(\phi_{ei}, \tau_{et}) & \phi_{ei} &= \alpha_0 + \alpha_1(\text{Trt}_i - 1) + \alpha_2 u^*_{0i} & \mu_{et} &= \alpha_0 + \alpha_1(t-1) \\ c_i \mid e_i &\sim \text{Normal}(\phi_{ci}, \tau_{ct}) & \phi_{ci} &= \beta_0 + \beta_1(\text{Trt}_i - 1) + \beta_2(e_i - \mu_e) & \mu_{ct} &= \beta_0 + \beta_1(t-1), \end{aligned}$$

where ϕ_{ei} and τ_e are the benefits *marginal* mean and precision, respectively, while ϕ_{ci} and τ_c are the costs *conditional* mean and precision, respectively. In this model, the ancillary parameters are $\xi_e = \tau_e$ and $\xi_c = \tau_c$ and both $g_e(\cdot)$ and $g_c(\cdot)$ are the identity function and so the two intercepts represent directly the population average parameters.

Note that, in this particular case, because we are using rescaled data on c_i, the population average cost also needs to be rescaled up by £1000 and thus $\mu_{ct} = 1000\,(\beta_0 + \beta_1(t-1))$.

This formulation is indeed fairly similar to that of Equations 5.3 and 5.4, with the notable improvement that we no longer assume independence across the outcomes, because of the inclusion of the term $\beta_1(\text{Trt}_i - 1)$ in the linear predictor for the location parameter of the conditional cost distribution.

While perhaps less intuitive, *at face value*, than a bivariate distribution, the modelling framework of Figure 5.3 has the advantage that the two components in which we factorise the joint distribution have lower dimension – we do not need to model a bivariate distribution, but two univariate ones.

What's so special about the Normal distribution?...

One of the nice features of the Normal distribution is that, given a joint, multivariate Normal for a K-dimensional vector $\boldsymbol{y} = (y_1, \ldots, y_K) \sim \text{Normal}_K(\boldsymbol{\mu}, \boldsymbol{\Sigma})$, then we can prove that all the resulting marginal and conditional distributions remain Normal. Specifically, in the bivariate case of interest in HTA

$$\begin{pmatrix} e \\ c \end{pmatrix} \sim \text{Normal}_2\left(\begin{pmatrix} \mu_e \\ \mu_c \end{pmatrix}, \begin{pmatrix} \sigma^2_e & \rho\sigma_e\sigma_c \\ & \sigma^2_c \end{pmatrix} \right)$$

we can prove that

$$e \sim \text{Normal}(\mu_e, \sigma_e) \quad \text{and} \quad c \mid e \sim \text{Normal}\left(\eta_c, \lambda_c\right),$$

where

$$\eta_c = \mu_c + \rho\frac{\sigma_c}{\sigma_e}(e - \mu_e)$$

is the *conditional mean* and

$$\lambda_c = \sqrt{(1-\rho^2)\sigma_c^2}, \tag{5.10}$$

is the *conditional standard deviation* for the costs, both defined as functions of the marginal means μ_e, μ_c, the marginal standard deviations σ_e, σ_c and the correlation coefficient ρ. Of course we can derive the other factorisation with a marginal for c and a conditional $e \mid c$, accordingly.

This property, specific to the Normal distribution, implies that the Normal/Normal MCF model is indeed equivalent to the SUR model.

The modelling assumptions detailed above can be encoded in the JAGS code below.

```
# Normal/Normal MCF - JAGS code
nn_mcf=function(){
  for (i in 1:N) {
    # Marginal model for the effects
    e[i] ~ dnorm(phi.e[i], tau.e[Trt[i]])
    phi.e[i] <- alpha0 + alpha1*(Trt[i]-1) + alpha2*u0star[i]
    # *Conditional* model for the costs
    c[i] ~ dnorm(phi.c[i], tau.c[Trt[i]])
    phi.c[i] <- beta0 + beta1*(Trt[i]-1) + beta2*(e[i]-mu.e[Trt[i]])
  }
  # Rescales the main economic parameters
  for (t in 1:2) {
    mu.e[t] <- alpha0 + alpha1*(t-1)
    # (NB costs need to be scaled up by 1000)
    mu.c[t] <- 1000*(beta0 + beta1*(t-1))
  }
  # Minimally informative priors on the regression coefficients
  alpha0 ~ dnorm(0,0.0001)
  alpha1 ~ dnorm(0,0.0001)
  alpha2 ~ dnorm(0,0.0001)
  beta0 ~ dnorm(0,0.0001)
  beta1 ~ dnorm(0,0.0001)
  beta2 ~ dnorm(0,0.0001)
  for (t in 1:2) {
  # PC-prior on the *marginal* sd with Pr(sigma_e>0.8) \approx 0.01
    sigma.e[t] ~ dexp(5.75)
    tau.e[t] <- pow(sigma.e[t],-2)
  # PC-prior on the *conditional* sd with Pr(lambda_c>2) \approx 0.5
    lambda.c[t] ~ dexp(0.35)
    tau.c[t] <- pow(lambda.c[t],-2)
  # Retrieves the correlation coefficients
    rho[t] <- beta2*sigma.e[t]/sigma.c[t]
  # And the *marginal* standard deviation for the cost
    sigma.c[t] <- sqrt(pow(lambda.c[t],2) + pow(sigma.e[t],2)*pow(beta2,2))
  }
}
```

Because of the underlying assumption of joint Normality, we can write down analytically and monitor the posterior distributions for the correlation coefficient rho[t] and the marginal cost standard deviation sigma.c[t], obtained using Equation 5.8 and combining it with Equation 5.10.

In reality, defining and monitoring rho[t] and sigma.c[t] is not essential – we can do it analytically in the bivariate Normal case and thus we show how to handle this in the code above. But, realistically, for the purposes of the HTA analysis, we do not care massively about them and could dispense with this extra computation.

The model is run using the following code.

```
# Runs JAGS in the background and stores the output in the element 'nn_mcf'
model$nn_mcf=jags(
  data=data,
  parameters.to.save=c(
    "mu.e","mu.c","alpha0","alpha1","alpha2","beta0","beta1","beta2",
    "sigma.e","sigma.c","lambda.c","rho"
  ),
  inits=NULL,n.chains=2,n.iter=5000,n.burnin=3000,n.thin=1,DIC=TRUE,
  # This specifies the model code as the function nn_mcf()
  model.file=nn_mcf
)

# Shows the summary statistics from the posterior distributions.
print(model$nn_mcf,digits=3,interval=c(0.025,0.5,0.975))
```

```
Inference for Bugs model at "/tmp/RtmpERtvsp/modeld78bd7ea2128e.txt",
 2 chains, each with 5000 iterations (first 3000 discarded)
 n.sims = 4000 iterations saved. Running time = 0.774 secs
             mu.vect sd.vect     2.5%      50%    97.5%  Rhat n.eff
alpha0         1.551   0.021    1.510    1.551    1.593 1.002  1400
alpha1        -0.006   0.039   -0.082   -0.006    0.069 1.001  2000
alpha2         1.281   0.073    1.138    1.280    1.424 1.001  2900
beta0          1.589   0.136    1.326    1.589    1.863 1.001  4000
beta1          1.003   0.413    0.205    1.002    1.829 1.002  1500
beta2         -1.199   0.324   -1.834   -1.196   -0.563 1.001  4000
lambda.c[1]    1.304   0.094    1.140    1.298    1.502 1.002  1100
lambda.c[2]    3.208   0.280    2.706    3.192    3.819 1.001  4000
mu.c[1]     1588.972 135.730 1326.442 1589.459 1862.958 1.001  4000
mu.c[2]     2591.987 393.036 1831.773 2595.672 3372.217 1.001  2800
mu.e[1]        1.551   0.021    1.510    1.551    1.593 1.002  1400
mu.e[2]        1.545   0.032    1.483    1.545    1.610 1.001  4000
rho[1]        -0.188   0.051   -0.285   -0.187   -0.087 1.001  4000
rho[2]        -0.101   0.031   -0.163   -0.099   -0.045 1.001  4000
sigma.c[1]     1.329   0.095    1.164    1.323    1.529 1.002  1100
sigma.c[2]     3.225   0.278    2.726    3.210    3.827 1.001  4000
sigma.e[1]     0.208   0.015    0.181    0.207    0.238 1.001  4000
sigma.e[2]     0.268   0.024    0.226    0.266    0.320 1.002  1300
deviance     664.245   4.514  657.519  663.542  675.146 1.001  3000

For each parameter, n.eff is a crude measure of effective sample size,
```

```
and Rhat is the potential scale reduction factor (at convergence, Rhat=1).

DIC info (using the rule: pV = var(deviance)/2)
pV = 10.2 and DIC = 674.4
DIC is an estimate of expected predictive error (lower deviance is better).
```

Looking at the summary table produced by JAGS, we can see that convergence and autocorrelation are not a problem. All $\hat{R}$ statistics are well below the rule-of-thumb threshold of 1.1 (see Section 2.3.2.1) and the effective sample size (Section 2.3.2.2) is generally close to the nominal one, for almost all the monitored nodes.

(Non-essential) Computed parameters in BUGS/JAGS

In fact, we do not even need to include the definition for the nodes `rho[t]` and `sigma.c[t]` in the JAGS model, because these are simply deterministic functions of other model parameters (`beta2`, `sigma.e[t]`, and `lambda.c[t]`). Thus, if we run the model by monitoring these key nodes, we can actually construct `rho[t]` and `sigma.c[t]` in R using simple algebra.

Note that BUGS/JAGS effectively adds a dimension to each node. So the node `beta2` is defined in the model code as a scalar, but because when processed by BUGS/JAGS we record `n.sims` simulations, then the resulting object turns into a vector with `n.sims` rows. Similarly, in the model code `lambda.c` is a vector with two elements (one for each treatment arm) and therefore when processed by BUGS/JAGS the element `model$nn_mcf$sims.list$sigma.e` is in fact a matrix with `n.sims` rows and 2 columns.

For this reason, when defining in R the new nodes `sigma.c` and `rho` we need to set them to matrices – and for convenience we can use the same dimension as `lambda.c`, as shown in the code below.

```
# Extracts the simulations from the BUGS object into R variables
lambda.c=model$nn_mcf$BUGSoutput$sims.list$lambda.c
sigma.e=model$nn_mcf$BUGSoutput$sims.list$sigma.e
beta1=model$nn_mcf$BUGSoutput$sims.list$beta1

# Defines the new variables -- note the dimensions!
sigma.c=rho=matrix(NA,nrow=nrow(lambda.c),ncol=ncol(lambda.c))

# Uses the simulated values to compute rho[t] and sigma.c[t]
for (t in 1:2) {
  sigma.c[,t]=sqrt(lambda.c[,t]^2 + (sigma.e[,t]^2*beta1^2))
  rho[,t]=beta1*sigma.e[,t]/sigma.c[,t]
}

# Summarises the results
colnames(sigma.c)=c("sigma.c[1]","sigma.c[2]")
colnames(rho)=c("rho[1]","rho[2]")
cbind(sigma.c,rho) |> bmhe::stats() |> round(digits=3)
```

```
            mean    sd  2.5% median 97.5%
sigma.c[1] 1.323 0.094 1.159  1.317 1.522
sigma.c[2] 3.221 0.279 2.719  3.207 3.827
```

```
rho[1]     0.158 0.065 0.031  0.157 0.288
rho[2]     0.084 0.036 0.016  0.083 0.157
```

As is possible to see in the summary table produced by R, the results are (of course!) identical with the ones reported directly by JAGS.

Most of the times, it does not really matter which way around we decide to make the algebraic calculation, However, it is perhaps good practice to leave all the non-essential non-MCMC computation to R, because BUGS/JAGS models scale up in computational complexity with the number of nodes defined. If the model is fairly quick to run, as in the present case, there really is not much difference; but for more structured models, it may be much more efficient to leave some of the computation back to R.

The correlation coefficients are estimated to be very small and with rather large variance. However, in frequentist parlance, they would be deemed to be "significant", because their posterior distribution has most of the mass below the threshold value of 0. This is consistent with the slight differences in the estimates for the conditional and the marginal standard deviations for the costs (`lambda.c` and `sigma.c`). These translate into slight differences in the estimates for the overall population average costs, although, on this occasion, these are fairly minor.

This is a reassuring feature of the MCF model – if there is no evidence of correlation in the data, we do not lose anything in comparison to the independence model of Example 5.2, because the resulting correlation is effectively set to 0, meaning that the two modules in Figure 5.3 become detached. If however, there is correlation in the data but we do not allow our model to pick it up we may end inducing important bias in our estimates.

Figure 5.4 shows a comparison of the Normal/Normal independent and the Normal/Normal MCF models. As is possible to see, the estimates for the model parameters are effectively identical – this is consistent with the discussion above, because with limited correlation, the two models more or less coincide.

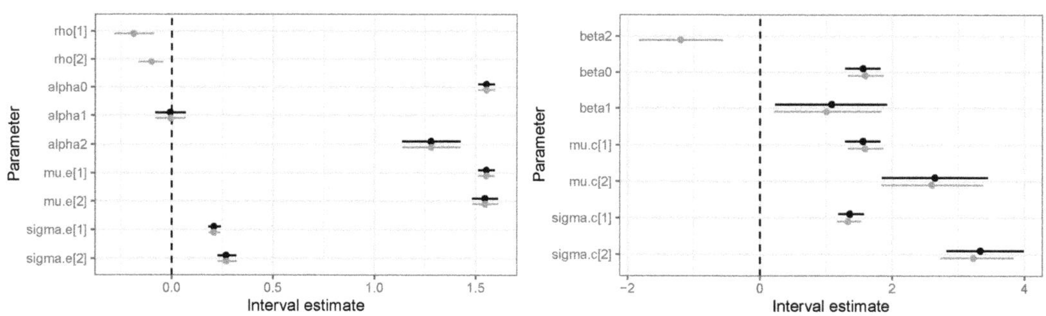

(a) (b)

Figure 5.4: Graphical summaries of the posterior distributions for the model parameters. The two panels collect parameters according to the range of their distributions, for better visualisation. The dots indicate the posterior means, while the lines expands to cover the 95% posterior intervals. Darker dots and lines indicate the Normal/Normal independence model, while lighter dots and lines indicate the Normal/Normal MCF model. For consistency in the visualisation, the parameters `mu.c[1]` and `mu.c[2]` are scaled down by a factor of 1000.

Using the structure described in Figure 5.3 it is possible to easily extend the Normal/Normal MCF model to virtually consider any combination of distributional assumptions for the costs and benefits. For example, we can assume a Gamma distribution to model skewed, positive costs, conditionally on a suitable measure of benefits; or a Beta distribution to model marginal benefits defined in terms of QALYs for a study where the time horizon is below 1 year – assuming there are no individuals with negative QALYs, implies that the range for the variable e would be between $(0, 1)$.

Example 5.4. *10TT (continued): Gamma/Gamma MCF model.* Figure 5.1 clearly shows that the empirical distributions for both costs and benefits are highly skewed. In addition, because the time horizon for the study is 24 months, the QALYs are naturally constrained to be below 2. For these reasons, it is a good idea to try and use non-Normal models.

One slight complication is that the QALYs show a rather large left skewness; in addition, a small number of individuals are associated with negative QALYs, indicating a very poor health state ("worse than death"). For these reasons, it is helpful to transform the original data, so that we can apply a simpler model. Following Gabrio et al. (2025), we define the transformation $e_i^* = (3 - e_i)$. This rescales the observed QALYs and turns the distribution into a right skewed one, which means we can appropriately use a Gamma distribution to model the sampling variability. We return to this point in Note 14 in Section 5.3.1.

With this, we can model:

$$\begin{aligned} e_i^* &\sim \text{Gamma}(\nu_e, \gamma_{ei}) & \log(\phi_{ei}) &= \alpha_0 + \alpha_1(\text{Trt}_i - 1) + \alpha_2 u_{0i}^* \\ c_i \mid e_i^* &\sim \text{Gamma}(\nu_c, \gamma_{ci}) & \log(\phi_{ci}) &= \beta_0 + \beta_1(\text{Trt}_i - 1) + \beta_2(e_i^* - \mu_e^*), \end{aligned}$$

where, because of the properties of the Gamma distribution, ϕ_{ei} indicates the marginal mean for the QALYs, while ν_e is the shape and $\gamma_{ei} = \nu_c/\phi_{ei}$ is the rate (see Section 1.2.3 and Equation 1.8, in particular). Similarly, ν_c is the shape and $\gamma_{ci} = \nu_c/\phi_{ci}$ is the rate of the conditional distribution for the costs given the benefits, with ϕ_{ci} representing the conditional mean.

The population average benefits and costs can be retrieved by back-transforming the linear predictors (using the exponential function)

$$\mu_e^* = \exp\left(\alpha_0 + \alpha_1(t-1)\right) \quad \text{and} \quad \mu_c = \exp\left(\beta_0 + \beta_1(t-1)\right),$$

though, of course, as we are still using rescaled data, in this instance the population average costs are computed as $\mu_c = £1000 \exp\left(\beta_0 + \beta_1(t-1)\right)$ – see again Note 14 in Section 5.3.1.

In terms of prior distributions, we keep the very vague, minimally informative priors for the regression coefficients – again, we could probably do better here, considering that both ϕ_{ei} and ϕ_{ci} are defined on a log scale and thus we are implying a very large range in the priors. Sensitivity analysis may be very important to this aspect.

As for the shape parameters ν_{et} and ν_{ct}, we specify again a PC prior. Generally speaking, it is more difficult to encode genuine prior knowledge on this scale (see the discussion in Section 1.2.3) and thus we start by including a fairly vague specification, where we assume that $\Pr(\nu_{et} > 30) = \Pr(\nu_{ct} > 30) \approx 0.01$, which implies an Exponential with rate $-\frac{\log(0.01)}{30} \approx 0.15$.

The modelling assumptions are mapped onto the JAGS code below.

```
# Gamma/Gamma MCF - JAGS code
gg_mcf=function(){
  for (i in 1:N) {
   # Marginal model for the *rescaled* effects
   estar[i] ~ dgamma(nu.e[Trt[i]], gamma.e[Trt[i],i])
   gamma.e[Trt[i],i] <- nu.e[Trt[i]]/phi.e[i]
   log(phi.e[i]) <- alpha0 + alpha1*(Trt[i]-1) + alpha2*u0star[i]
   # Conditional model for the costs
   c[i] ~ dgamma(nu.c[Trt[i]], gamma.c[Trt[i],i])
   gamma.c[Trt[i],i] <- nu.c[Trt[i]]/phi.c[i]
   log(phi.c[i]) <- beta0 + beta1*(Trt[i]-1) + beta2*(estar[i]-mustar.e[Trt[i]])
  }
  # Rescales the main economic parameters
  for (t in 1:2) {
   mustar.e[t] <- exp(alpha0 + alpha1*(t-1))
   mu.e[t] <- 3 - mustar.e[t]
   # (NB costs need to be scaled up by 1000)
   mu.c[t] <- 1000*exp(beta0 + beta1*(t-1))
  }
  # Minimally informative priors on the regression coefficients
  alpha0 ~ dnorm(0,0.0001)
  alpha1 ~ dnorm(0,0.0001)
  alpha2 ~ dnorm(0,0.0001)
  beta0 ~ dnorm(0,0.0001)
  beta1 ~ dnorm(0,0.0001)
  beta2 ~ dnorm(0,0.0001)
  # PC prior on the shape parameters
  # assume that Pr(nu.e>30) = Pr(nu.c>30) \approx 0.01
  for (t in 1:2) {
    nu.e[t] ~ dexp(0.15)
    nu.c[t] ~ dexp(0.15)
  }
}
```

Notice that in the code above we first define the variable `mustar.e` to indicate the population average QALYs *on the rescaled version* and then back-transform to the original scale by simply using the command `mu.e[t] <- 3 - mustar.e[t]`. This is possible because the transformation applied to the original data is linear and thus it holds for the expectations

$$e^* = 3 - e \quad \Rightarrow \quad \mathrm{E}[e^*] = \mathrm{E}[3 - e] = 3 - \mathrm{E}[e] \quad \Rightarrow \quad \mathrm{E}[e] = 3 - \mathrm{E}[e^*].$$

We return to this point in Section 5.2.3 and Note 14 below, as well as later in Chapter 11.

In order to run the model, we need to slightly modify the `data` list, to include the new variable `estar` (the rescaled QALYs).

```
# Defines the rescaled QALYs in the data list and remove the old version
data$estar=3-data$e

# Runs JAGS in the background and stores the output in the element 'gg_mcf'
model$gg_mcf=jags(
```

```
  data=data,
  parameters.to.save=c(
    "mu.e","mustar.e","mu.c","alpha0","alpha1","alpha2","beta0",
    "beta1","beta2","nu.e","nu.c"
  ),
  inits=NULL,n.chains=2,n.iter=5000, n.burnin=3000,n.thin=1,DIC=TRUE,
  # This specifies the model code as the function gg_mcf()
  model.file=gg_mcf
)

# Shows the summary statistics from the posterior distributions.
print(model$gg_mcf,digits=3,interval=c(0.025,0.5,0.975))
```

```
Inference for Bugs model at "/tmp/RtmpERtvsp/modeld78bd21d7d50c.txt",
 2 chains, each with 5000 iterations (first 3000 discarded)
 n.sims = 4000 iterations saved. Running time = 10.918 secs
             mu.vect sd.vect     2.5%      50%    97.5%  Rhat n.eff
alpha0         0.347   0.015    0.319    0.347    0.377 1.003   620
alpha1         0.012   0.027   -0.041    0.011    0.064 1.005   390
alpha2        -0.823   0.055   -0.929   -0.823   -0.713 1.001  4000
beta0          0.407   0.078    0.259    0.407    0.564 1.001  4000
beta1          0.429   0.146    0.152    0.430    0.711 1.001  4000
beta2          0.938   0.192    0.580    0.933    1.329 1.001  2800
mu.c[1]     1507.357 118.122 1295.520 1502.736 1758.003 1.001  4000
mu.c[2]     2325.120 286.992 1821.647 2306.301 2957.591 1.002  2400
mu.e[1]        1.585   0.021    1.542    1.585    1.624 1.003   610
mu.e[2]        1.568   0.032    1.502    1.569    1.629 1.003   810
mustar.e[1]    1.415   0.021    1.376    1.415    1.458 1.003   620
mustar.e[2]    1.432   0.032    1.371    1.431    1.498 1.003   860
nu.c[1]        1.819   0.231    1.384    1.811    2.300 1.003   940
nu.c[2]        1.147   0.178    0.831    1.139    1.520 1.001  4000
nu.e[1]       47.328   6.870   34.873   46.936   61.845 1.002   890
nu.e[2]       29.705   5.119   20.534   29.405   40.509 1.001  3900
deviance     480.202   5.071  472.413  479.522  491.862 1.001  4000

For each parameter, n.eff is a crude measure of effective sample size,
and Rhat is the potential scale reduction factor (at convergence, Rhat=1).

DIC info (using the rule: pV = var(deviance)/2)
pV = 12.9 and DIC = 493.1
DIC is an estimate of expected predictive error (lower deviance is better).
```

Again, convergence and autocorrelation seem under control from the summary statistics. In this case, however, the model accounting for skewness in the data suggest a lower estimate for the average costs, in comparison to the two Normal/Normal models shown above. The "correct-scale" population average QALYs, i.e. the nodes `mu.e[1]` and `mu.e[2]`, show also some differences with respect to the Normal/Normal models, although they are more aligned.

The computational effort required to run the Gamma/Gamma MCF is, unsurprisingly, much larger, relatively speaking, than for the two Normal/Normal models – it takes about 11 seconds to run (not enough to go and make a coffee, but still more expensive in terms of running time than the simpler Normal models).

5.2.3 Non-linearity and posterior predictive estimation

If we have available a set of simulations from the (posterior) distribution of a parameter ψ, say in the vector $\left(\psi^{(1)},\ldots,\psi^{(S)}\right)$, then we can use these to retrieve a set of simulations from the (posterior) distribution of any function $\theta = g(\psi)$ simply applying the inverse transformation and compute a vector of simulations from the (posterior) distribution for θ as

$$\left(\theta^{(1)} = g^{-1}\left(\psi^{(1)}\right),\ldots,\theta^{(S)} = g^{-1}\left(\psi^{(S)}\right)\right).$$

This works because we propagate the full uncertainty in ψ (through the S simulations) directly onto the distribution of θ and it is the basic principle of Monte Carlo simulation (see Section 1.2.4).

The problem is more complicated when we apply a non-linear transformation to a variable for which we do *not* have directly simulations to characterise the underlying uncertainty. Consider for example an observed variable y, which we transform as $y^* = g(y)$, for some non-linear function $g(\cdot)$. Suppose also that $\text{E}[Y^*] = \theta$. In this situation,

$$\text{E}[Y] = \text{E}[g^{-1}(Y^*)] \neq g^{-1}\left(\text{E}[Y^*]\right) = g^{-1}(\theta),$$

i.e. if the function $g(\cdot)$ is not linear, we cannot take it out of the integral that defines the expected value.

To give a more tangible example, consider $y^* = \log(y)$, where y is a variable representing skewed and positive costs and we model $y^* \sim \text{Normal}(\eta,\lambda)$ – technically, this is equivalent to assuming $y \sim \text{log-Normal}(\eta,\lambda)$, as defined in Equation 1.9. Suppose further that we have obtained a set of simulations from the posterior distribution of the mean $\eta \mid y^*$ and standard deviation $\lambda \mid y^*$ (both defined on the log scale), say $\left(\eta^{(1)},\ldots,\eta^{(S)}\right)$ and $\left(\lambda^{(1)},\ldots,\lambda^{(S)}\right)$.

The objective is to estimate the mean on the normal scale, $\text{E}[Y]$. In this case, however, because the transformation $g(\cdot) = \log(\cdot)$ is non-linear, simply rescaling the simulated values by applying $g^{-1}(\cdot) = \log^{-1}(\cdot) = \exp(\cdot)$ does not directly target the quantity of interest, i.e. the mean of the costs on the natural scale, as exemplified by the following chain of relationships

$$\text{E}[Y] = \text{E}[\exp(\log(Y))] = \text{E}[\exp(Y^*)] \neq \exp\left(\text{E}[Y^*]\right) = \exp\left(\text{E}[\log(Y)]\right) = \text{median}(Y).$$

To overcome this problem, in a Bayesian context we can simply resort to a further layer of simulation based on the posterior predictive distribution. In a nutshell, this amounts to obtaining a Monte Carlo sample for the variable in question, starting from simulated values of the model parameters on the transformed scale.

In the example above, we can use each of the S simulated values $\left(\eta^{(1)},\ldots,\eta^{(S)}\right)$ and $\left(\lambda^{(1)},\ldots,\lambda^{(S)}\right)$ to generate N draws from the (predictive) distribution of y^*, as

$$\begin{array}{lcl} y_1^{*(1)}, y_2^{*(1)}, \ldots, y_N^{*(1)} & \sim & \text{Normal}\left(\eta^{(1)}, \lambda^{(1)}\right) \\ y_1^{*(2)}, y_2^{*(2)}, \ldots, y_N^{*(2)} & \sim & \text{Normal}\left(\eta^{(2)}, \lambda^{(2)}\right) \\ & \vdots & \\ y_1^{*(S)}, y_2^{*(S)}, \ldots, y_N^{*(S)} & \sim & \text{Normal}\left(\eta^{(S)}, \lambda^{(S)}\right). \end{array}$$

Now that we have a full characterisation of the uncertainty in y^* for all the simulated combinations of the parameters, we can use the samples from the predictive on y^* to back-transform to the original scale, by simply applying the inverse function $g^{-1}(\cdot)$

$$\begin{array}{lcl} y_1^{(1)} = \exp\left(y_1^{*(1)}\right), & \ldots, & y_N^{(1)} = \exp\left(y_N^{*(1)}\right) \\ y_1^{(2)} = \exp\left(y_1^{*(2)}\right), & \ldots, & y_N^{(2)} = \exp\left(y_N^{*(2)}\right) \\ & \vdots & \\ y_1^{(S)} = \exp\left(y_1^{*(S)}\right), & \ldots, & y_N^{(S)} = \exp\left(y_N^{*(S)}\right). \end{array}$$

These, in turn, can be used to compute an empirical summary, for instance the mean as

$$\begin{array}{lcl} \mu^{(1)} & = & \frac{1}{N}\left(y_1^{(1)} + y_2^{(1)} + \ldots + y_N^{(1)}\right) \\ \mu^{(2)} & = & \frac{1}{N}\left(y_1^{(2)} + y_2^{(1)} + \ldots + y_N^{(2)}\right) \\ & \vdots & \\ \mu^{(S)} & = & \frac{1}{N}\left(y_1^{(S)} + y_2^{(S)} + \ldots + y_N^{(S)}\right) \end{array}$$

and the sample $\left(\mu^{(1)},\ldots,\mu^{(S)}\right)$ now does characterise the distribution of the function of interest on the natural scale, in this case $\text{E}[Y]$.

We return to similar (but subtly and fundamentally distinct!) arguments in the context of g-computation for population adjustment in Section 11.3.2.

Gamma vs log-Normal distribution

The log-Normal distribution described above is another good candidate to describe the sampling variability or uncertainty for variables whose natural range is positive and skewed – typical examples in HTA include total resource costs, or, in some cases, HRQL-related measures.

Figure 5.5a shows the densities for a Gamma(ν,γ) and a log-Normal(η,λ). These are constructed so that in both cases the mean and standard deviations on the natural scale are, respectively, $\mu = 8$ and $\sigma = 5$. In particular, we can use the properties of the log-Normal distribution to see that the natural-scale can be linked to the original-scale parameters through the relationship

$$\eta = \log(\mu) - \frac{1}{2}\log\left(1+\frac{\sigma^2}{\mu^2}\right) \quad \text{and} \quad \lambda = \sqrt{\log\left(1+\frac{\sigma^2}{\mu^2}\right)} \tag{5.11}$$

and thus plugging in the values $\mu = 8$ and $\sigma = 5$ into Equation 5.11 gives $\eta = 1.915$ and $\lambda = 0.574$. Similar reasoning applied to Equation 1.8 allows us to derive $\nu = 2.56$ and $\gamma = 0.32$.

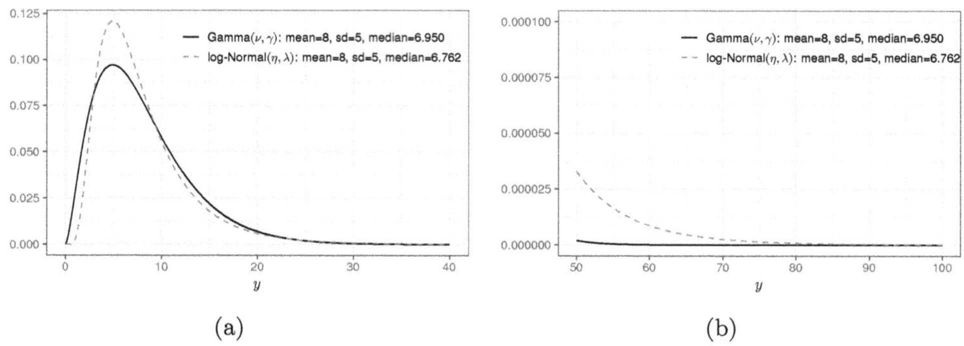

Figure 5.5: This plot shows the density for a log-Normal and a Gamma distributions with similar "natural" parameters. Panel (a) shows a larger range along both axes and from a cursory inspection, the two distributions look extremely close. In Panel (b), however, which focuses on the higher range along the x–axis, it is possible to see that the log-Normal has much fatter tails.

While the shape of the Gamma and log-Normal distribution tends to be superficially similar, there is an important difference. By the mathematical properties of the two distributions, the log-Normal tends to have much heavier tails, meaning that it tends to assign higher probability to very large values of the underlying variable, as is obvious in Figure 5.5b.

This may be seen as an attracting feature, in case we want to safeguard from the theoretically justified possibility of having very large values (e.g. for the cost associated with a given treatment), even without having observed any in the data.

Generally speaking, however, this often implies that the Gamma is a safer option to model variables such as costs, limiting the potential impact of too large ranges in the estimates (Thompson and Nixon, 2005).

When we can write down the algebraic relationships linking the natural-scale to the original-scale parameters analytically then posterior predictive Monte Carlo estimation is not necessary – given simulations for (η, λ), we can simply rescale them properly and obtain simulations for the relevant parameter. For instance, to retrieve samples from the distribution of the natural scale variable y in the example above, we simply need to invert the relevant relationship in Equation 5.11 and compute

$$\mu = \exp\left(\eta + \frac{1}{2}\lambda^2\right)$$

directly using the output of our model.

Example 5.5. *10TT (continued): Gamma/Gamma MCF model – posterior predictive estimation.* We can compute the estimates for the population average benefits using posterior predictive Monte Carlo simulation, using the following R code.

```
# Extracts the relevant parameters from the JAGS object
nu.e=model$gg_mcf$BUGSoutput$sims.list$nu.e
mustar.e=model$gg_mcf$BUGSoutput$sims.list$mustar.e

# Compute the "average" rate
rate=nu.e/mustar.e

# Posterior predictive estimation for the mean on the original scale
# 1. defines the number of MC simulations for the outcome
N=4000
# 2. defines the dimension of the object 'mu' in which to store the means
mu=matrix(NA,nrow=nrow(rate),ncol=2)
# 3. loops over the simulations for 'nu.e' and 'rate'
for (i in 1:nrow(nu.e)) {
  for (t in 1:2) {
# Simulate 'mcsim' values of estar, for the current value of the parameters
    estar=rgamma(N,shape=nu.e[i,t],rate=rate[i,t])
# Computes the mean for the *inverse transformation*
    mu[i,t]=3-estar |> mean()
  }
}

# Computes the summary statistics
colnames(mu)=c("mu.e[1]","mu.e[2]")
mu |> bmhe::stats()
```

```
              mean          sd     2.5%   median    97.5%
mu.e[1] 1.584524 0.02130020 1.542437 1.584747 1.625502
mu.e[2] 1.567492 0.03260136 1.500650 1.568376 1.629143
```

As is possible to see, the posterior predictive version of this calculation aligns with the one provided directly in the JAGS model – but of course, in case of non-linear transformations for the outcomes, it would be necessary to either perform the back-transformation analytically, or by a similar numerical process as the one highlighted here.

5.3 Model selection

As shown throughout Section 5.2, there may be several formulations for our model, particularly in terms of "structural" assumptions, i.e. the way in which we describe both the sampling variability and the epistemic uncertainty about the model parameters. Sometimes, this is immaterial, because, at the end of the process, the inference is basically identical (just as in the case of the models in Examples 5.2 and 5.3). In general, however, the results will be sensitive to the structural choices and assumptions we make and thus it is natural to compare the performance of the models we have used, in order to select the "best" one.

Note 13: All models are wrong

In reality, we can never select the "best" model, at least not in absolute terms, as suggested by the famous statistical aphorism "*All models are wrong but some are useful*" (Box, 1979).

The deeper meaning of George Box' quote is that the real aim of statistical modelling is not so much to find a hidden "truth", but rather to update and, hopefully, reduce the uncertainty we have in our current understanding of complex phenomena, which we often struggle to even approximate to a reasonable degree.

Nonetheless, we can use statistical tools to assess the performance of competing model specifications, in order to narrow down even further our uncertainty and present results that are as consistent and robust as possible.

More importantly, we also note here that the idea presented in this section do not just apply to the case where ILD are available – assessing the impact of structural assumptions (e.g. using the tools described below) is an important part of *any* statistical modelling exercise and should be applied more widely.

5.3.1 Deviance Information Criterion (DIC)

One of the most popular tools to assess model fit and perform model selection in a Bayesian context is the *Deviance Information Criterion* (DIC, Spiegelhalter et al., 2002a). The DIC is based on the model deviance, defined as

$$D(\boldsymbol{\theta}) = -2 \log \mathcal{L}(\boldsymbol{\theta} \mid \boldsymbol{y}). \tag{5.12}$$

In isolation, a model's deviance is meaningless, because the scale on which the likelihood is defined varies with different models and parameterisations – see Note 14 below. Thus, reporting the value of a single model's deviance does not give information on its performance. Comparatively, however, it can be used to assess how well a given model fits the observed data, with respect to an alternative one. Models associated with a lower deviance fit the observed data better.

Similarly to other information criteria, e.g. the *Akaike* Information Criterion (AIC, Akaike, 1974) or the *Bayesian* Information Criterion (BIC, Schwarz, 1978), the DIC is designed to safeguard against the phenomenon of *overfitting* (which occurs when a model with a large number of parameters tends to do extremely well for the data at hand, but generally struggles to adapt to new/different data) by adding a penalty for model complexity.

Formally, in its original definition, the DIC is constructed as

$$\text{DIC} = \underbrace{\overline{D(\boldsymbol{\theta})}}_{\texttt{"dbar"}} + p_D = \underbrace{D(\bar{\boldsymbol{\theta}})}_{\texttt{"dhat"}} + 2p_D, \tag{5.13}$$

where:

$$\begin{aligned}\overline{D(\boldsymbol{\theta})} = \text{E}\left[D(\boldsymbol{\theta})\right] &= \int -2 \log \mathcal{L}(\boldsymbol{\theta} \mid \boldsymbol{y}) p(\boldsymbol{\theta} \mid \boldsymbol{y}) d\boldsymbol{\theta} \\ &\approx \frac{1}{S}\sum_{s=1}^{S} -2 \log \mathcal{L}(\boldsymbol{\theta}^{(s)})\end{aligned}$$

is the *average model deviance* (averaged over the posterior distribution of the model parameters, which can be approximated using a sample of S draws $\boldsymbol\theta^{(1)},\ldots,\boldsymbol\theta^{(S)} \sim p(\boldsymbol\theta \mid \boldsymbol y)$ obtained from the MCMC process);

$$D(\overline{\boldsymbol\theta}) = D(\mathrm{E}[\boldsymbol\theta \mid \boldsymbol y]) = -2\log\mathcal{L}\left(\int \boldsymbol\theta p(\boldsymbol\theta \mid \boldsymbol y)d\boldsymbol\theta\right)$$
$$\approx -2\log\mathcal{L}\left(\frac{1}{S}\sum_{s=1}^{S}\boldsymbol\theta^{(s)}\right)$$

is the *model deviance calculated in correspondence of the average value of the model parameters* (which, again, can be approximated using the simulations from the MCMC process); and

$$p_D = \overline{D(\boldsymbol\theta)} - D(\overline{\boldsymbol\theta}) \tag{5.14}$$

is the *penalty for model complexity*. This is the version used by `BUGS` when calculating the DIC – as evident by the note at the bottom of the outcome of the `print(mbugs,...)` instruction in Section 3.3. Equation 5.14 has an interesting direct interpretation as an estimate of the number of free parameters in the model, a quantity usually referred as "*effective number of model parameters*" – see Section 6.2 as well as Spiegelhalter et al. (2002a) and Lunn et al. (2013) for more details on this, in the context of hierarchical models.

Note 14: Deviance and rescaled data

Technically, the dataset used to fit the two Normal/Normal models of Examples 5.2 and 5.3 is slightly different than the one used to fit the Gamma/Gamma MCF of Example 5.4; this is due to the rescaling applied to define $e_i^* = 3 - e_i$.

Fortunately, *in this case*, we can rely on a combination of two factors: firstly, the underlying Normal sampling distribution is symmetric; and secondly, the transformation applied to the data is *affine* (i.e. a linear transformation that does not need to preserve the origin), which means that the shape of the likelihood function is unchanged.

To fix ideas, let us consider the simple case of one observation $y \sim \text{Normal}(\mu, \sigma)$: using Equation 1.4, the likelihood function is

$$\mathcal{L}(\mu, \sigma \mid y) = \frac{1}{\sigma}\exp\left(-\frac{1}{2}\left(\frac{y-\mu}{\sigma}\right)^2\right)$$

and thus the deviance is

$$D(\mu,\sigma) = -2\log\mathcal{L}(\mu,\sigma \mid y) = -2\left(-\log(\sigma) - \frac{1}{2}\left(\frac{y-\mu}{\sigma}\right)^2\right).$$

Using basic probability theory, we get that $y^* = (3-y) \sim \text{Normal}(3-\mu,\sigma) = \text{Normal}(\mu^*,\sigma)$ and thus

$$D(\mu^*,\sigma) = -2\log\mathcal{L}(\mu^*,\sigma \mid y^*) = -2\left(-\log\sigma - \frac{1}{2}\left(\frac{y^*-\mu^*}{\sigma}\right)^2\right)$$
$$= -2\left(-\log\sigma - \frac{1}{2}\left(\frac{(3-y)-(3-\mu)}{\sigma}\right)^2\right) = D(\mu,\sigma).$$

We could re-run the two Normal/Normal models on the exact same data (i.e. using e_i^* instead of e_i, throughout), but while this would change the parameter estimates, it would not modify the computed value for the model deviance in the two Normal/Normal models and hence the DIC. Consequently, we can simply compare the three models using the DICs computed above and summarised in Table 5.3.

Notice however that other transformations or different distributional assumptions would break this property and thus comparing models based on different data would *not* be appropriate, in that case.

For instance, using standard probability theory, if $y \sim \text{Gamma}(\text{shape} = \nu, \text{rate} = \gamma)$, then rescaling the data by a factor κ implies that $y^* = y/\kappa \sim \text{Gamma}(\nu, \kappa\gamma) = \text{Gamma}(\nu, \gamma^*)$. Using Equation 1.3, we can derive the likelihood associated with the Gamma distribution and thus

$$D(\nu, \gamma) = -2 \log \mathcal{L}(\nu, \gamma \mid y) = -2 \left(\nu \log \gamma - \log \Gamma(\nu) + (\nu - 1) \log y + \gamma y\right)$$

but, substituting $y^* = y/\kappa$ and $\gamma^* = \kappa\gamma$ we obtain

$$\begin{aligned} D(\nu, \gamma^*) &= -2 \log \mathcal{L}(\nu, \gamma^* \mid y^*) \\ &= -2 \left(\nu \log \gamma - \log \Gamma(\nu) + (\nu - 1) \log y + \gamma y - \log \kappa\right) \neq D(\nu, \gamma). \end{aligned}$$

In the general case with n observations, this implies that $D(\nu, \gamma) = D(\nu, \gamma^*) + 2n \log \kappa$. Thus, even if in theory we could simply use the original scale cost data to apply the Gamma/Gamma model of Example 5.4, if we want to compare it with the two Normal models in Examples 5.2 and 5.3 by means of the DIC, we *must* use the same cost data in all three models, because rescaling by £1000 makes the deviance off by a factor of $2n \log \kappa = 2(167 \log 1000) = 2307.19$ in the Gamma/Gamma model.

Despite its success and popularity in applied work, the DIC has been subject to substantial criticism – some of the main limitations are described in Plummer (2008), as well as in the extensive discussion of the original paper by Spiegelhalter et al. (2002a).

Among these, one of the most cited is the fact that p_D (and hence the whole DIC) is, in general, not invariant to re-parameterisations of the model. To counter this issue, Gelman et al. (2013) suggest a slightly different definition for the penalty

$$p_V = \frac{1}{2} \text{Var}\left[D(\boldsymbol{\theta})\right], \tag{5.15}$$

which has the advantage of being invariant to re-parameterisations of the model and non-negative. This is the version used by `JAGS`, as reported at the bottom of the output for the `print(mjags,...)` command in Section 3.3 as well as in the outputs of all `print()` commands in the examples above.

p_V vs p_D

Somewhat confusingly, earlier versions of the `R2jags` package still indicated the computed value for p_V with the general terminology `pD`. `R2jags` would highlight in the summary table produced by the `print()` method that the computation was performed using Equation 5.15, but the naming convention was still confusing.

This behaviour has changed in version `0.8-9` (released in October 2024), since which `R2jags` explicitly distinguishes between `pV` (the default calculation) and `pD`, which is computed using the method described by Plummer (2008) and using in the background the function `rjags::dic.samples()` – this is a slightly different version than the original one defined by Spiegelhalter et al. (2002a), although it usually provides near-identical results.

Equation 5.14 has the obvious advantage of being extremely easy to compute, once the deviance is monitored. In addition, in the case of weak prior information, it also approximates the effective number of model parameters. When the prior is not dominated by the likelihood, however, this result does not hold and the penalty can vary in ranges that are more complex to analyse. This implies that the scale of the penalty and thus of the DIC may be different when using BUGS (i.e. p_D), as opposed to the default specification of JAGS based on p_V.

5.3.2 Computing p_D manually

Irrespective of the software used to perform the MCMC analysis, we can still compute the penalty p_D by using the resulting simulations to estimate $\overline{D(\boldsymbol{\theta})}$ and $D(\overline{\boldsymbol{\theta}})$.

The first one is easy to obtain as the mean of the simulated values for the deviance. For instance, considering the model in Example 5.4, this can be easily extracted from the JAGS object, as we show below.

As for $D(\overline{\boldsymbol{\theta}})$, this is a bit more involved, because we first need to extract the mean value of all the model parameters and then compute the full likelihood function associated with these values.

In the case of the model in Example 5.4 this can be done using the following code. First we consider the part of the model that deals with the effects.

```
# 1. Model for the effects
# Extracts the shape parameter
nu.e=c(
  model$gg_mcf$BUGSoutput$summary["nu.e[1]","mean"],
  model$gg_mcf$BUGSoutput$summary["nu.e[2]","mean"]
)
# Extracts the regression coefficients
alpha0=model$gg_mcf$BUGSoutput$summary["alpha0","mean"]
alpha1=model$gg_mcf$BUGSoutput$summary["alpha1","mean"]
alpha2=model$gg_mcf$BUGSoutput$summary["alpha2","mean"]
# Computes the linear predictor
trt=data$Trt-1
u0=data$u0star
log.phi.e=alpha0 + alpha1*trt + alpha2*u0
# Computes the overall mean (needed for the costs)
mustar.e=numeric()
for (t in 1:2) {
  mustar.e[t]=exp(alpha0 + alpha1*(t-1))
}
# Computes the rate parameter
gamma.e=numeric()
for (i in 1:data$N) {
  gamma.e[i]=nu.e[data$Trt[i]]/exp(log.phi.e[i])
```

```
}
# Computes the likelihood contribution from each observation
lik.e=-2*dgamma(data$estar,shape=nu.e[data$Trt],rate=gamma.e,log=TRUE)
```

The R code effectively replicates the constructions described for the JAGS model to use the mean value of the shape parameter nu.e and the linear predictor log.phi.e to derive the rate parameter gamma.e.

We then use the R built-in function dgamma() to compute the likelihood given the observed data data$estar and the shape and rate parameters computed at the average value. Note that this code computes the full likelihood, including any constant that does not depend on the parameters.

Technically, dgamma() returns the density of a Gamma distribution using Equation 1.2, given the value of the parameters. In the calculation here, however, we use always the same fixed (observed) data data$estar, but vary the parameters, thus constructing a likelihood, rather than a sampling distribution – and, incidentally, this is the same strategy used by BUGS when computing p_D.

The option log=TRUE computes the likelihood on the log scale and by multiplying it by -2 we obtain the individual contribution for the deviance with respect to the effects.

We can replicate this computation for the part of the model that deals with the costs, as in the code below.

```
# 2. Model for the costs
# Extracts the shape parameter
nu.c=c(
  model$gg_mcf$BUGSoutput$summary["nu.c[1]","mean"],
  model$gg_mcf$BUGSoutput$summary["nu.c[2]","mean"]
)
# Extracts the regression coefficients
beta0=model$gg_mcf$BUGSoutput$summary["beta0","mean"]
beta1=model$gg_mcf$BUGSoutput$summary["beta1","mean"]
beta2=model$gg_mcf$BUGSoutput$summary["beta2","mean"]
# Computes the linear predictor
log.phi.c=beta0 + beta1*(trt) + beta2*(data$estar-mustar.e[data$Trt])
# Computes the rate parameter
gamma.c=numeric()
for (i in 1:data$N) {
  gamma.c[i]=nu.c[data$Trt[i]]/exp(log.phi.c[i])
}
# Computes the likelihood contribution from each observation
lik.c=-2*dgamma(data$c,shape=nu.c[data$Trt],rate=gamma.c,log=TRUE)
```

The objects lik.e and lik.c are vectors of length 167 – one value for each individual in the data.

Once we have an estimate for these, we can simply sum them up to obtain an estimate for $D(\overline{\boldsymbol\theta})$, which, in accordance with BUGS parlance, we indicate as dhat in the code below. Together with the estimate for $\overline{D(\boldsymbol\theta)}$, indicated as dbar and obtained by simply extracting the average for the posterior distribution of the deviance, we can simply compute p_D and the DIC, according to Equations 5.14 and 5.13, using the code below.

```
# 3. Finally computes pD & DIC
# Computes the average model deviance
dbar=model$gg_mcf$BUGSoutput$summary["deviance","mean"]
# Computes the deviance at the average value for the parameters
dhat=sum(lik.e) + sum(lik.c)
# Computes pD
pD=dbar-dhat
# Computes DIC
DIC=dbar+pD
```

The computed values are $p_D = 10.13$ and DIC $= 490.3$, which in this case are fairly similar to the estimates based on the calculation of p_V, provided by JAGS (which can be found in the summary table in Example 5.4), although this is not necessarily always the case.

Note 15: Computing the likelihood using built-in JAGS functions

Of course, it is always possible to obtain the log-likelihood using the simulations for the model parameters and R commands, at the point of post-processing the output of the JAGS model.

However and conveniently, there is a built-in facility to generate a node that contains the individual contributions to the (log)likelihood, directly in the JAGS script.

For every distribution `dxxxx` that is available for sampling, JAGS has also a function `logdensity.xxxx()`, which takes as arguments the data and the relevant parameters to compute the resulting log-density, which in turns constitutes the full form of the likelihood function (see Note 3 in Section 1.2).

For example, if we consider a simple linear regression model, we can create the following JAGS code

```
model=function() {
  # Model for the data and linear predictor
  for (i in 1:n) {
    y[i] ~ dnorm(mu[i], tau)
    mu[i] <- X[i,] %*% beta
  # Computes the log-likelihood for the model
    log.lik[i] <- logdensity.norm(y[i], mu[i], tau)
  }
  # Prior distributions
  for (k in 1:K) {
    beta[k] ~ dnorm(0,0.001)
  }
  sigma ~ dexp(0.1)
  tau <- pow(sigma,-2)
}
```

to embed the basic assumptions and add a node `log.lik[i]`, which, for each observation `i` automatically computes the individual contribution to the overall log-likelihood. We expand on this in Example 5.7.

While with a bit of coding and maths to obtain the relevant values for the deviance we can always post-process a JAGS object and obtain an estimate for p_D, we do not necessarily need to do so and instead obtain an approximation to the value of p_D as would be computed by BUGS (and thus a more direct estimate of the number of effective parameters) using the function `dic.samples()` from the `rjags` package (which is automatically loaded when `R2jags` is). For instance, we can use code such as

```
rjags::dic.samples(object$model,n.iter=1000,type="pD")
```

where `object` is a `R2jags` object (e.g. `mjags` above) and `n.iter` is the number of iterations to be used to make the computation. When `type=pD` (which is the default), the element `penalty` in the output object is an approximation to p_D.

In addition, since version `0.8-6`, `R2jags` embeds this calculation in the call to the function `jags()`, where it is possible to specify an input `pD=TRUE`. If that is the case, then `R2jags` will first run the model and then `dic.samples()` to compute the penalty p_D, which is stored in the resulting `JAGS` object, alongside the default p_V, as we demonstrate in Example 5.6.

5.3.3 Using DIC to compare models

Technically speaking, a full-on, proper Bayesian analysis concerned with model selection would work by identifying a set of finite and exhausting models $\mathcal{M} = (\mathcal{M}_1, \ldots, \mathcal{M}_H)$, where each of the models is indexed by a set of parameters $\boldsymbol\theta$ and a suitable prior distribution $p(\boldsymbol\theta \mid \mathcal{M}_h)$. In addition to this "standard" framework, we would add a prior distribution $p(\mathcal{M}_h)$ for each of the alternative models – this would indicate the contextual assessment of model $\mathcal{M}_h$ being the "true" one.

Under this framework, we would use the observed data $\boldsymbol y$ and estimate

$$p(\mathcal{M}_h \mid \boldsymbol y) \propto p(\mathcal{M}_h) \int p(\boldsymbol y \mid \boldsymbol\theta, \mathcal{M}_h) p(\boldsymbol\theta \mid \mathcal{M}_h) d\boldsymbol\theta,$$

which would then be used to compute a weighted average for any function of the parameters over the space of models.

While this approach is perfectly aligned with the Bayesian machinery, it has the important limitations of *i*) requiring that *all* possible models are completely specified and given a prior probability; and *ii*) that the set $\mathcal{M}$ does include the "true" model. This is usually a very tall order – most of the times, we only have a very limited and far from exhaustive number of models that we can possibly use, which presents a major limitation to the fully-fledged Bayesian framework (see Lunn et al., 2013, sec. 8.3.3 for further discussion).

To overcome this issue, if we have two or more models *based on the exact same data*, we can use the DIC to provide a ranking and assess whether differences in model fit are "substantial" across the various models – notice that a meaningful comparison is not possible for models using different data, because, by definition, the likelihood function (which is conditional on the observed data) would be different – with the caveats discussed in Note 14, above.

Focussing on AIC, Burnham and Anderson (1998) propose a heuristic rule of thumb to compare models based on information criteria and Spiegelhalter et al. (2002a) map this onto an evaluation based on DIC. Specifically, for a set of H competing models, we can compute the absolute difference in DIC between the $h-$th model and the one associated with the lowest DIC

$$\Delta\text{DIC}_h = \mid \min_h(\text{DIC}_h) - \text{DIC}_h \mid \qquad (5.16)$$

and then values for $\Delta\text{DIC}_h < 2$ indicate that model h deserves some consideration, while differences in the range [3–7] indicate less support towards model h and, in line with Burnham and Anderson (2002) discussion based on AIC, differences exceeding 10 indicate no support for the $h-$th model.

Example 5.6. *10TT (continued): model selection.* Comparing the models in Example 5.2 and in Example 5.3 we can see from the summary tables that they have rather similar DIC values: 686 and 674, respectively. While the estimates are materially indistinguishable (as evident from Figure 5.4), according to the rule-of-thumb described above, the Normal/Normal MCF provides a much better fit to the data, as its DIC is over 10 points lower than that of the Normal/Normal independent model.

If we include in the mix the model in Example 5.4, the situation becomes even more clear-cut, as the DIC for the Gamma/Gamma MCF version is substantially lower, with a computed value of 493 – that is a difference of over 200 points with respect to the two versions of the Normal/Normal model, indicating a much better fit for the Gamma/Gamma MCF.

Especially in the absence of genuine information in the prior distributions, the computed value for p_V generally tends to agree with the value that could be obtained for p_D. In this case, for Gamma/Gamma MCF model, $p_V = 12.9$, which is slightly higher than those for the Normal/Normal models, respectively obtained at 9.1 and 10.2. In this particular case, all the p_V values are reasonably aligned with the nominal number of fundamental parameters, which is 9 (`alpha0`, `alpha1`, `alpha2`, `beta0`, `beta1`, `sigma.e[1]`, `sigma.e[2]`, `sigma.c[1]` and `sigma.c[2]`) for the model in Example 5.2, 10 (with `beta2` in addition to the ones above) for the model in Example 5.3 and 10 (`alpha0`, `alpha1`, `alpha2`, `beta0`, `beta1`, `beta2`, `nu.e[1]`, `nu.e[2]`, `nu.c[1]` and `nu.c[2]`) for the model in Example 5.4.

As mentioned above, more generally we can directly compute p_D from `R2jags` by adding the option `pD=TRUE` to the call to the function `jags()`. As all the models above have reached reasonable convergence, we can keep the other optional argument `n.iter.pd` to its default (1000 extra simulations) and re-run the three models. For instance, for the Normal/Normal independence model, the revised call to `jags()` would be as in the following code.

```
# Re-runs the model adding the option pD=TRUE
model$nn_indep=jags(
  data=data,
  parameters.to.save=c(
    "mu.e","mu.c","alpha0","alpha1","alpha2","beta0","beta1","sigma.e","sigma.c"
  ),
  inits=NULL,n.chains=2,n.iter=5000,n.burnin=3000,n.thin=1,DIC=TRUE,
  # This specifies the model code as the function nn_indep()
  model.file=nn_indep,
  # Adds the computation for pD
  pD=TRUE
)

# Shows the summary table, including the estimate for pD
print(model$nn_indep,digits=3,interval=c(0.025,0.5,0.975))
```

```
Inference for Bugs model at "/tmp/RtmpERtvsp/modeld78bd3abfa7c1.txt",
 2 chains, each with 5000 iterations (first 3000 discarded)
 n.sims = 4000 iterations saved. Running time = 0.664 secs
             mu.vect sd.vect    2.5%     50%    97.5% Rhat n.eff
alpha0         1.552   0.021   1.510   1.552    1.592 1.001  4000
alpha1        -0.007   0.039  -0.083  -0.007    0.069 1.003   670
alpha2         1.278   0.072   1.138   1.279    1.420 1.001  3800
beta0          1.562   0.135   1.303   1.558    1.828 1.001  4000
beta1          1.087   0.433   0.223   1.093    1.946 1.001  2500
```

Table 5.3: Model selection via DIC, using the two versions – the first one based on p_V and the second based on p_D. The values reported for p_V are those obtained in Examples 5.2, 5.3 and 5.4, based on the original model runs

Model	p_V	DIC $= p_V + \overline{D(\boldsymbol{\theta})}$	p_D	DIC $= p_D + \overline{D(\boldsymbol{\theta})}$
Normal/Normal independent	9.13	686	9.21	686
Normal/Normal MCF	10.19	674	10.16	674
Gamma/Gamma MCF	12.86	493	10.53	490

```
mu.c[1]     1562.243 134.882 1302.603 1557.503 1828.056 1.001  4000
mu.c[2]     2649.017 412.371 1822.148 2650.565 3456.258 1.002  1900
mu.e[1]        1.552   0.021    1.510    1.552    1.592 1.001  4000
mu.e[2]        1.544   0.033    1.482    1.544    1.609 1.003   680
sigma.c[1]     1.357   0.096    1.180    1.353    1.559 1.001  3500
sigma.c[2]     3.332   0.295    2.821    3.308    3.955 1.002  1200
sigma.e[1]     0.207   0.015    0.181    0.206    0.239 1.002  4000
sigma.e[2]     0.267   0.023    0.227    0.265    0.318 1.002  4000
deviance     676.670   4.236  670.367  675.973  686.903 1.001  4000

For each parameter, n.eff is a crude measure of effective sample size,
and Rhat is the potential scale reduction factor (at convergence, Rhat=1).

DIC info (using the rule: pV = var(deviance)/2)
pV = 9.0 and DIC = 685.6
DIC info (using the rule: pD = Dbar-Dhat, computed via 'rjags::dic.samples')
pD = 9.2 and DIC = 685.9
DIC is an estimate of expected predictive error (lower deviance is better).
```

The summary table now includes at the bottom the values for p_D and the revised DIC – notice that, because JAGS needs to re-runs the model to compute p_D, the DIC associated with it is computed based on a new (possibly slightly different) distribution of the deviance, although if the model is at convergence, the discrepancy is minimal. For the same reason, the reported values for p_V and DIC are also slightly different to the ones in Example 5.2, but these differences are only down to Monte Carlo error (due to the new MCMC run used to construct this table).

We can do the same for all three models considered here. The resulting values for the model fitting statistics are presented in Table 5.3. As mentioned above, the Normal/Normal independent model is the one with the worst performance, according to the DIC, with values that are over 10 points higher than for the Normal/Normal MCF and almost 200 points above the Gamma/Gamma MCF, confirming its better performance over the others. For the Gamma/Gamma MCF, the value computed by `R2jags::jags()` is also close (but not identical, again due to simulation error) to the one we obtained manually in Section 5.3.2.

What if?...

Incidentally, if we included some substantial information in the prior for the shape of the effects, in the Gamma/Gamma MCF model of Example 5.4, e.g. $\nu_{et} \sim$

Exponential(6), to encode the assumption that $\Pr(\nu_{et} > 0.5) \approx 0.05$, then we would get estimates for the DIC of 798, for p_V of 132.7 and for p_D of 11.1.

Because of the gross mis-specification for the shape parameter, not only would this change the scale of the estimate for p_V, but also the ordering of the three models – this new version of the Gamma/Gamma MCF would have worse performance than the two Normal/Normal models!

5.3.4 Other information criteria

As mentioned above, the DIC is *not* the only (or necessarily the best) way of assessing model fitting and, in fact, several alternatives have been proposed; Gelman et al. (2013, ch. 7) present a few, including the *Watanabe Applicable Information criterion* (WAIC), as well as procedures such as *leave-one-out cross validation* (LOO-CV), which are perhaps considered more "modern" measures of predictive accuracy. These are similar to DIC as they use a penalty to discount a measure of model fit. However, instead of directly on the likelihood, they are based on the posterior predictive distribution, given the observed data.

Formally, for each observation $i = 1, \ldots, n$, we define the *log pointwise predictive density* (lpd) as

$$\begin{aligned}\text{lpd} &= \sum_{i=1}^{n} \log p(y_i \mid \boldsymbol{y}) = \sum_{i=1}^{n} \log \int p(y_i \mid \boldsymbol{\theta}) p(\boldsymbol{\theta} \mid \boldsymbol{y}) d\boldsymbol{\theta} \\ &= \sum_{i=1}^{n} \log \text{E}_{\boldsymbol{\theta}\mid\boldsymbol{y}} \left[p(y_i \mid \boldsymbol{\theta}) \right] \\ &\approx \sum_{1=1}^{n} \log \frac{1}{S} \sum_{s=1}^{S} p\left(y_i \mid \boldsymbol{\theta}^{(s)}\right)\end{aligned}$$

and

$$\text{WAIC} = -2\text{lpd} + 2p_W,$$

where p_W is the penalty. There are different choices for the definition of p_W, but a simple and effective one is to consider

$$\begin{aligned}p_W &= \sum_{i=1}^{n} \text{Var}_{\boldsymbol{\theta}\mid\boldsymbol{y}} \left[\log p(y_i \mid \boldsymbol{\theta}) \right] \\ &\approx \sum_{i=1}^{n} \frac{1}{S-1} \sum_{s=1}^{S} \left[\log p\left(y_i \mid \boldsymbol{\theta}^{(s)}\right) - \frac{1}{S} \sum_{s=1}^{S} \log p\left(y_i \mid \boldsymbol{\theta}^{(s)}\right) \right]^2.\end{aligned} \tag{5.17}$$

The penalty can be interpreted similarly to p_D, as a measure of "effective number of parameters".

These computations are implemented in the `R` package `loo` (Vehtari et al., 2024), which can be used to compute the WAIC, as well as the LOO-CV, which is an estimate of out-of-sample predictive, where the lpd is modified to consider $\log p(y_i \mid \boldsymbol{y}_{-i})$. More details are presented in Vehtari et al. (2017) and Gelman et al. (2013).

Example 5.7. *Computing the WAIC using the* `loo` *package.* We can slightly modify the Gamma/Gamma MCF model to include the computation of the individual log-likelihood contribution, which we can then use to compute WAIC and LOO. As discussed in Note 15 above, it is sufficient to add a single command to the model code function defined in Example 5.4

```
gg_mcf_waic=function(){
  for (i in 1:N) {
    ...
    # Computes the individual contributions to the log-likelihood
    log.lik[i] <- logdensity.gamma(estar[i], nu.e[Trt[i]], gamma.e[Trt[i],i]) +
                  logdensity.gamma(c[i], nu.c[Trt[i]], gamma.c[Trt[i],i])
  }
  ...
}
```

to include a node `log.lik[i]`, which sums the contributions to the likelihood from both cost and effects data. We can run the model, e.g. using the following `R` code

```
m_waic=jags(
  data=data,parameters.to.save=c("log.lik"),model.file=gg_mcf_waic,
  inits=NULL,n.chains=2,n.iter=5000, n.burnin=3000,n.thin=1,DIC=TRUE
)
```

and then use the simulated values for the node `log.lik` (which consist of `n.sims`=4000 simulations for each of the 167 individual observations) to feed into the `loo` functions and compute the WAIC, for example as in the following `R` code.

```
# Prints the WAIC
loo::waic(m_waic$BUGSoutput$sims.list$log.lik)
```

```
Computed from 4000 by 167 log-likelihood matrix.

          Estimate   SE
elpd_waic   -245.3 21.3
p_waic        10.2  1.4
waic         490.6 42.5

3 (1.8%) p_waic estimates greater than 0.4. We recommend trying loo instead.
```

The first quantity returned by this function is an estimate of the *expected* log pointwise predictive density, defined as

$$\text{elpd} = \text{E}_{Y_i}\left[\sum_{i=1}^{n} \log p(y_i \mid \boldsymbol{y})\right] = \sum_{i=1}^{n} \int \tilde{p}(y_i) \log p(y_i \mid \boldsymbol{y}) dy_i,$$

where $\tilde{p}(\cdot)$ is the unknown distribution representing the "true" data-generating process for an observation y_i. The elpd is a measure of predictive accuracy for the n data points, taken one at a time and is estimated as $\widehat{\text{elpd}} = \text{lpd} - p_W$; this is the quantity labelled as `elpd_waic`, above.

The computed value for the WAIC and p_W are fairly close to the ones obtained using DIC and p_D (see Table 5.3). In this particular case, `loo()` returns a warning: as is obvious by Equation 5.17, the penalty is computed by summing over all the individual n contributions and the fact that for some observations p_W exceeds the arbitrarily chosen threshold of 0.4 may pose some concerns around the reliability in the overall estimate (see Vehtari et al., 2017 for more details on diagnostics for the WAIC).

For this reason, `loo()` suggests moving to the more robust LOO-CV approach, which we can obtain using the following `R` commands.

```
# Prints the LOO-CV
loo::loo(m_waic$BUGSoutput$sims.list$log.lik)
```

```
Computed from 4000 by 167 log-likelihood matrix.

         Estimate   SE
elpd_loo   -245.4 21.3
p_loo        10.3  1.4
looic       490.8 42.6
------
MCSE of elpd_loo is 0.1.
MCSE and ESS estimates assume independent draws (r_eff=1).

All Pareto k estimates are good (k < 0.7).
See help('pareto-k-diagnostic') for details.
```

The estimates are effectively identical and in fact, the LOO suggests that the estimates are consistent (see Vehtari et al., 2017 for more details on how Pareto smoothed importance sampling is used to improve the efficiency of the LOO estimate).

5.3.5 Model averaging

One possible way to reconcile the uncertainty over distributional assumptions (cfr. also the discussion in Section 4.3.4) is to consider a form of "model averaging". Here, instead of simply presenting a measure of model fitting with a view to selecting the "best" option (as in Table 5.3), the idea is to instead use the model fitting statistics to derive weights and then construct a "meta-model", which combines the feature of all the options being considered.

Expanding on a suggestion based on AIC in Burnham and Anderson (2002), as well as related work in Jackson et al. (2009), Baio (2012) proposes to weigh each of the H competing models using weights determined as

$$w_h = \frac{\exp(-0.5\Delta\text{DIC}_h)}{\sum_{h=1}^{H}\exp(-0.5\Delta\text{DIC}_h)}, \tag{5.18}$$

with ΔDIC_h defined in Equation 5.16.

The underlying implication is that the weight for the $h-$th model decreases steeply with the increase in the absolute difference between its DIC and the one associated with the minimum DIC – and effectively vanishes to 0 as ΔDIC_h approaches 10, as shown in Figure 5.6 (in the case of two models being compared) and in line with Section 5.3.3.

In order to construct the model average, we can simply multiply the MCMC simulations for the main parameters or computed quantities of interest for each of the H models being considered by the respective weights in Equation 5.18. We demonstrate this computation in Example 5.6. Note that the analysis in Figure 5.6 suggests that constructing the model average is only useful if there is substantial uncertainty among at least two of the H options, because otherwise the weights will be very small and thus the model average will be almost entirely driven by the best fitting model (for example as in Example 5.6).

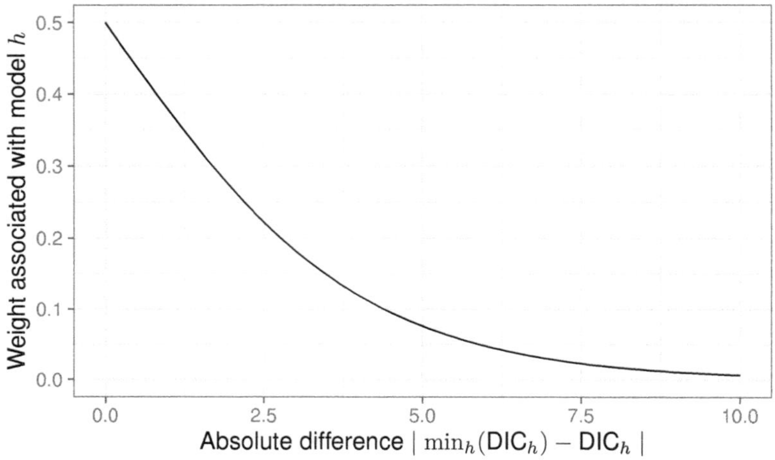

Figure 5.6: The relationship between a model weight and its absolute difference with the model associated with the lowest DIC, assuming these are the only models under consideration.

5.4 Cost-effectiveness modelling

As discussed in Chapter 4, the statistical model is the most fundamental building block for the process of HTA, but once we have the estimates for the relevant parameters, we still need to post-process them to propagate the underlying uncertainty all the way to the decision process.

In the context of ILD and especially in the case of HTA alongside trial data, the model parameters are very close to the actual economic quantities, necessary for the HTA evaluation – typically we retrieve directly full estimates for the population average benefit and costs, in each treatment arm and these are simply combined to obtain the quantities (Δ_e, Δ_c), upon which we base the decision making, e.g. by computing summary measures such as the ICER and EIB, as well as performing the uncertainty analysis, as detailed in Chapter 4.

Example 5.8. *10TT (continued): cost-effectiveness analysis.* We can post-process the outcome by accessing directly the simulations from the `BUGS` model, for instance stored in the object `model$sims.list`. For instance, we could construct the relevant variables (Δ_e, Δ_c) as

```
delta_e=model$nn_indep$BUGSoutput$sims.list$mu.e[,2]-
  model$BUGSoutput$sims.list$mu.e[,1]
delta_c=model$nn_indep$BUGSoutput$sims.list$mu.c[,2]-
  model$BUGSoutput$sims.list$mu.c[,1]
```

and then we could use these to, for instance, plot the Cost-Effectiveness plane.

Alternatively (and, perhaps, more efficiently), we can use the `R` package `BCEA` (Baio et al., 2025a). This is a rather simple package, really, which codes up a set of operations to be performed on objects given as input by the user, representing simulations from the distribution of the population average cost and benefits[2].

This means we would only need to feed the simulations to the function `bcea()` to then produce a range of standardised output for the economic evaluation. For instance, we could use the following `R` code.

```
# Load 'BCEA'
library(BCEA)
# Defines a list of labels for the interventions
interventions=c("Standard","Active intervention")
# Sets the reference (t=2=intensive case management)
ref=2

# 1. Normal/Normal independent
# Defines the variables for effects and costs
eff=model$nn_indep$BUGSoutput$sims.list$mu.e
cost=model$nn_indep$BUGSoutput$sims.list$mu.c
# Runs BCEA
m_nn_indep=bcea(
  eff=eff,cost=cost,interventions=interventions,ref=ref
)

# 2. Normal/Normal MCF
# Defines the variables for effects and costs
eff=model$nn_mcf$BUGSoutput$sims.list$mu.e
cost=model$nn_mcf$BUGSoutput$sims.list$mu.c
# Runs BCEA
m_nn_mcf=bcea(
  eff=eff,cost=cost,interventions=interventions,ref=ref
)

# 3. Gamma/Gamma MCF
# Defines the variables for effects and costs
eff=model$gg_mcf$BUGSoutput$sims.list$mu.e
cost=model$gg_mcf$BUGSoutput$sims.list$mu.c
# Runs BCEA
m_gg_mcf=bcea(
  eff=eff,cost=cost,interventions=interventions,ref=ref
)
```

Figure 5.7 shows the cost-effectiveness plane with overlaid a contour for the joint posterior distribution of (Δ_e, Δ_c) – these figures can be obtained using the `contour2()` function from `BCEA`.

As is possible to see (and consistently with the discussion detailed throughout this chapter), the two Normal/Normal models of Examples 5.2 and 5.3 provide similar results. Figures 5.7a and 5.7b show more or less the same picture, with the larger dot in the middle of the

[2]In reality, as far as `BCEA` is concerned, the inputs do not *have* to come from a full Bayesian analysis and thus represent samples from the joint posterior distributions. As long as simulations are provided (e.g. from a bootstrap procedure, in a frequentist approach), the user can call the main `BCEA` function and obtain the post-processed results. `BCEA` will silently judge the user, in that case, though.

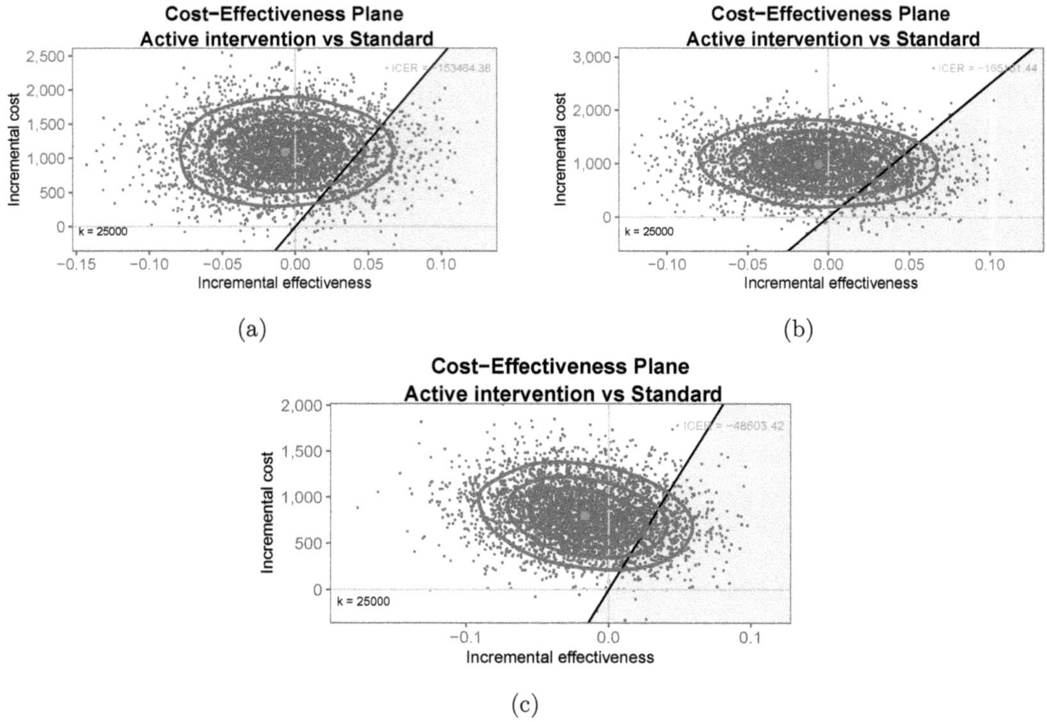

Figure 5.7: The contour plot overlaid on the cost-effectiveness plane. Panel (a) shows the cost-effectiveness plane for the Normal/Normal independent model, while panel (b) presents the results for the Normal/Normal MCF. The two are virtually identical. Panel (c) shows a different picture and interpretation, for the Gamma/Gamma MCF model.

contour representing the ICER that, albeit numerically slightly different, is firmly placed outside the "sustainability area". In both cases, we would conclude that the intervention is *not* cost-effective, for the default threshold of £25 000 per QALY, although there seems to be some uncertainty, based on the proportion of points that lay below the cost-effectiveness threshold line. As for the Gamma/Gamma MCF, this result is generally confirmed, while the ICER is numerically different.

These results are even more obvious when looking at the CEACs displayed in Figure 5.8 and obtained using the `BCEA` function `ceac.plot()`. Generally speaking, when a `BCEA` object is constructed through the call to the function `bcea()`, as shown above, then it is possible to apply various plotting and summary methods by simply using it as the main parameter for a given function. For instance, the command `ceac.plot(m_nn_indep)` plots the CEAC for the Normal/Normal independent model.

More importantly, if in the call to any `BCEA` plotting method we specify the option `graph=gg` (= `ggplot`) for the graphical engine, then the resulting objects can be manipulated further, taking advantage of the `ggplot2` capabilities. For instance, Figure 5.8 is obtained using the following code.

```
# Plots the CEAC with the 'ggplot' graphical engine and saves the graphs to the
# R objects 'p1', 'p2' and 'p3'
```

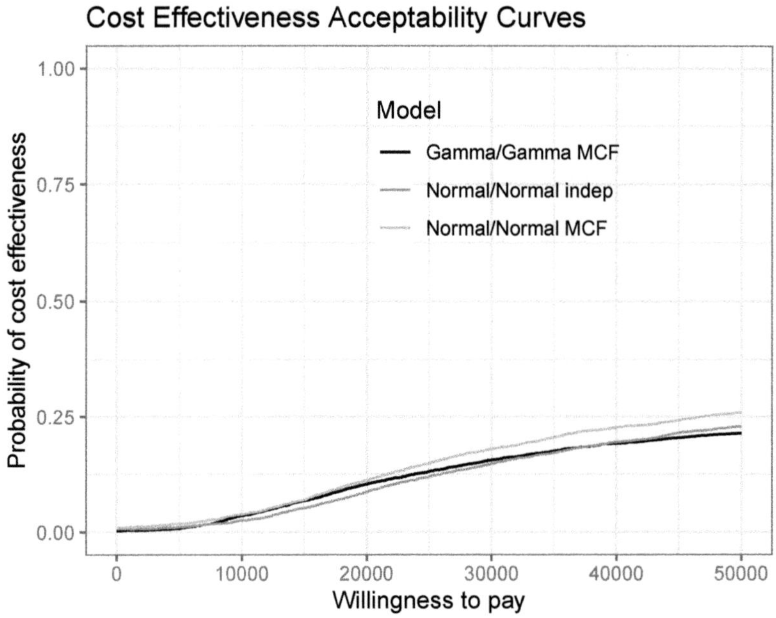

Figure 5.8: The Cost-Effectiveness Acceptability Curves for the three models described in the chapter.

```
p1=ceac.plot(m_nn_indep,graph="gg")
p2=ceac.plot(m_nn_mcf,graph="gg")
p3=ceac.plot(m_gg_mcf,graph="gg")

# Post-processes the graphs to superimpose the three CEACs
# First stack the underlying data (extracted from the three 'ggplot' objects)
# And associate each with a 'model' variable
p1$data |> mutate(model="Normal/Normal indep") |>
  bind_rows(p2$data |> mutate(model="Normal/Normal MCF")) |>
  bind_rows(p3$data |> mutate(model="Gamma/Gamma MCF")) |>
# Then use 'ggplot' to make the actual plot using the three original datasets
# but different colours for each model
  ggplot(aes(k,ceac,color=model)) + geom_line() +
# And then provide further customisation
  xlab("Willingness to pay") + ylim(0,1) +
  ylab("Probability of cost effectiveness") +
  labs(title="Cost Effectiveness Acceptability Curves",color="Model") +
  theme(
    legend.position="inside",legend.position.inside=c(.6,.75),
    legend.background=element_blank()
  ) + scale_color_manual(values=c("#000000","#1F77B4","#FF7F0E"))
```

All CEACs in Figure 5.8 have consistently a low value (well below 0.5), which is only relatively sensitive to the choice of the willingness to pay threshold along the x–axis, indicating that, in this particular occasion, there is clear evidence (and little uncertainty) about the fact that, conditionally on the model assumptions, the new intervention is *not* cost-effective.

The optimal decision is then to keep the standard of care, which can also be assessed using the summary() method from BCEA. For instance, when applied to the Gamma/Gamma MCF model, this would return the following output.

```
summary(m_gg_mcf)
```

```
Cost-effectiveness analysis summary

Reference intervention:  Active intervention
Comparator intervention: Standard

Standard dominates for all k in [0 - 50000]


Analysis for willingness to pay parameter k = 25000

                     Expected net benefit
Standard                            38083
Active intervention                 36870

                                   EIB  CEAC   ICER
Active intervention vs Standard -1212.7 0.131 -48603

Optimal intervention (max expected net benefit) for k = 25000: Standard

EVPI 65.734
```

We can also use the models simulations to perform a structural uncertainty analysis, combining them into a "model average", based on weights determined by the respective DICs, as described in Section 5.3.5. We could do this manually, first constructing the weights according to Equation 5.18, then multiplying them by the objects eff and cost for each of the three alternative models and finally adding the results together and feeding them to BCEA, to obtain the model average output, say m_avg.

More simply, we can use the BCEA function struct.psa(), which runs exactly these operations in the background.

```
# Defines a list with the simulations for the effects
effects=list(
  model$nn_indep$BUGSoutput$sims.list$mu.e,
  model$nn_mcf$BUGSoutput$sims.list$mu.e,
  model$gg_mcf$BUGSoutput$sims.list$mu.e
)
# Defines a list with the simulations for the costs
costs=list(
  model$nn_indep$BUGSoutput$sims.list$mu.c,
  model$nn_mcf$BUGSoutput$sims.list$mu.c,
  model$gg_mcf$BUGSoutput$sims.list$mu.c
)
# Defines a list of models
models=list(
  "nn-indep"=model$nn_indep,"nn-mcf"=model$nn_mcf,"gg-mcf"=model$gg_mcf
)
```

```
# Finally runs struct.psa to compute the model average
m_avg=struct.psa(
  models,effects,costs,ref=ref,interventions=interventions
)
```

The object m_avg is for all intents and purposes similar to the various BCEA objects created above (and, in fact, it *also* is in the class bcea, which means that it can access all the same methods and functions as the three BCEA fits above). In addition, however, it also contains a few more outputs (and the additional class struct.psa).

We can visualise the weights associated with each of the three models considered using the following command.

```
# Shows the weights for each of the three models, in the order with which
# we have passed them in the 'models' list
m_avg$w
```

```
    nn-indep       nn-mcf       gg-mcf
1.426740e-42 3.171575e-40 1.000000e+00
```

Unsurprisingly, here the third model dominates, with a weight of effectively 1. This is of course consistent with Figure 5.6 and Table 5.3: we already know that the Gamma/Gamma MCF is way superior in terms of model fitting, as assessed by the DIC. We can check this also by creating the summary for the model average,

```
summary(m_avg)
```

```
Cost-effectiveness analysis summary

Reference intervention:  Active intervention
Comparator intervention: Standard

Standard dominates for all k in [0 - 50000]


Analysis for willingness to pay parameter k = 25000

                    Expected net benefit
Standard                           38083
Active intervention                36870

                                EIB  CEAC   ICER
Active intervention vs Standard -1212.7 0.131 -48603

Optimal intervention (max expected net benefit) for k = 25000: Standard

EVPI 65.734
```

which looks identical to the one produced above for the Gamma/Gamma MCF alone. Of course, in cases where competing models based on the same data showed closer fit, the model average would be a mixture of its individual components and would be much more worthy of reporting.

5.5 Conclusions

This chapter has focused on the analysis of individual-level data, e.g. coming from HTA alongside a RCT. We have discussed the "standard" framework of analysis, often based on unrealistic simplifying assumptions, such as independence between costs and benefits and underlying Normality. We have also showed how a Bayesian approach is able to naturally and relatively simply relax these assumptions, especially through the "Marginal/Conditional" factorisation.

We have also considered various other important aspects of ILD modelling, including assessment of model fitting and its use to make model selection choices. We have also explored suitable measures such as the DIC, which will also be used later in the book.

In the next chapter, we present a different background for HTA modelling, in which the data do not provide information at the individual-level, but rather are obtained using summary statistics, perhaps coming from systematic literature review.

6

Aggregated level data and evidence synthesis

6.1 Introduction

In Chapter 5 we have discussed models to deal with the nuances of correlated, non-symmetrical, bounded individual-level data – this situation often arise when HTA evaluations are conducted alongside randomised clinical trials. In that situation, often we consider the single source of evidence to inform the economic modelling.

However, robust healthcare decisions should involve a wider process that considers all costs and benefits, over a patients lifetime (e.g. beyond the time horizon of a randomised study), as well as being evidence-based, reflecting all the relevant sources of information. Of course, limiting ourselves to data from a single RCT has several disadvantages, in general.

First, we may fail to capture longer-term costs/benefits, which manifest well beyond the duration of an experimental study, for example in case of rare side-effects, which are unlikely to occur in a limited sample size, but become more visible as the follow-up and relevant target population increase.

Second, randomised studies often do not generalise to other populations/settings. This is particularly relevant because, by necessity, RCTs have exclusion and inclusion criteria that may not apply to the general population in which a given intervention is eventually rolled out. Thus, the conclusions of an HTA evaluation based exclusively on RCT data may simply not be relevant for the economic decision-making process.

Finally, the one randomised study we have available (perhaps because we are working closely with the sponsor and hence are able to directly access the ILD) may not be the only relevant source of evidence and perhaps not even the most relevant comparison: for instance, very often RCTs are conducted on a pairwise comparison against placebo. While this is good for the purpose of market authorisation, placebo is never one of the options in the real world and cost-effectiveness need to be measured against all other *active* interventions that are available for a given disease – we return to this point in Chapters 7 and 11.

For these reasons, it is usually important to expand the sources of data to all relevant evidence, using transparent, reproducible and specific processes (often termed "systematic literature review", SLR), which is a cornerstone of the vast majority of HTA evaluations (see among others Welton et al., 2012; Grant and Di Tanna, 2025).

More importantly, when doing so, we are extremely unlikely to access individual-level data for *all* the relevant studies. In reality, while it is still possible that we access a full ILD for a specific source, for all the others we would have only access to summary statistics, derived by published literature.

DOI: 10.1201/9781003771050-6

6.2 Meta-analysis of aggregated summaries from RCTs

In this section, we describe the process of *evidence synthesis*, using various modelling assumptions and a running example, based on data reported in the form of "number of occurrence for the event under study out of number of individuals observed" (i.e. binary data).

Of course, there is no reason why this should always be the case – and in principle, we can extend the modelling framework to account for other assumptions in terms of how we represent the sampling variability in the data.

Example 6.1. *Magnesium (adapted and expanded from Spiegelhalter et al., 2004).* In the late 1980s and throughout the early 1990s, much research has been devoted to investigating the effect of intravenous magnesium sulphate in reducing the risk of acute myocardial infarction, especially by preventing serious arrhythmia.

A series of relatively small and potentially non-definitive studies have been conducted throughout the decade 1984-1994, mostly indicating a positive effect, with a marked reduction of the odds of death, until the very large ISIS-4 trial seemingly reversed this finding and actually indicated a lack of any meaningful effect. Table 6.1 shows the data collected in $S = 16$ studies, in terms of the number of deaths out of the total number of people observed in the placebo and magnesium arms.

Table 6.1: The summary statistics for the 16 trials of Magnesium vs Placebo

			Placebo		Magnesium	
ID	Name	Year	Deaths (r_1)	Total (n_1)	Deaths (r_2)	Total (n_2)
1	Morton	1984	2	36	1	40
2	Rasmussen	1986	23	135	9	135
3	Smith	1986	7	200	2	200
4	Abraham	1987	1	46	1	48
5	Felstedt	1988	8	148	10	150
6	Shechter	1989	9	56	1	59
7	Ceremuzynski	1989	3	23	1	25
8	Bertschat	1989	1	21	0	22
9	Singh	1990	11	75	6	76
10	Pereira	1990	7	27	1	27
11	Shechter 1	1991	12	80	2	89
12	Golf	1991	13	33	5	23
13	Thorgersen	1991	8	122	4	130
14	LIMIT-2	1992	118	1157	90	1159
15	Shechter 2	1995	17	108	4	107
16	ISIS-4	1995	2103	29 039	2216	29 011

As seen above, data are reported for the magnesium trials as counts indicating the number of "events" (in this case, deaths), out of the overall sample size included in each study. Thus, we can model for study s in arm t (for $t = 1$: placebo or $t = 2$: magnesium)

$$r_{st} \sim \text{Binomial}(\pi_{st}, n_{st}) \tag{6.1}$$

and then construct a suitable model for the underlying study- and arm-specific probability of death, e.g. using logistic regression. The most general form for the linear predictor is

$$\text{logit}(\pi_{st}) = \alpha_s + \delta_s(\text{Trt}_{st} - 1)\,[+\ldots], \tag{6.2}$$

where $\text{Trt}_{st} = 1, 2$ is a treatment arm indicator for study s and arm t, with 1 indicating placebo and 2 the magnesium arm. Here, α_s is a baseline (rescaled) probability of death for study s, while δ_s is an incremental effect that is activated only for the magnesium arm – in the case of a logistic regression, this is measured in terms of a *log odds ratio* (log OR)

$$\delta_s = \log \text{OR} = \log\left(\frac{\pi_{s2}}{1-\pi_{s2}} \Big/ \frac{\pi_{s1}}{1-\pi_{s1}}\right),$$

describing how much more (or less) likely individuals in the magnesium arm are to die, in comparison to the individuals in the placebo arm. Similarly to Section 5.2, the notation $[+\ldots]$ indicates that we may or may not add other covariates to the linear predictor.

Note 16: Absolute vs relative effects

Head-to-head studies (whose results are typically the summaries obtained by SLRs) are designed to provide *relative* effects, i.e. how much better is the active treatment, when compared to placebo. Depending on the scale on which the analysis is performed, the actual nature of the summary can vary. For instance, in the case of binary outcomes (as in Table 6.1) and logistic regression, we would estimate a log odds ratio; in a linear regression, the estimate would be a mean difference; or in a survival model, we may target a hazard ratio (see Chapter 8 for more details).

On the other hand, the full economic evaluation is likely to be interested in the *absolute* effects, i.e. what is the actual benefit provided by a given intervention. Examples include a probability of occurrence (e.g. π_{st} in Equation 6.1), mean scores, or event rates.

Relative effects are typically more generalisable than absolute effects, but the latter are more specific to the HTA problem. Thus, the goal is to apply relative effects to reference absolute effect to obtain absolute treatment effects. For instance, if we have an estimate for a baseline mean score, say μ_0 (which applies to the "untreated" population) and we can obtain a measure of mean difference, say δ, then we can retrieve an estimate for the mean score in the treated population as

$$\mu_1 = \mu_0 + \delta. \tag{6.3}$$

Similarly, in a simple logistic regression context the parameters (θ_0, θ_1) represent the probability of experiencing the event under study for the general and the treated population, respectively. If we define $\text{odds}_0 = \theta_0/(1-\theta_0)$ and $\text{odds}_1 = \theta_1/(1-\theta_1)$, then we can use the relationship

$$\log \text{odds}_1 = \log \text{odds}_0 + \log \text{OR}$$

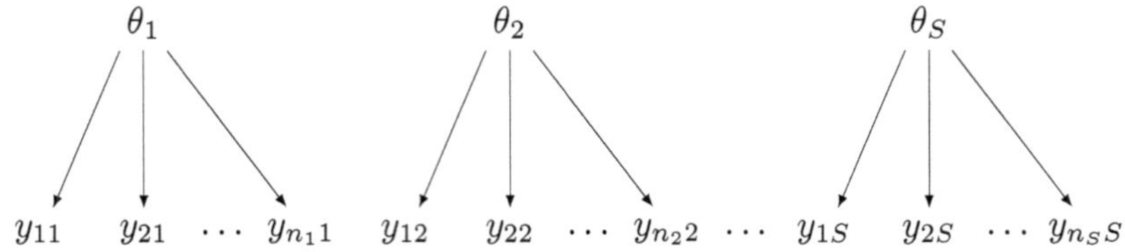

Figure 6.1: A DAG representation of the assumptions underlying the no pooling model. Each study can be used to inform a study-specific parameter only and no borrowing of information happen across studies.

or, equivalently (and perhaps more intuitively)

$$\text{logit}(\theta_1) = \text{logit}(\theta_0) + \log \text{OR} \tag{6.4}$$

and then, given an estimate for logit(θ_0) and a log OR, we can obtain an estimate for the absolute effect in the treated population logit(θ_1), which we can scale back as a probability using the inverse logit transformation

$$\theta_1 = \frac{\exp\left(\text{logit}(\theta_0) + \log \text{OR}\right)}{1 + \exp\left(\text{logit}(\theta_0) + \log \text{OR}\right)}.$$

Of course, we need to fully propagate the uncertainty in the relative to the absolute effect to perform the full economic evaluation (including the uncertainty analysis). In this case, being Bayesian makes life easier, because, once a posterior distribution is available for the quantities in the right-hand side of Equation 6.3 or Equation 6.4, the deterministic relationships automatically determine a full posterior probability for the left-hand side terms.

Given the formulation of Equations 6.1 and 6.2, applying the inverse logit transformation yields:

$$\pi_{st} = \begin{cases} \dfrac{\exp(\alpha_s\,[+\ldots])}{1 + \exp(\alpha_s\,[+\ldots])} & \text{for the placebo arm } (t = 1) \\[2ex] \dfrac{\exp(\alpha_s + \delta_s\,[+\ldots])}{1 + \exp(\alpha_s + \delta_s\,[+\ldots])} & \text{for the magnesium arm } (t = 2). \end{cases}$$

Under this general structure, we can encode different assumptions on the mechanism for the data-generating process and the resulting judgement about the relationships among the data and the model parameters.

6.2.1 No-pooling

At one extreme, we may deem the S studies to be so different that it would be inappropriate to pool them together. Figure 6.1 shows a general graphical representation of this modelling assumption, in form of a DAG (see Section 1.1).

Here, the observed data are represented at the bottom of the graph and labelled as $\boldsymbol{y}_s = (y_{1s}, y_{2s}, \ldots, y_{n_s s})$, for each of the $s = 1, \ldots, S$ groups (say, studies) considered. Generally speaking, while each study will be based on individual-level data such as $\boldsymbol{y}_s$, in reality, when working with evidence synthesis we are more likely to actually access only a summary, for

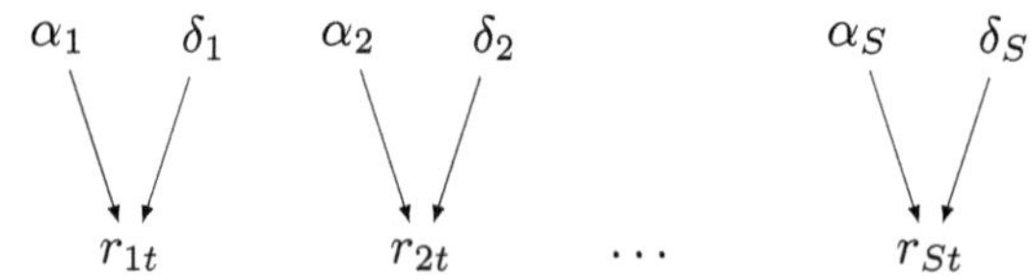

Figure 6.2: The DAG for the no pooling assumption, in the magnesium example.

instance the total count for the occurrence of the event under study, r_s, in the magnesium example.

In Figure 6.1, each study is assumed to follow a data-generating process that depends on a specific parameter (in this case, labelled as $\theta_1, \theta_2, \ldots, \theta_S$). Effectively, there is no connection whatsoever across the S studies and the data in each of them contribute solely to the estimate of the study-specific parameter, an assumption encoded by $\theta_1, \ldots, \theta_S \overset{iid}{\sim} p(\cdot)$.

In the magnesium example, this assumption amounts to modelling α_s and δ_s *independently*

$$\alpha_s, \delta_s \overset{iid}{\sim} \text{Normal}(0, sd), \tag{6.5}$$

for some suitable value of the standard deviation *sd*.

Figure 6.2 is a specific version of the more general Figure 6.1, with reference to the magnesium example. Note that we explicitly include in the DAG representation the core parameters (α_s, δ_s), of which the probabilities π_{st} are just transformations nodes that are defined as deterministic function – in fact, we could write the model in Equation 6.1 as

$$r_{st} \sim \text{Binomial}(\underbrace{\text{logit}^{-1}(\alpha_s + \delta_s(\text{Trt}_{st} - 1))}_{\pi_{st}}, n_{st}).$$

However, for ease of representation, we omit from the DAG the constant Trt_{st}.

The model with "no-pooling" is not very helpful for the purpose of evidence synthesis, but it may be the most appropriate, for instance if we have some knowledge to deem (some of) the studies *fundamentally* different.

6.2.2 Complete pooling

At the other extreme, we may be willing to assume that all the studies are generated by the exact same mechanism and thus they share a common effect. A generalised version of this assumption can be shown graphically in Figure 6.3. Here, all the data points across the S studies depend on a single, common parameter θ – this model is often referred to as "fixed effects", particularly in a non-Bayesian context.

In this case, all the data are connected (and thus, in principle, strongly dependent) through the single DGP that we are assuming. This is of course the most useful assumption in terms of pooling and producing a precise estimate of the parameter θ. However, of course, complete pooling does represent a very strong modelling formulation, which is often difficult to defend dogmatically, as studies may embed inevitable heterogeneity (by design, measurements, inclusion/exclusion criteria, etc.).

In the case of the magnesium example, the complete pooling model is characterised by the assumption that

$$\delta_s = d \quad \text{for all } s = 1, \ldots, S. \tag{6.6}$$

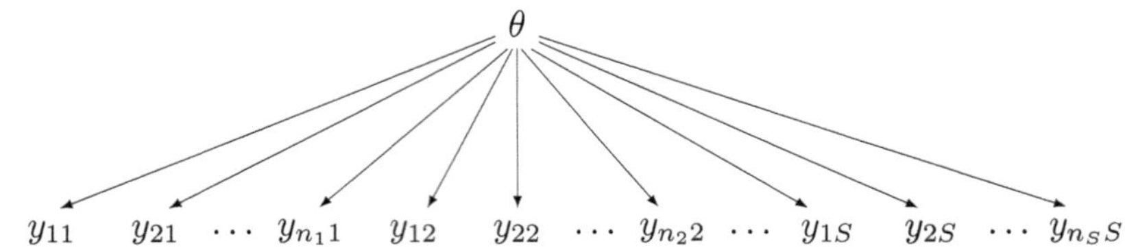

Figure 6.3: A DAG representation of the assumptions underlying the complete pooling model. All studies are assumed to be generated by a single process and therefore they all inform the one parameter.

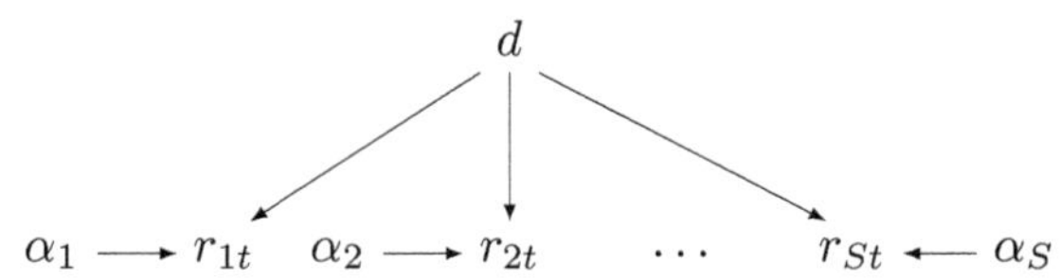

Figure 6.4: The DAG for the complete pooling assumption, in the magnesium example.

Figure 6.4 shows the DAG for this modelling assumption. Here, technically, the α_s parameters are in fact specified for each different study; however, they essentially represent some "background noise" (i.e. the baseline for the probability of death) and the key parameter is the treatment effect d, which is assumed to be just one and common across all studies.

6.2.3 Partial pooling (hierarchical models)

An intermediate situation is represented by the assumption of partial pooling, sometimes referred to as "random effects". In a more general case, partial pooling can be depicted as in Figure 6.5, which can be seen as a compromise between the representations of Figures 6.1 and 6.3.

In each of the S studies, the data $\boldsymbol{y}_1, \boldsymbol{y}_2, \ldots, \boldsymbol{y}_S$ are assumed to be generated by study-specific parameters $\theta_1, \theta_2, \ldots, \theta_S$, exactly as in Figure 6.1. However, in the spirit of Fig-

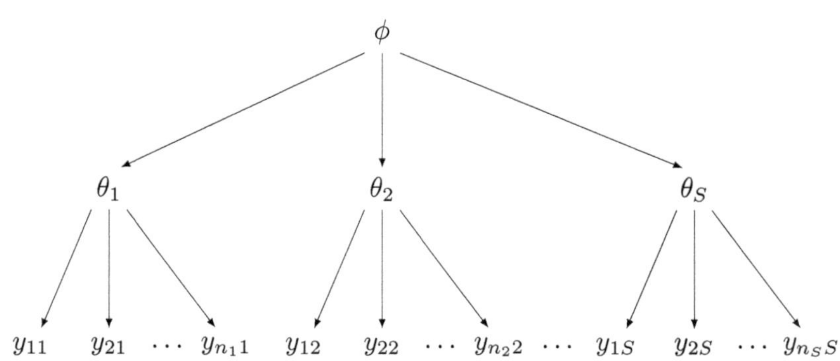

Figure 6.5: A DAG representation of the assumptions underlying the partial pooling model. Each study can be used to inform a study-specific parameter. These set of study-specific parameters are supposed to be generated by a common data-generating process, governed by the hyper-parameters, which implies borrowing of information across studies.

ure 6.3, the study-specific parameters are also assumed to be subject to a common data-generating process, which is governed by a "*hyper-parameter*", indicated as ϕ in Figure 6.5.

Generally speaking, this implies a factorisation of the overall prior distribution as

$$p(\theta_1, \ldots, \theta_S, \phi) = p(\phi) \prod_{s=1}^{S} p(\theta_s \mid \phi).$$

Fixed vs random effects

In a Bayesian context, the distinction between *fixed* and *random* effects is not very helpful – in fact, perhaps even a bit confusing. In both cases, within a Bayesian framework, the relevant parameters are random, in the sense that we associate a probability distribution with them, to describe our uncertainty before seeing the data.

The real difference between the two models is in fact in the assumption we make for the distribution – following the phrasing suggested by Gelman and Hill (2007), in the former case, we use an "unstructured" approach, where the study-specific effect is assumed to be "fixed" across all the studies (i.e. there is a single d parameter, in the magnesium case); in the latter, we use a rather "structured" approach, where the various study-specific parameters are modelled using a common data-generating process.

For this reason, a better terminology (especially from a Bayesian perspective) would be to identify the two model specifications as "structured" vs "unstructured" effects (as opposed to "random" vs "fixed" effects).

This slightly more complex model formulation is often referred to as "hierarchical" or "multilevel", to highlight the fact that we have several layers in our model. The evidence from the data will directly inform the study-specific parameters; however, because of the common "ancestor" ϕ, learning something about one of the study-specific parameter will allow us to also learn some information about all the others.

This process is sometimes referred to as "borrowing information" and it is particularly relevant if, for instance, one of the studies is small. In that case, the estimate for the corresponding parameter θ_s is likely to be very imprecise, because of the lack of information in the data. However, through the implied correlation with all the other elements of the study-specific vector $\boldsymbol{\theta}$, we can get a more precise estimate, by "borrowing" the information provided by the other studies. We return to this point in Section 6.2.7.

Under this setting, for the magnesium example, we would model

$$\begin{aligned} \delta_s &\sim \text{Normal}(d, \sigma_\delta) \\ d &\sim \text{Normal}(0, sd) \\ \sigma_\delta &\sim p(\sigma_\delta), \end{aligned} \tag{6.7}$$

for a fixed value sd and a suitable prior distribution $p(\sigma_\delta)$.

Figure 6.6 shows the DAG for partial pooling with specific reference to the magnesium example. To keep the parallel with Figure 6.5, here $\boldsymbol{\theta} = (\boldsymbol{\alpha}, \boldsymbol{\delta})$ and $\boldsymbol{\phi} = (d, \sigma_\delta)$ are the hyper-parameters.

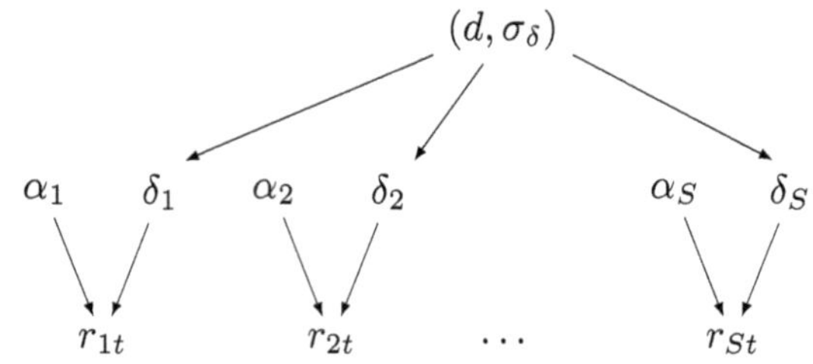

Figure 6.6: The DAG for the partial pooling assumption, in the magnesium example.

6.2.4 Exchangeability

An important implication of considering a hierarchical structure is the assumption of *exchangeability* across the study-specific parameters. From the technical point of view, exchangeability is a rather complex concept, first introduced by the work of Bruno de Finetti in the 1930s, although the definitive references for this are perhaps the later textbooks by de Finetti (1974) and Bernardo and Smith (1999).

Formally, a sequence of random variables $(y_1, \ldots, y_n)$ is *judged* to be exchangeable if our degree of belief in the occurrence of that sequence does not depend on the order in which the variables are observed. For example, considering $n = 3$ binary variables taking values $(0, 1)$, exchangeability implies that

$$\Pr(Y_1 = 1, Y_2 = 0, Y_3 = 1) = \Pr(Y_1 = 0, Y_2 = 1, Y_3 = 1) = \Pr(Y_1 = 1, Y_2 = 1, Y_3 = 0).$$

More pragmatically, a judgement of exchangeability implies that the variables under consideration are assumed to be *similar*, or to put it in a more technical way, that they are generated by a common process, which is governed by common random parameters.

Example 6.2. *Pasta consumption and exchangeability (based on Gelman et al., 2013).* Data are available from the 2012 International Pasta Organisation Annual Survey (yes: that *is* a real thing!) on the annual average per-capita pasta consumption (in kg).

You are told that 9 European countries have been selected and the average consumption of pasta has been recorded; these values are indicated as $y_1, \ldots, y_9$. Notice that, at this stage, you do not know which countries have been selected for this study.

The concept of exchangeability can be explained making reference to "ignorance". In the data, as currently provided, there is nothing for you to distinguish what the country associated with y_1 may be, as opposed to that associated with y_9, say.

We probably know something about the underlying target population, for instance that, generally speaking, European countries like pasta and make large use of it in their diets. But, for now, there is nothing in the data for us to be able to "tell which one is which". Consequently, for the moment at least, it is probably reasonable to assume exchangeability, under this set up.

Imagine now that, out of the original 9 countries, we randomly select 8 and the actual observed results are the following (in kg):

$$4.4, 8.1, 6.6, 7.3, 8.1, 9.3, 7.5, 4.1.$$

Should this modify our assessment of exchangeability (or lack thereof)? And what should our best estimate of the value for the ninth European country, that has not been selected at this stage be?

The actual data (which now we get to see, at least partially) show some variability. There is a range of values, with some higher than others, but we may still assume that this is down to sampling variability and that all the observed values are drawn from a common data-generating process. In the absence of any other information, we may take the mean of the observed values (6.92kg per capita) as the "best estimate" for the missing country.

Now, suppose we are told that the 9 countries are: France, Latvia, Hungary, Portugal, Switzerland, Italy, Lithuania, Croatia, Germany – note that the order in which this information is presented is *not* the same in which the data are given. At this stage, we still do not know for which country the data have not been presented. Should this change your assessment of exchangeability (or lack thereof)?

Now we know that Italy is part of the sample and we may know how crazy Italians are about pasta. Thus, perhaps this may change your judgement – we may now think that the largest observed value is actually Italy, which means we would be able to distinguish one of the y-s from the others.

Or, perhaps, we may now be willing to stipulate that the missing value is Italy, which again would mean we would be able to tell some values apart from the others. Perhaps, at this stage, *conditionally on all the information you now have*, exchangeability would be broken and you may not be willing to assume it anymore.

Drum roll...

Incidentally, the "hidden" country was, in fact, Italy, where in 2012 the average consumption was a whopping 26kg per capita!

The main distinction between complete and partial pooling can be visualised in Figure 6.7. Figure 6.7a shows that, under complete pooling, we are assuming a single, "fixed" true overall effect, θ; each study produces some observed results y_s, which are subject to some random error, representing a deviation from the true overall mean, θ.

In Figure 6.7b, conversely, each study is characterised by a trial-specific effect θ_s (the dashed vertical lines) and the study specific results (again described by the solid dots) are also subject to random errors with respect to that trial-specific effect. These, in turn, are drawn from a common distribution, whose mean ϕ represents the overall pooled estimate.

Example 6.3. *Magnesium (continued): no-pooling analysis.* Assuming no other covariate is available or relevant, we could assume some very vague priors (i.e. $sd \to \infty$) on the regression coefficients α_s and δ_s, defined in Equation 6.5. In the presence of large data, this would be, most likely, immaterial.

However, it would also be overly cautious and rather unnecessary – we are modelling the probability of death in the two arms *on the logit scale.* At face value, priors such as $\alpha_s \sim \text{Normal}(0, sd = 4)$ may look too restrictive and potentially bringing too much information in the analysis. Looking more closely, however, this actually implies a large variability,

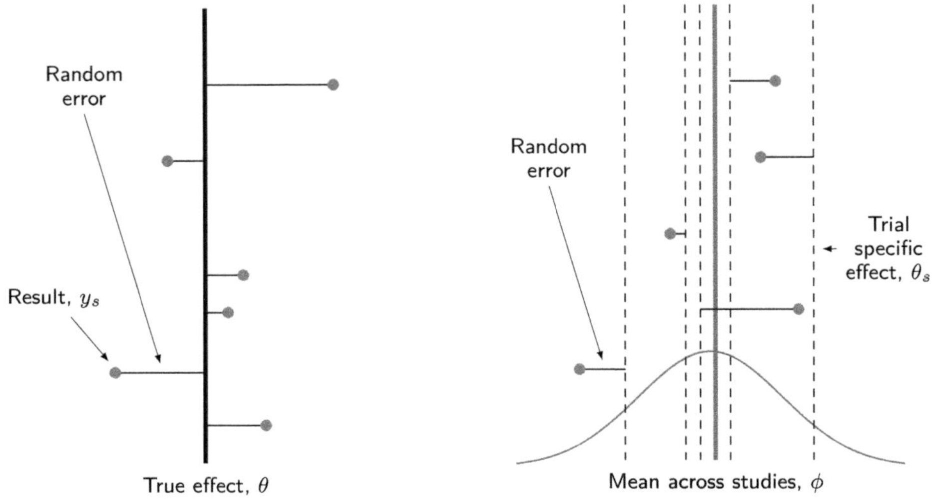

(a) Complete pooling. (b) Partial pooling.

Figure 6.7: Distinction between the complete and partial pooling model. In panel (a), every study is used to estimate the single common parameter, while in panel (b) each study provides a noisy measurement for the overall treatment effect, which is in fact generated by a probabilistic process.

given the scale in which they are defined. We can check this using forward sampling (see Section 1.2.6), with the following code.

```
# Simulates 10000 values from the prior alpha_i ~ Normal(0,sd=4)
tibble(alpha=rnorm(10000,0,4)) |>
  # Rescales to probabilities applying inverse logit
  mutate(pi=exp(alpha)/(1+exp(alpha))) |> select(pi) |>
  # Uses 'bmhe' to summarise the simulations
  bmhe::stats()
```

```
        mean        sd         2.5%    median     97.5%
pi 0.4975282 0.3974699 0.0003924477 0.4956394 0.9996017
```

As is possible to see, the distribution for the resulting parameter `pi`, the probability that a random individual in the placebo arm dies, effectively spans the whole $[0; 1]$ range.

Similarly, the parameters δ_s represent the log OR for magnesium treatment, i.e. indicate how much more or less likely a random individual is to die if they are treated with magnesium, instead of placebo. We could go overboard and assume a very vague distribution, say $\delta_s \sim \text{Normal}(0, sd = 1000)$, so as to remove any bias in favour of the active treatment and "let the data speak for themselves".

However, this is also a rather silly assumption, because we would be implying a ridiculous prior on the resulting OR, with extremely high and implausible values being given a large amount of probability, in the prior. Already assuming $sd = 2$ would imply a large range, when suitably rescaled.

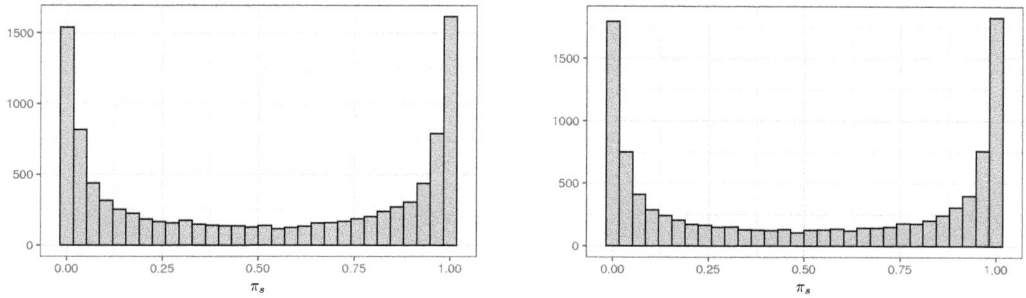

(a) $\pi_s = \text{logit}^{-1}(\alpha_s)$.

(b) $\pi_s = \text{logit}^{-1}(\alpha_s + \delta_s)$.

Figure 6.8: Prior distributions for the underlying probability of death in the treatment arms of the magnesium evidence synthesis.

```
# Simulates 10000 values from the prior alpha_i ~ Normal(0,sd=4),
# and delta_i ~ Normal(0,sd=2)
tibble(alpha=rnorm(10000,0,4),delta=rnorm(10000,0,2)) |>
  # Rescales to probabilities applying inverse logit
  mutate(pi=exp(alpha+delta)/(1+exp(alpha+delta))) |> select(pi) |>
  # Uses 'bmhe' to summarise the simulations
  bmhe::stats()
```

```
        mean        sd         2.5%    median     97.5%
pi 0.5063376 0.4098462 0.0001353949 0.5208656 0.9998531
```

Once again, when rescaled to the probability range, the distribution for `pi`, which in this case represents the probability of death for a random individual treated with magnesium, does effectively cover the whole [0; 1] range, indicating that even a seemingly informative prior, in this particular case, is vague enough. Figures 6.8a and 6.8b show the resulting prior for each of the π_s, in the placebo and treatment arm, respectively – as is possible to see these distribution resemble closely the Jeffreys' prior discussed in Note 5 in Example 2.5 and shown in Figure 2.10.

Crucially, we allow for sufficient mass at either end of the range (i.e. towards 0 or 1), which should be able to safeguard against marked heterogeneity in the individual studies estimates.

Note 17: The parachute effect

While we do not want to impose too strong priors on the "treatment effect", there is much information that we can use to restrict the reasonable range of a log OR.

For instance, consider an experiment in which we test the effectiveness of parachutes, when jumping off a flying plane. We define our outcome Y as 0 if the individual jumps off the plane and dies and 1 if they survive. The treatment is measured through X_i, taking value 1 if individual i is given a parachute and 0 otherwise.

In a situation such as this, we may expect the treatment to have a very large effect – almost everyone with a parachute can be reasonably expected to survive, while almost (or probably just!) everyone without one is most likely to die. So if we define $\theta_1 = \Pr(Y = 1 \mid X = 1)$ and $\theta_0 = \Pr(Y = 1 \mid X = 0)$, we could reasonably estimate something like $\theta_1 = 0.9$ and $\theta_0 = 0.1$ (the actual numbers are irrelevant – but the magnitude is important and arguably realistic). Thus, in this case the OR would be

$$\begin{aligned} \text{OR} &= \frac{\theta_1}{1-\theta_1} \Big/ \frac{\theta_0}{1-\theta_0} \\ &= \frac{0.9}{1-0.9} \Big/ \frac{0.1}{1-0.1} \\ &= \frac{0.9}{0.1} \Big/ \frac{0.1}{0.9} = 9 \Big/ \frac{1}{9} = 81. \end{aligned} \tag{6.8}$$

This means that people with a parachute are 81 times more likely to survive the jump off the plane than those without a parachute. This massive OR comes about, of course, because of the assumptions we are making about such a large treatment effect – almost everyone without the parachute dies, while almost everyone with survives. In a case such as this, we may be prepared to believe a very large OR. But in most cases, interventions do **not** have such dramatic effects. And thus, it is reasonable to imagine that ORs greater than 3 or perhaps 4 are already relatively unlikely to be observed in practice!

We can write down the JAGS code for the no-pooling assumption as below.

```
no_pooling=function(){
  for(s in 1:S) {
  # Sampling distributions
    r1[s] ~ dbin(pi1[s], n1[s])
    r2[s] ~ dbin(pi2[s], n2[s])
    logit(pi1[s]) <- alpha[s]
    logit(pi2[s]) <- alpha[s] + delta[s]
  # Baselines (NB: sd=4 => precision = 0.0625)
    alpha[s] ~ dnorm(0,0.0625)
  # Study-specific treatment effects (sd=2 => precision = 0.25)
    delta[s] ~ dnorm(0,0.25)
  }
}
```

We can then run the model using R2jags – notice that we specify a function inits() which randomly generates initial values for alpha and delta. In this case, we choose a vector of 16 random draws from a Normal$(0, 1)$. This is not essential (and we could leave the generation of the initial values to JAGS, as we have done in all the examples in Section 5.2), but it is helpful to have the option, particularly for model that are a bit more complex.

Moreover, we use a relatively large number of simulations (10 000) and apply thinning of 1 every 4 simulations (so as to save 4000 iteration at the end of the process) – we do this to combat potential issues with autocorrelation, which we can expect, since we are assuming that each study is modelled independently with no possibility of "borrowing information" from the others. Thus, small studies or those where information is very sparse (e.g. study number 8, where there have been only 1 death in total, with very small sample sizes) will be harder to estimate, given the lack of definitive evidence in the data.

```
# Defines the data list
data=list(r1=r1,r2=r2,n1=n1,n2=n2,S=nrow(trials))

# Initialises the object 'model' as a list to store all the results
model=list()

# Stores the JAGS output
model$no_pooling=jags(
  data=data,
  parameters.to.save=c(
    "alpha","delta"
  ),
  inits=function(){
    list(alpha=rnorm(16,0,.5),delta=rnorm(16,0,.5))
  },n.chains=2,n.iter=10000,n.burnin=2000,n.thin=4,DIC=TRUE,
  model.file=no_pooling
)
```

We can visualise the diagnostic measures for the model, using the `bmhe::diagplot()` function (and customising it using `ggplot2` facilities), as shown in Figure 6.9.

```
# Rhat
bmhe::diagplot(model$no_pooling)

# n.eff
# Highlights all parameters where n.eff < 10% of the nominal sample size (400)
bmhe::diagplot(model$no_pooling,what = "n.eff",label=TRUE) +
  geom_hline(yintercept=400, linetype="dashed") +
  annotate("rect",xmin=-Inf,xmax=Inf,ymin=-Inf,ymax=400,alpha=0.2,fill="gray70")

# Traceplots for selected nodes (below 10% of the nominal number of simulations)
bmhe::traceplot(
  model$no_pooling,parameter=which(
    model$no_pooling$BUGSoutput$summary[,"n.eff"]<400
  ) |> names()
)
```

Figure 6.9a generally indicates satisfactory convergence for the model – looking at the $\hat{R}$ statistic, almost all nodes have values below the cutoff of 1.1. Even with thinning and a long run, autocorrelation seems to impact quite a few parameters, for which the effective sample size is rather low. Figure 6.9b shows the value of the effective sample size for each of the model parameters – we have highlighted in the grey area the few ones with ESS below 10% of the nominal sample size (i.e. 400).

There are not very many of them and thus, on this occasion, we may still be satisfied with the convergence of the model, although perhaps we may want to run for an even longer number of iterations or test different specifications for the priors. This is confirmed by the analysis of the traceplots for these nodes, which is depicted in Figure 6.10, in which all seem reasonably mixing, despite the larger autocorrelation.

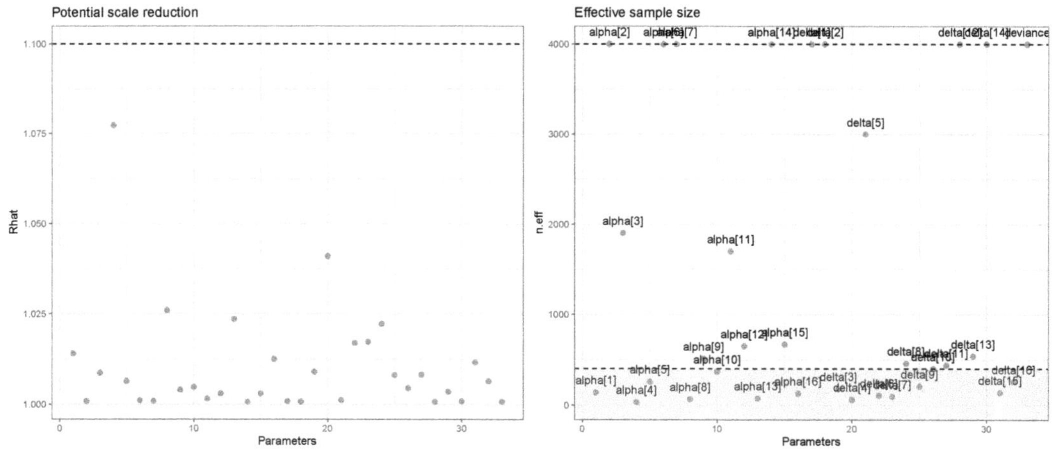

(a) $\hat{R}$. (b) n_{eff}.

Figure 6.9: Model diagnostics for the no-pooling evidence synthesis.

> **The art of setting priors**
>
> Notice that there is nothing special whatsoever to the values of 4 and 2 for the standard deviations of α_s and δ_s – these choices should be dictated by contextual knowledge, as well as subject to substantial sensitivity analysis.
>
> For example, we could use a "lazy" option and set priors for $\alpha_s, \delta_s \stackrel{iid}{\sim} \text{Normal}(0, sd = 100)$. In this case, for most parameters, the choice of priors would not make a difference – not to in a tangible fashion, anyway. However, it is likely that the node `delta[8]` would struggle to converge, if we used a very wide, "non-informative" prior.
>
> This is not entirely surprising: study number 8 (Bertschat) in Table 6.1 has very low numbers of observed deaths (only 1 in the placebo arm and none in the magnesium arm, in correspondence of very small sample sizes too). For this reason, the estimate for the log OR parameter δ_8 can be highly unstable, particularly if we do not "help" by suggesting a reasonable range in the prior, given that we take every study as separate in the no-pooling model.

Example 6.4. *Magnesium (continued): complete-pooling analysis.* We can code up the model in Equations 6.1 and 6.6 into the following `JAGS` code. Notice that we use here the following prior specification: $\alpha_s \sim \text{Normal}(0, sd = 4)$ and $d \sim \text{Normal}(0, sd = 2)$, in line with the model used in Example 6.3.

```
complete_pooling=function() {
  for(s in 1:S) {
  # Sampling distributions
    r1[s] ~ dbin(pi1[s], n1[s])
    r2[s] ~ dbin(pi2[s], n2[s])
  # Model
    logit(pi1[s]) <- alpha[s]
    logit(pi2[s]) <- alpha[s] + d
```

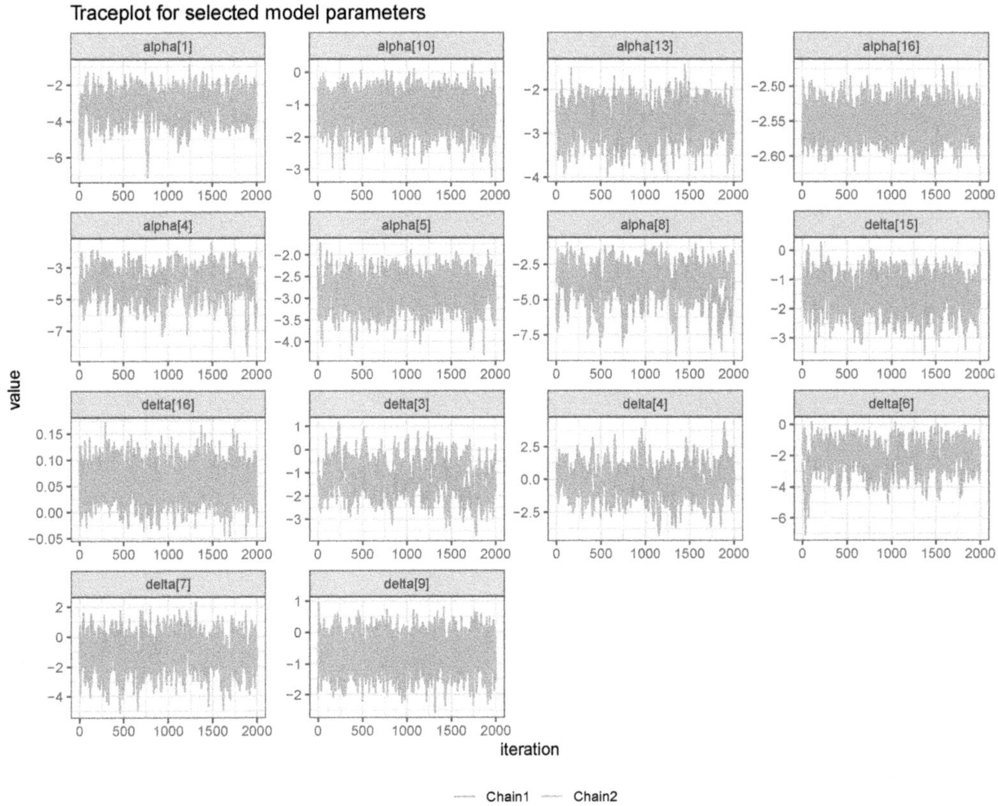

Figure 6.10: Traceplots for the nodes associated with $n_{eff} < 400$ (=10% of the nominal number of iterations saved).

```
  # Baselines
    alpha[s] ~ dnorm(0,0.0625)
  }
  # Priors
  d ~ dnorm(0,0.25)
  OR <- exp(d)
}
```

In addition, now that we have a (rather strong) form of pooling across the various studies, we are able to produce an overall measure of treatment effect. We can simply rescale the parameter d by exponentiating it to obtain an overall OR – the node `OR` indicates the odds ratio for magnesium treatment, or, in other words, a measure of how more likely a random individual is to die if they are treated with magnesium, rather than with placebo.

The model is run using code all but identical to that shown in Example 6.3 – we just change the name of the output to the object `model$complete_pooling` and point the execution of `JAGS` to the function describing the relevant model, `model.file=complete_pooling` in this case. We use again a relatively long run with 40 000 iterations and thinning of 18, to limit the impact of autocorrelation.

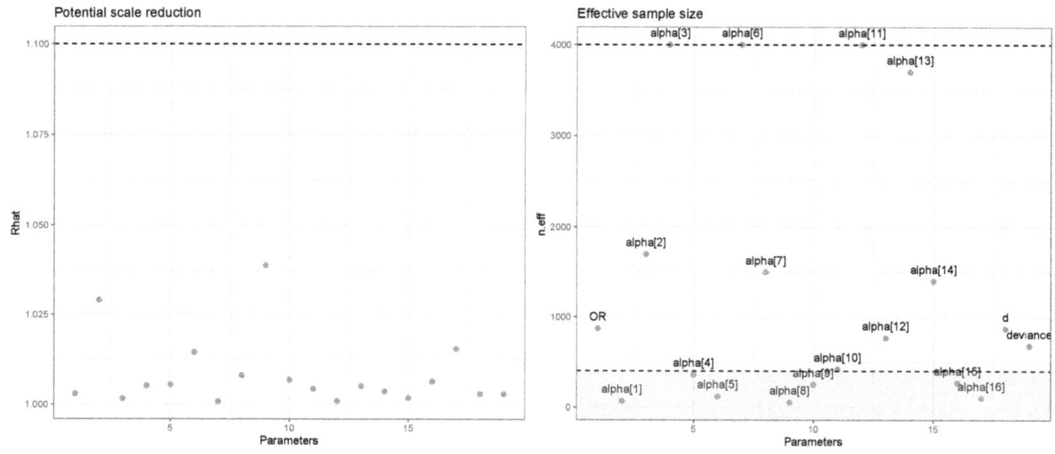

(a) $\hat{R}$. (b) n_{eff}.

Figure 6.11: Model diagnostics for the complete pooling evidence synthesis.

Figure 6.11 shows graphical summaries for the model diagnostics – again, with the selected model specification, convergence is reached (according to the threshold of 1.1 for the $\hat{R}$ statistic) for all nodes. There are a few that are still subject to some substantial autocorrelation – this time only 7 (`alpha[1]`, `alpha[4]`, `alpha[5]`, `alpha[8]`, `alpha[9]`, `alpha[15]` and `alpha[16]`) are below the cutoff of 10% of the nominal sample size, again set at 4000 iterations, but, all in all, we may be satisfied with the model convergence.

Example 6.5. *Magnesium (continued): partial-pooling analysis.* We complete the range of models for the magnesium trials fitting the hierarchical version of Equation 6.7. In this case, we still keep the prior for $\alpha_s \sim \text{Normal}(0, sd = 4)$, implying a precision of 0.0625. As for the structured effects δ_s, we model their standard deviation using a PC prior, encoding the assumption that $\Pr(\sigma_\delta > 1) \approx 0.1$, giving an Exponential(2.31) – see Example 2.5. Finally, the pooled estimate d, which represents the mean around which all the δ_s are distributed, is given a minimally informative prior $\text{Normal}(0, sd = 2)$.

Notice also that, this time, we are able to produce two different pooled summaries. The first one is the same as in Example 6.4, i.e. the pooled OR $= \exp(d)$. The second is based on the predictive distribution of the treatment effects δ_s – this can be interpreted as the prediction for an entirely new study, assumed exchangeable with the 16 analysed thus far. Exponentiating the node `delta.pred` would provide an estimate of the OR for this new study.

The model is defined in the following `R` code

```
partial_pooling=function(){
   for(s in 1:S) {
 # Sampling distributions
   r1[s] ~ dbin(pi1[s], n1[s])
   r2[s] ~ dbin(pi2[s], n2[s])
 # Model
   logit(pi1[s]) <- alpha[s]
```

```
    logit(pi2[s]) <- alpha[s] + delta[s]
  # Baselines
    alpha[s] ~ dnorm(0,0.0625)
  # Random Effects
    delta[s] ~ dnorm(d, prec)
  }
  # Priors
  d ~ dnorm(0,0.25)
  # Pr(sigma.delta>1) \approx 0.1
  sigma.delta ~ dexp(2.31)
  prec <- pow(sigma.delta,-2)
  # Summaries
  OR <- exp(d)
  delta.pred ~ dnorm(d, prec)
}
```

and can be run using code similar to the one used for the previous models. We store the output in an object `model$partial_pooling` and set `model.file=partial_pooling`.

Similarly to the previous analyses, we can check the diagnostics using Figure 6.12.

This time convergence is really not an issue – all nodes show values for $\hat{R}$ well below 1.1 and none of the nodes has an effective sample size that is below 10% of the nominal one. The information is shared across all the studies, through the hierarchical structure.

The model code and discussion above highlights how the partial pooling is effectively a bigger version of the model for evidence synthesis, which includes as special cases the two extremes of no- and complete pooling. In fact, from the model in Equation 6.7 we can derive the complete pooling by setting

$$\delta_s \sim \text{Normal}(d, \sigma_\delta = 0)$$

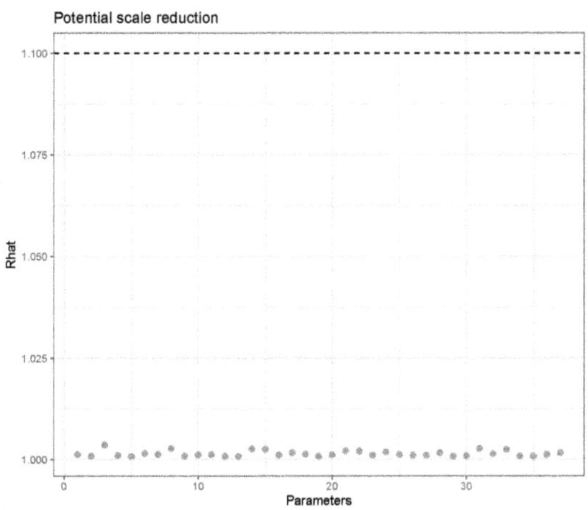

(a) $\hat{R}$

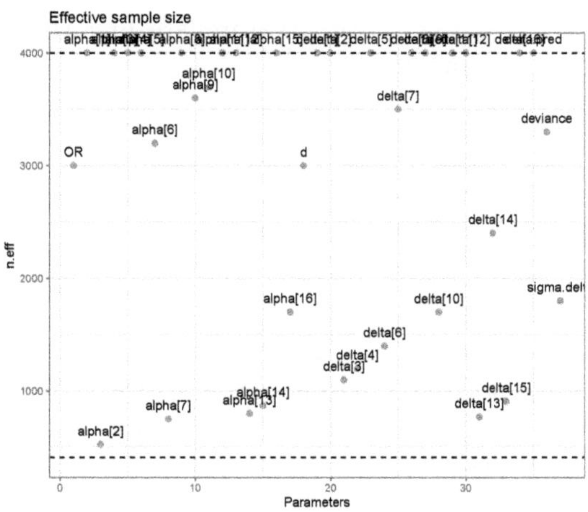

(b) n_{eff}

Figure 6.12: Model diagnostics for the partial pooling evidence synthesis.

— if the standard deviation in the distribution of the structured effects is 0, then there is no variability across them and so each one of them is identical with their mean, d, exactly as in Equation 6.6.

Similarly, if we set

$$\delta_s \sim \text{Normal}(d, \sigma_\delta \to \infty)$$

then the variations across the structured effects are so large that each δ_s is different from the others and, crucially, they become unrelated – just like in Equation 6.5.

6.2.5 When should we use hierarchical models?

Intuitively, the discussion above suggests that we probably are better off at least testing a hierarchical version of the model: if the data provide no evidence for pooling, then the model will respond by estimating $\sigma_\delta \to \infty$; if on the other hand, the data indicate little or no heterogeneity, then, in the posterior, $\sigma_\delta \to 0$. The strong assumptions encoded in either of the two extreme versions of the model are much less flexible.

Of course, if we only have a small number of groups (e.g. studies) to pool across, then using hierarchical models becomes a bit more complicated, because we would have very little information to estimate the standard deviation σ_δ. Gelman and Hill (2007) suggest that we need at least 3 groups for a "vanilla" hierarchical model to work – this is of course sensible, because with only 2 data points, any estimate for a standard deviation is highly unstable.

From a purely Bayesian perspective, however, even low number of groups does not pose an impossibility to the use of partial pooling – this simply means that the information present in the data is sparse and, as such, in order to have consistent inference, we need to complement it with strong prior assumptions. More importantly, generally speaking, we need to be careful when setting models for the standard deviation of the "random effects" – unless we have a large amount of data over a large number of groups, we probably will not be able to get away with lazy, vague priors.

For instance, a model with $\sigma_\delta \sim \text{Uniform}(0, K)$ for some constant K is often suggested and used in applied work. Again, this may work well if there is enough information in the data and, more importantly, if this information is strong enough to "travel against the arrow" in Figure 6.5 – there is a long way from the evidence in the bottom layer of the DAG (the data $y_{1s}, y_{2s}, \ldots, y_{n_s s}$) to update first the "level 1" parameters $(\theta_1, \ldots, \theta_S)$ and then the hyper-parameter ϕ.

A subtle artifact of using this modelling structure with insufficient data/groups is that, in the posterior, σ_δ will tend to push to the upper range of the Uniform. Thus, in the absence of firm evidence, a model with this prior will probably have a posterior for the standard deviation of the hyper-parameter highly concentrated towards K – but note that, of course, no matter what the data say, a Uniform prior will not allow the posterior to have any mass outside of the range ($[0; K]$, in this case).

The PC prior that we have used in Example 6.5 is certainly a good compromise, because while not implying unduly strength in the prior, it manages to stabilise the inference and does allow for values that are larger than where most of the mass is, in the prior. We thus recommend the use of this formulation and discourage other options, such as the conjugate vague $\text{Gamma}(\varepsilon, \varepsilon)$ on the precision scale, for a small constant ε (say 0.001), or the $\text{Uniform}(0, K)$ for the standard deviation – see Note 18 below, for a more detailed discussion.

Another useful alternative is the Half Cauchy model with location $\mu = 0$ and scale λ, suggested by (Gelman, 2006), which is often implemented as the default in `Stan`. This is equivalent to modelling

$$\sigma_\delta \sim \text{Cauchy}(\mu = 0, \lambda)\mathbb{I}(0, \infty),$$

where, in general

$$y \sim \text{Cauchy}(\mu, \lambda) \quad \Rightarrow \quad p(y \mid \mu, \lambda) = \pi\lambda \left(1 + \left(\frac{y-\mu}{\lambda}\right)^2\right)^{-1} \tag{6.9}$$

(with the Half Cauchy, we restrict the expression in Equation 6.9 to $\mathbb{R}^+$, as we are modelling a standard deviation) – see Example 7.3 for more detailed discussion. Gelman and Hill (2007, p. 428) also provide more details on the definition and use of Half Cauchy distributions in hierarchical models.

Note 18: The problem with Gamma priors on the precision

A Gamma(α, β) prior on the precision (defined as in Equation 1.2) implies

$$\sigma^2 \sim \text{Inverse-Gamma}(\alpha, \beta) \quad \Rightarrow \quad p(\sigma^2) = \frac{\beta^\alpha}{\Gamma(\alpha)} \sigma^{-2(\alpha+1)} \exp\left(-\frac{\beta}{\sigma^2}\right) \tag{6.10}$$

– we can derive this applying the change of variable rule in Equation 1.14 with $\sigma^2 = 1/\tau$. As $(\alpha, \beta) \to 0$, this becomes a proper version (i.e. it still integrates to 1 over the range of σ^2) of the Jeffreys' prior $p(\sigma^2) \propto \frac{1}{\sigma^2}$ (see the general discussion in Note 5 in Example 2.5).

Together with the fact that a Gamma is conjugated for a precision (see Equation 2.9 and Example 2.7), this has made Equation 6.10 a popular choice to give a conjugate, vague prior to model precisions/variances, often used uncritically in applied work, especially early on in the `BUGS` revolution of the 1990s.

In the context of hierarchical modelling, however, Gelman (2006) has shown that there are some potential pitfalls to this particular choice. Applying again Equation 1.14, we can derive the implied prior on the scale of the standard deviation, using the following relationships:

$$\sigma = \frac{1}{\sqrt{\tau}} \Rightarrow \tau = \frac{1}{\sigma^2} = \sigma^{-2},$$

which imply that

$$\begin{aligned}
\left|\frac{\partial \sigma^{-2}}{\partial \sigma}\right| = \left|-2\sigma^{-3}\right| = 2\sigma^{-3} \Rightarrow p(\sigma) &= \frac{\beta^\alpha}{\Gamma(\alpha)} \sigma^{-2(\alpha-1)} \exp\left(-\frac{\beta}{\sigma^2}\right) 2\sigma^{-3} \\
&= \frac{2\beta^\alpha}{\Gamma(\alpha)} \sigma^{-(2\alpha+1)} \exp\left(-\frac{\beta}{\sigma^2}\right) \\
&\propto \sigma^{-(2\alpha+1)} \exp\left(-\frac{\beta}{\sigma^2}\right).
\end{aligned}$$

This formulation tends to have extremely heavy right tail, which in turn implies that very large values of σ are highly probable. When data are directly observed to estimate the variance parameter, this may not matter much. But in the case of hierarchical models, the parameter of interest (e.g. σ_δ) is only informed *indirectly* by the data – see Figure 6.5, which may lead to unintended (and dangerous) consequences.

This is because the use of (an approximation to) the Jeffreys' formulation for the precision means that, while we do not mean to imply a strong prior near 0 (and thus towards large values for the variance (see the discussion in Note 5 in Example 2.5), the Bayesian machinery takes this information at face value and the standard deviation may be unduly pulled towards large values, implying excess of heterogeneity – cfr. Section 6.2.5.

We can easily check using Monte Carlo forward sampling, as with the following code.

```
# Simulates from the prior for the precision
tau=rgamma(10000,shape=0.001,rate=0.001)
# Computes tail-area probabilities
sum(tau>0.001)/length(tau)
```

```
[1] 0.0141
```

Under this formulation for the precision, there is very, very little chance of exceeding values as small as 0.001! Consequently, as the whole distribution for the precision is highly concentrated towards 0, the resulting distribution for σ will exhibit a large number of large values and thus a model based on this assumption will often infer a very large standard deviation, even when the data show little support to it.

Conversely, while still allowing to control for the amount of mass placed above a certain threshold, e.g. in our case $\Pr(\sigma_\delta > 1)$, using a Half-Cauchy or a PC prior tends to spread the mass over a large enough range of possible values, while leaving the posterior free to move towards specific values, given the support from the data. In addition to this, by being directly defined on the scale of interest, it is easier to include even minimal information and thus we prefer and recommend it, at least as a default choice.

6.2.6 Model selection

As we have seen in Section 5.3, one simple criterion to perform model selection, or at any rate, to assess the performance of competing models in terms of fitting to the same data, is to use the DIC. Because in all the examples above, we have used 2 chains to run the Gibbs sampling via `JAGS`, this is automatically computed and stored, together with the penalty.

We can extract the penalty and the DIC from an object `x` generated by a call to `R2jags::jags()` simply calling the elements `x$BUGSoutput$pD` and `x$BUGSoutput$DIC`. For the three models stored in the elements of the object `model`, created in Example 6.3 and then populated in Examples 6.4 and 6.5, the resulting values are presented in Table 6.2.

As is possible to see, the values are substantially different across the three models – the partial pooling model has values for the DIC smaller than for the other two models. This

Table 6.2: The values for the DIC and the penalty p_V (see Equation 5.15), together with $\overline{D(\boldsymbol{\theta})}$ and its standard deviation, for the three models described above.

Model	p_V	DIC	$\mathrm{E}\left[D(\boldsymbol{\theta})\right]$	$\mathrm{sd}\left[D(\boldsymbol{\theta})\right]$
No-pooling	30.20	177.93	147.74	7.77
Complete pooling	16.14	211.14	195.00	5.69
Partial pooling	26.38	173.47	147.10	7.26

indeed indicates a better performance of the hierarchical model, particularly against the complete pooling model.

Ultimately, the analysis of Table 6.2 strongly suggests that the partial pooling model should be used here, to cope with the inherent heterogeneity across the studies. We can also compute the penalty as p_D (as in Equation 5.14), which provides a more direct assessment of the amount of correlation across the structured effects, which the model is able to detect.

6.2.7 Borrowing information

Intuitively, the no-pooling model of Example 6.3 has a nominal number of parameters equal to the sum of the number of α_s parameters and the number of δ_s parameters, resulting in $16+16=32$. This is because they are the only parameters included in the model and there is no sharing of information/correlation implied.

At the other extreme, the complete pooling model of Example 6.4 has 16 α_s parameters in addition to the pooled effect, d and thus, in total, 17 parameters, nominally.

For the partial pooling model of Example 6.5, things are a bit more complicated: there are 16 α_s, as well as, *nominally*, 16 δ_s in addition to the pooled log OR, d, the predicted log OR (d_{pred}) and the standard deviation of the structured effects σ_δ. At face value, we thus have 35 parameters. However, because we are implying correlation across the δ_s, through the hierarchical structure, the number of *effective* parameters (which is estimated by p_D – but, in general, not by p_V; recall the discussion in Section 5.3) is generally reduced. The amount of "shrinkage", i.e. how many effective parameters are saved by the hierarchical structure, is a measure of how much correlation the model is able to pick up.

Counting the number of stochastic nodes

Notice that when running `R2jags::jags()`, if the option `quiet` is set to `FALSE`, which is the default, a very helpful summary message is printed out at the point of compiling the model – this is when `JAGS` converts the model file into a DAG (see Section 3.1.1). For example, for the partial pooling model this would look like the following,

```
Compiling model graph
   Resolving undeclared variables
   Allocating nodes
Graph information:
   Observed stochastic nodes: 32
   Unobserved stochastic nodes: 35
   Total graph size: 156

Initializing model
```

which reports the number of modelled data (`Observed stochastic nodes`) as well as the number of "face-value" parameters (`Unobserved stochastic nodes`).

Example 6.6. *Magnesium (continued): analysis and model comparison.* As discussed in Section 5.3, we can compute an approximation to the version of the penalty defined in Equation 5.14 using the function `rjags::dic.samples()`, which returns the estimated p_D (`penalty`) and the resulting DIC (`Penalized deviance`) – notice however, that we can

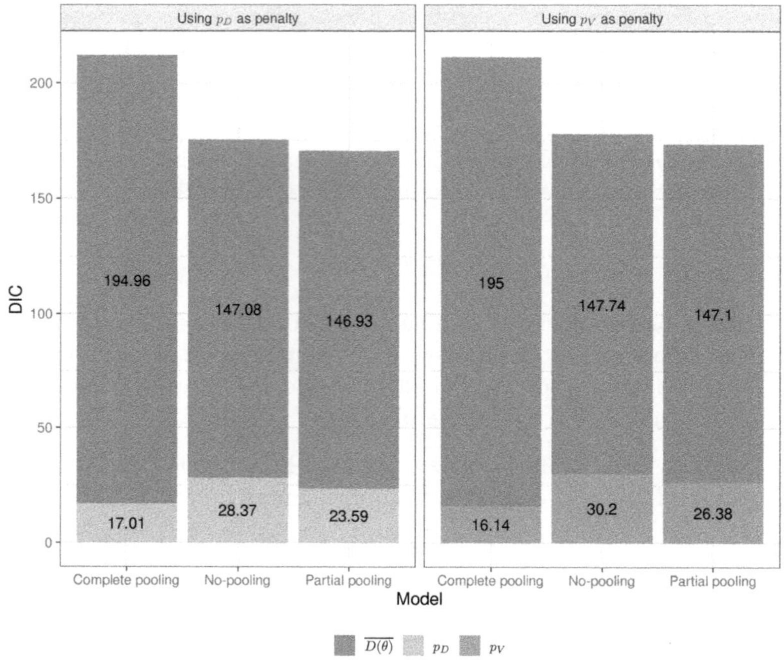

Figure 6.13: Total value for the DIC, portioned into the mean deviance, $\overline{D(\boldsymbol{\theta})}$ and the model penalty for the three models.

compute both versions of the penalty by adding the input `pD=TRUE` to the call to the function `R2jags::jags()`.

Figure 6.13 shows the overall value for the DIC for the three models, partitioned into the contribution of the average deviance, $\overline{D(\boldsymbol{\theta})}$ and the estimate of the effective number of parameters, p_D. As it is often (but not necessarily always) the case, the estimates for p_V and p_D are fairly aligned with very minimal numerical differences.

The value of p_D for the partial pooling model indicates that the effective number of parameters (23.59) is substantially lower than the nominal one (35), by effect of the implied correlation and borrowing of information among the δ_s. This is also in line with p_V, as reported in Table 6.2.

Note 19: Model averaging

In line with the discussion in Section 5.3.5, instead of simply selecing the "best" model, we could instead use the resulting values for the DIC to combine them, in a model average-framework. We can use the following `R` code to determine the weights associated with each of the three versions of the model described above.

```
# Extracts the DIC values from the list 'model'
dic=unlist(lapply(model,function(x) x$BUGSoutput$DIC))
# Computes the absolute difference in DIC vs the model with lowest value
delta.dic=abs(min(dic)-dic)
# Computes the weights
(exp(-.5*delta.dic)/sum(exp(-.5*delta.dic))) |> format(scientific=FALSE)
```

```
         no_pooling    complete_pooling     partial_pooling
"0.097032364701307" "0.000000005975042" "0.902967629323651"
```

First, we extract the value of the DIC from each of the three models, stored in the list `model`; then we construct the values for ΔDIC_h for each of the $H = 3$ options and then apply Equation 5.18 to compute the weights.

As is possible to see, in this case, the mixture is a bit more meaningful: the partial pooling model still drives the model average (with a weight of around 0.9); however, because the difference in DIC between the partial pooling and the complete pooling is around 4.5, in line with Figure 5.6, the latter has a non-negligible weight of around 0.1.

Table 6.3 shows some summary comparison of the complete vs partial pooling model. Interestingly, when assuming no heterogeneity in the trials, the effect of magnesium disappears – the OR is virtually 1 and the 95% interval is relatively narrow and spanning across 1. This is highly influenced by the ISIS-4 trial, which is by far the largest and with a result at odds with most of the other trials.

When allowing for the possibility of heterogeneous effects with the partial pooling model, the results change dramatically, with magnesium now being substantially protective. The posterior mean OR of death is 0.43 (i.e. an average reduction in the odds of death of around 57%) and the entire 95% interval is below 1.

Figure 6.14 shows an analysis of the magnesium effect across the three models. In some cases, the estimates for the log OR from the no- and partial pooling are fairly similar – that is the case for trials with large sample size. However, for those with weaker evidence (e.g. δ_4), the no-pooling model shows much larger uncertainty. This is because the estimate is based only on that small study, while for the partial pooling model, it benefits from the information coming from the other larger studies.

As mentioned above, another interesting point is that the complete pooling model is highly influenced by ISIS-4, which is by far the largest study. The estimate for d is pooled towards the estimate for δ_{16}. However, the partial pooling model mitigates this and the posterior distribution for d is more balanced and influenced by the combined evidence present in the other 15 trials.

Finally, we also show the estimate for the predictive distribution δ_{pred}: unsurprisingly, this is more or less centred around the same mean as d, but with larger variance. This is because the best estimate for a future trial is essentially given by the average of what has been observed so far – but we are more uncertain because the new study has not been observed yet.

Figure 6.15 shows the amount of "shrinkage" – that is the phenomenon whereby the estimates are pulled towards the grand mean (d). Again, for smaller study, the amount of

Table 6.3: Summary statistics for the evidence synthesis of the magnesium studies, for the complete and partial pooling models

Model	OR (95% interval)	Between study sd (σ_δ)	$\overline{D(\boldsymbol{\theta})}$	p_D	DIC
Complete pooling	1 (0.95; 1.07)	—	195.0	17.01	212.01
Partial pooling	0.43 (0.25; 0.64)	0.61 (0.32; 1.03)	147.1	23.59	170.69

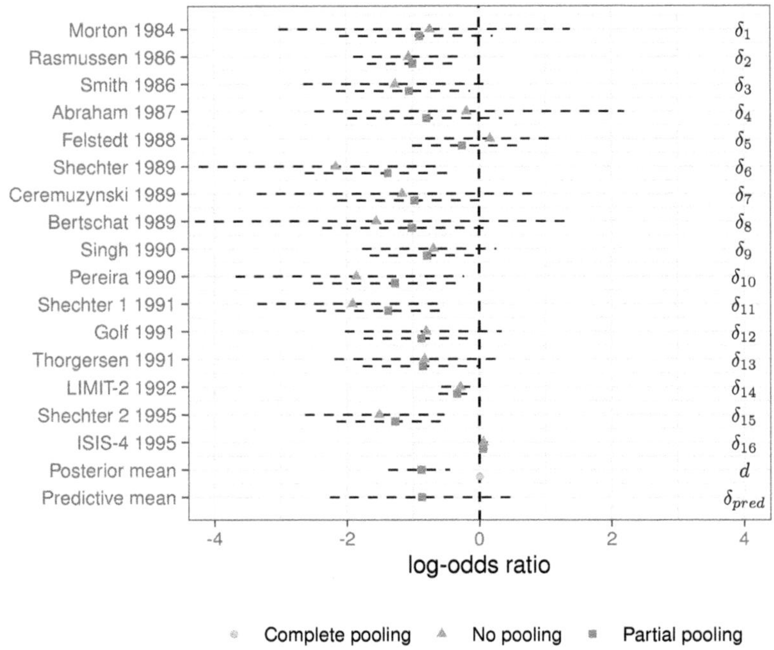

Figure 6.14: Comparison of the three versions of the model in terms of posterior estimates for the log OR. The dots represent the posterior mean, while the dashed segments indicate the 95% posterior intervals.

pulling is larger – it is possible to see that the arrow from the no- to the partial pooling for, say, study number 4 (which only has around 50 individuals in each arm) is much longer than for, say, study number 16 (ISIS-4), for which there is basically no difference in the two estimates.

6.3 Evidence synthesis and economic modelling

We can use the principles described above and extend the statistical modelling to the actual economic evaluation, by further combining the estimates for the model parameters so as to obtain relevant measures of population average benefit and costs.

Generally speaking, when the inputs are made by ALD, the process can be divided into the following steps. First, we build a population level model, for example using decision trees or Markov models (see Chapter 9), to represent the "natural history of the disease". This is typically a simplified version of the underlying reality, which we use to describe how individuals may be affected by a given disease.

Again, in general terms, there is no reason why the actual data might not comprise of a combination of individual- and aggregated-level data: for instance, we may have access to a full dataset (as in Example 5.1 and throughout Chapter 5) that can inform some of the

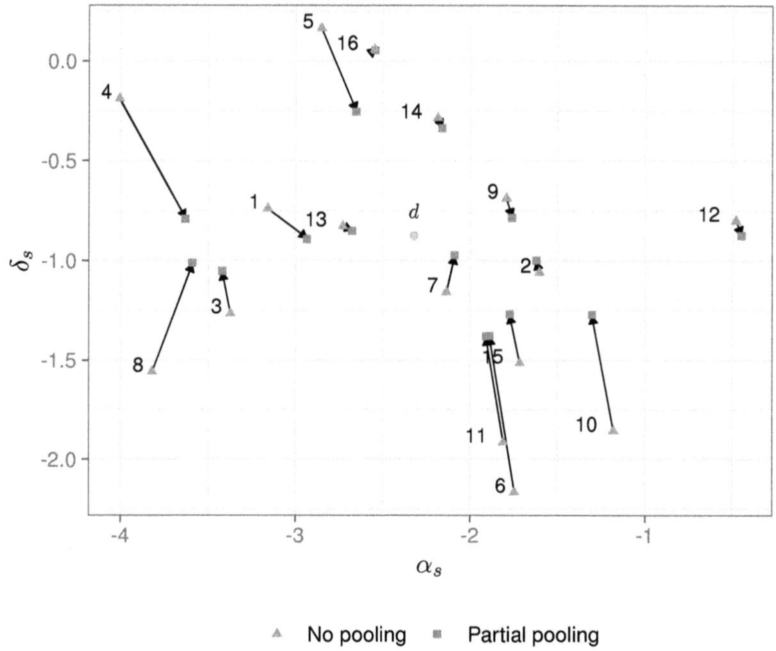

Figure 6.15: Posterior means for the model parameters. The dot labelled as d is the grand-mean estimated from the partial pooling model. The arrows indicate the amount of shrinkage induced by the partial pooling model, in comparison to the no pooling model.

relevant parameters, but only summary statistics for others. Even more realistically, we may have access to a number of studies that we can use to inform our final estimate and then propagate the resulting uncertainty all the way to the decision process, as we demonstrate in Example 6.7.

Example 6.7. *Influenza (adapted and expanded from Cooper et al., 2004).* Neuraminidase inhibitors (NIs) are a class of antiviral drugs that provide additional potential strategies for the control of influenza. The objective of this analysis is to build an economic model to determine the cost-effectiveness of the prophylaxis with NI, compared to a "status quo" in which no other treatment is available. Figure 6.16 shows a decision tree, in which we assume that the only relevant uncertainty is about whether people can be infected by influenza or not. Depending on the treatment that they are given, this happens with different probabilities (say, p_2 under the active treatment arm, or p_1, in case the prophylaxis is not applied/available).

In reality, the underlying clinical pathways may be much more complicated – for instance, here, we do not consider complications, other adverse events, etc., but, in line with Cooper et al. (2004), do limit the analysis to this much simplified version of the problem.

Evidence synthesis for the relative effectiveness of NIs

Cooper et al. (2004) consider a number of $S = 6$ randomised trials comparing the use of NIs against no prophylaxis to reduce the incidence of influenza (specifically the A and B types) during an epidemic.

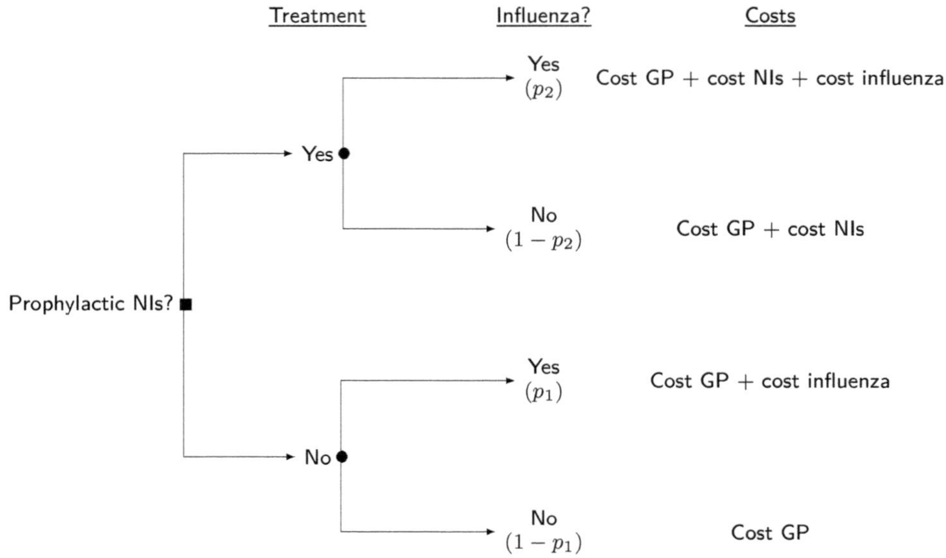

Figure 6.16: A decision tree describing the influenza problem. In the extremely simplified situation, individuals may or may not get influenza (with probability p_2 and p_1 in the case where prophylactic NIs are or are not available) and the costs accrue accordingly.

The data are shown in Table 6.4 and can be modelled in a similar way to the ones used in Example 6.1, i.e. $r_{st} \sim \text{Binomial}(\pi_{st}, n_{st})$, for $s = 1, \ldots, S = 6$ studies and $t = 1, 2$ treatment arms. The linear predictor is modelled as

$$\text{logit}(\pi_{s1}) = \alpha_s \qquad \text{and} \qquad \text{logit}(\pi_{s2}) = \alpha_s + \delta_s,$$

where α_s is a study-specific log event (i.e. baseline risk of influenza) rate in the placebo group, while δ_s is the study-specific log OR, quantifying the effect of the prophylaxis.

Table 6.4: The original data from the $S = 6$ studies on the relative effectiveness of NIs prophylaxis, considered in Cooper et al. (2004). The full list of studies is also presented in Turner et al. (2003)

		Placebo		NIs	
Study	Age group	Total n_1	Cases r_1	Total n_2	Cases r_2
Monto et al. (1999)	18-64	554	34	553	11
Hayden et al. (2000)	5+	423	40	414	7
Kaiser et al. (2000)	13-65	144	9	144	3
Hayden et al. (1999)	18-65	268	19	268	3
Hayden et al. (1999)	18-65	251	6	252	3
Welliver et al. (2001)	12-85	462	34	493	4

We slightly modify the original analysis in Cooper et al. (2004) and complete our evidence synthesis model with the following assumptions:

$$\begin{aligned}\alpha_s &\sim \text{Normal}(0, \text{sd} = 10)\\ \delta_s &\sim \text{Normal}(\mu_\delta, \sigma_\delta)\\ \mu_\delta &\sim \text{Normal}(0, \text{sd} = 10)\\ \sigma_\delta &\sim \text{Exponential}(\lambda_\delta).\end{aligned}$$

In this specification, the baseline risk α_s are modelled independently (no-pooling), while the treatment effect δ_s is modelled using partial pooling; thus, OR $= \exp(\mu_\delta)$ represents the pooled OR overall relative treatment effect.

Evidence synthesis for the underlying probability of influenza in the adult population

In addition to the S head-to-head comparisons for NIs vs placebo, there are data from $H = 9$ randomised studies in which the control arm (placebo) can be used to measure the incidence of influenza among healthy adults, in terms of number of observed cases $\boldsymbol{y} = (y_1, \ldots, y_H) = (0, 6, 5, 6, 25, 18, 14, 3, 27)$ over the total sample size $\boldsymbol{m} = (m_1, \ldots, m_H) = (23, 241, 159, 137, 519, 298, 137, 24, 132)$.

Again, we slightly modify the model originally presented in Cooper et al. (2004) and assume $y_h \sim \text{Binomial}(\theta_h, m_h)$ with

$$\begin{aligned}\text{logit}(\theta_h) = \beta_h &\sim \text{Normal}(\mu_\beta, \sigma_\beta)\\ \mu_\beta &\sim \text{Normal}(0, \text{sd} = 10)\\ \sigma^2_\beta &\sim \text{Exponential}(\lambda_\beta).\end{aligned}$$

Rescaling μ_β allows us to obtain an estimate of the pooled baseline probability of influenza infection for a random individual of the general population, i.e. in case no treatment is available, i.e.

$$p_1 = \frac{\exp(\mu_\beta)}{1 + \exp(\mu_\beta)} \quad \Leftrightarrow \quad \text{logit}(p_1) = \mu_\beta.$$

Pooling all background information

In the model described above, the parameters α_s and β_h are modelled as two separate and independent processes: in the case of the baseline risks for the S head-to-head studies, we apply no-pooling, while we pool together the other H studies to estimate the background probability of influenza $p_1 = \text{logit}^{-1}(\mu_\beta)$.

We could use a slightly different version of the model, in which also the baseline risk α_s are modelled using partial pooling across the S studies, which could be achieved by assuming the following structure

$$\begin{aligned}\alpha_s &\sim \text{Normal}(\mu_\alpha, \sigma_\alpha)\\ \mu_\alpha &\sim \text{Normal}(0, \text{sd} = 10)\\ \sigma_\alpha &\sim \text{Exponential}(\lambda_\alpha).\end{aligned}$$

In this case, we would also estimate a pooled background risk of influenza (μ_α). This specification would relax the original assumption that the S head-to-head studies are effectively too heterogeneous in their definition of the placebo arm (and hence not pooled at all), while allowing for some shrinkage in the estimates for the α_s parameters. Even in this case, however, the parameters α_s and β_h would be modelled separately.

On the one hand, this separation may be justified, for instance if we think that there may be strict inclusion criteria for the S head-to-head studies that perhaps do not really match those that characterise the H studies from which we gather evidence to estimate the baseline probability p_1. Perhaps, the head-to-head studies are very specific and therefore we do not want to use them to inform a parameter that is supposed to work at the general population level.

On the other hand, we may in fact think that, in reality, the $(S + H)$ studies are all fairly similar, at least in their definition of the placebo arm and, if that is the case, we may be willing to actually model α_s and β_h as exchangeable – in other words to assume that they have a common data-generating process, e.g.

$$\alpha_s, \beta_h \sim \text{Normal}(\mu_\beta, \sigma_\beta).$$

If this assumption is reasonable, we would probably gain some precision in the resulting estimate for p_2, because it would be based on a larger number of data points. Of course, if the two sets of studies are actually quite heterogeneous, we may not be willing to assume exchangeability among the main parameters and be better off modelling them separately (although as exchangeable within the two modules).

We can combine the two modules and apply the estimated treatment effect (OR) from the first evidence synthesis to the baseline probability p_1, estimated in the second module. As by definition the OR is the ratio of two probability odds, e.g. $\dfrac{p_2}{1-p_2} = \text{OR}\dfrac{p_1}{1-p_1}$, then taking logs on both sides we obtain

$$\begin{aligned}\text{logit}(p_2) = \log\left(\frac{p_2}{1-p_2}\right) &= \log\left(\text{OR}\frac{p_1}{1-p_1}\right) \\ &= \log\text{OR} + \log\left(\frac{p_1}{1-p_1}\right) \\ &= \log\text{OR} + \text{logit}(p_1).\end{aligned}$$

In a Bayesian context, this of course means that we propagate the uncertainty in the estimates for OR and p_1 all the way to the implied posterior distribution for p_2.

Baseline-risk adjustment

The original model in Cooper et al. (2004) considers a slightly different structure for the evidence synthesis on the S head-to-head trials, where the linear predictor for the treatment arm is

$$\text{logit}(\pi_{s2}) = \alpha_s + \delta_s^* + \gamma(\alpha_s - \bar{\alpha}).$$

In this formulation, the study-specific log OR is then $\delta_s = \delta_s^* + \gamma(\alpha_s + \bar{\alpha})$, where $\delta_s^* \sim \text{Normal}(\mu_\delta, \sigma_\delta)$ is a study-specific treatment effect, while $\gamma(\alpha_s - \bar{\alpha})$ is used to adjust for differences in the study-specific background risk. In this model, μ_δ is the pooled treatment effect – this is obtained for a hypothetical study in which the baseline risk is identical to the underlying average and thus the term $(\alpha_s - \bar{\alpha})$ is 0.

While, in general, this adjustment may be important and reduce bias (Welton et al., 2012, pp. 107–109), when the underlying data are reasonably consistent, there may not be any material difference, in practice.

Cost and benefit parameters

Following Cooper et al. (2004), we consider that the course of prophylaxis assumes 6 weeks of daily treatment at a cost of £2.4 per day and thus, assuming VAT at 17.5%, a total $c^{NI} = £118.44$, as well as a fixed cost $c^{GP} = £19$ for a GP visit. As indicated in Figure 6.16 and in line with the original analysis in Cooper et al. (2004), we assume that even in the case where NIs are not prescribed, there is a background GP visit (and hence a cost of c^{GP} even in the bottom branch of the decision tree).

As for the cost of treating a case of influenza (including GP visits, outpatient visits and inpatient stays but not time off work, for adults), we should account for the individual variance. Official resource use data suggest that the average total cost is £16.78 and a standard deviation of £2.34. We can use these values to define an informative prior to model the total cost of treatment for influenza, for example using $c^{Inf} \sim \text{Normal}(\text{mean} = 16.78, \text{sd} = 2.34)$.

Technically, the Normal distribution is not the most appropriate for a quantity that must be positive, but given the values for the mean and standard deviation, the chance of this quantity being negative is effectively non-existent – and to be precise, this can be computed as `pnorm(0,16.78,2.34)=0`, which for all intents and purposes *is* 0.

The final element included in the model is the average duration of the influenza infection. Cooper et al. (2004) models this as $l \sim \text{log-Normal}(\mu_l, \sigma_l)$, where the mean and standard deviation (μ_l, σ_l) are selected so that on the natural scale the mean is 8.2 and the standard deviation is 2 days. We can use the function `lognPar()` from the package `bmhe` to map the natural scale values to the log scale

```
mu.l=bmhe::lognPar(8.2,2)$mulog
sigma.l=bmhe::lognPar(8.2,2)$sigmalog
```

and the resulting values are computed at $\mu_l = 2.0752411$ and $\sigma_l = 0.2403875$.

`JAGS` modelling and analysis

The modelling assumptions described above can be embedded in the code listed below. Notice that we use a PC prior Exponential(1.65) for all the standard deviations of the structured effects α_s, β_h and δ_s, to imply $\Pr(\sigma_\alpha > 1) = \Pr(\sigma_\beta > 1) = \Pr(\sigma_\delta > 1) \approx 0.2$ (see Section 2.2.3). In line with the discussion of Section 6.2.5, we avoid the use of the Gamma(0.001, 0.001) for the various precisions τ_δ, which was used in the original model of Cooper et al. (2004)

Another difference in our setup is for the prior selected for μ_β, which in the original formulation has a very large value for the standard deviation (1 000 000). We change this too to a value of 10 – the underlying parameter is modelled on the logit scale and a standard deviation of 10 still implies a very large variance, when rescaled to the probability range $[0; 1]$.

```
influenza=function() {
  # 1. Evidence synthesis of relative effectiveness vs placebo
  for (s in 1:S) {
```

```
    # Placebo arm
    r1[s] ~ dbin(pi1[s],n1[s])
    logit(pi1[s]) <- alpha[s]
    # NIs arm
    r2[s] ~ dbin(pi2[s],n2[s])
    logit(pi2[s]) <- alpha[s] + delta[s]
    # Study-specific baseline probability of influenza (logit scale)
    alpha[s] ~ dnorm(0,0.1)
    # Study-specific log-OR for NIs
    delta[s] ~ dnorm(mu.delta,tau.delta)
  }
  # Pooled log-OR for NIs vs placebo
  mu.delta ~ dnorm(0,0.1)
  # Prior on the sd of delta[s]
  sigma.delta ~ dexp(1.65);   tau.delta <- pow(sigma.delta,-2)
  # Pooled log-OR for NI vs placebo
  or <- exp(mu.delta)

  # 2. Evidence synthesis for incidence of influenza
  for (h in 1:H) {
    y[h] ~ dbin(theta[h],m[h])
    logit(theta[h]) <- beta[h]
    beta[h] ~ dnorm(mu.beta,tau.beta)
  }
  # Pooled influenza incidence among adults (with no NIs) on the logit scale
  mu.beta ~ dnorm(0,0.1)
  # Prior on the sd of beta[h]
  sigma.beta ~ dexp(1.65);   tau.beta <- pow(sigma.beta,-2)

  # 3. Probability of influenza with and without NIs
  # Rescaled pooled probability of influenza without NIs
  logit(p1) <- mu.beta
  # Rescaled probability of influenza with NIs
  logit(p2) <- logit(p1) + mu.delta

  # 4. Outcomes
  # Model for the costs of treating influenza (prec = 1/2.34^2 = 0.1826)
  c.inf ~ dnorm(16.78,0.1826)
  # Duration of infection (prec = 1/0.2403^2 = 17.3051)
  l ~ dlnorm(2.075,17.3051)
}
```

We can then construct a data list using the values in Table 6.4 and for the variables $\boldsymbol{y}$, $\boldsymbol{m}$, H and S and then call the function `jags()` to run the model and save the output in the object `flu`, say. We use 25 000 iterations, with a burn-in of 5000 and thinning of 1 every 10 iterations, to limit the potential impact of autocorrelation.

The resulting estimates are shown in the table below.

```
Inference for Bugs model at "/tmp/RtmpRoDBAn/modelf8d70fdc9ab7.txt",
 2 chains, each with 25000 iterations (first 5000 discarded), n.thin = 10
```

```
n.sims = 4000 iterations saved. Running time = 1.218 secs
         mu.vect sd.vect   2.5%    25%     50%     75%   97.5% Rhat n.eff
c.inf     16.816   2.333 12.246 15.207  16.796  18.382  21.347 1.001  4000
l          8.213   1.955  5.016  6.816   7.997   9.402  12.669 1.001  4000
or         0.210   0.058  0.119  0.171   0.204   0.240   0.342 1.002  1200
p1         0.062   0.019  0.032  0.049   0.059   0.071   0.104 1.001  4000
p2         0.014   0.006  0.006  0.010   0.013   0.016   0.028 1.002  2000
deviance 102.777   6.010 92.897 98.518 102.121 106.340 116.505 1.001  4000

For each parameter, n.eff is a crude measure of effective sample size,
and Rhat is the potential scale reduction factor (at convergence, Rhat=1).

DIC info (using the rule: pV = var(deviance)/2)
pV = 18.1 and DIC = 120.8
DIC info (using the rule: pD = Dbar-Dhat, computed via 'rjags::dic.samples')
pD = 15.3 and DIC = 117.7
DIC is an estimate of expected predictive error (lower deviance is better).
```

The diagnostic measures are satisfactory for all the major nodes included in the analysis. In particular, we see that the baseline pooled probability of influenza is estimated at 0.062 with a 95% posterior interval [0.032; 0.104], whereas the probability of infection in the NIs prophylaxis arm is estimated at a much lower value 0.014 with a 95% posterior interval [0.006; 0.028].

We can also run the version of the model in which α_s and β_h are modelled as exchangeable (i.e. pooling together *all* the information on the background risk of influenza) – this is easy to do by simply ensuring that the two sets of parameters have the same data-generating process, e.g. by modifying the code above to `alpha[s] ~ dnorm(mu.beta,tau.beta)`. Figure 6.17 shows a comparison of the results for the main model parameters (p_1, p_2, OR).

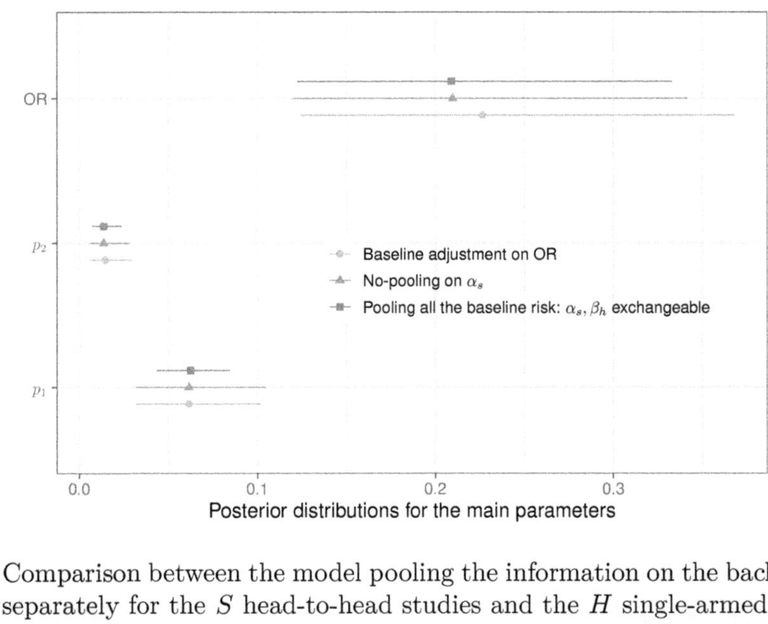

Figure 6.17: Comparison between the model pooling the information on the background risk of influenza separately for the S head-to-head studies and the H single-armed studies and the model pooling all the information together. In this case, the differences are minimal.

As is possible to see, in this particular case, the two versions of the model do not differ substantially. The model pooling all the available information in the background risk of influenza (labelled as "α_s, β_h exchangeable" in Figure 6.17) tends to produce slightly more precise estimates for p_1. This is due to the fact that the two sets of studies are indeed probably quite comparable. Conversely, the estimates for the OR are slightly more variable in the base-case analysis where α_s and β_h are not pooled together, but they are still fairly aligned.

Figure 6.17 also displays the results for the model adjusting for the baseline risk in the S head-to-head studies – in this case, the posterior distribution for the OR is shifted to the right, with a slightly larger average value. However, these differences do not appear material, which is consistent with the fact that a posterior 95% interval of $[-2.18; 0.65]$ is estimated for the parameter γ; as it spans across 0, this indicates that the effect of the baseline adjustment is "non-significant".

Even in terms of model fitting, the three versions described here have very minimal differences: in terms of DIC, the computed values are 117.7, 117.8 and 118.4 for the base-case, pooling for all the baseline risk and baseline risk adjustment versions.

Post-processing and economic evaluation

In order to fully quantify the costs and benefits of the two alternative strategies, we need to also consider further quantities. Assuming that l is the length of the influenza infection, c^{GP} is the cost of a preliminary GP visit to issue the prescription of NIs, c^{NI} is the total cost for the prophylactic NIs and c^{Inf} is the cost of treating influenza, given the structure of the problem described in Figure 6.16, the population average outcomes are:

$$\mu_{e1} = -lp_1 \qquad \text{and} \qquad \mu_{e2} = -lp_2 \tag{6.11}$$

for the clinical effectiveness, which we simplistically measure here as "the number of days required to clear the infection", without any specific reference to utilities[1] (with longer duration being worse – hence the negative sign); and

$$\begin{aligned} \mu_{c1} &= (1-p_1)c^{GP} + p_1\left(c^{GP} + c^{Inf}\right) \\ \mu_{c2} &= (1-p_2)\left(c^{GP} + c^{NI}\right) + p_2\left(c^{GP} + c^{Inf} + c^{NI}\right), \end{aligned} \tag{6.12}$$

for the costs – it is easy to follow the pathways in the decision tree of Figure 6.16 and work out what the resulting cost would be overall.

We can post-process the output of the Bayesian modelling to construct the main economic summaries, as defined in Equations 6.11 and 6.12, using the following R code

```
# Define the variables 'mu.e' and 'mu.c' as empty matrices with 'n.sims'
# rows (one per each MCMC simulation) and 2 columns (one per treatment arm)
n.sims=flu$BUGSoutput$n.sims
mu.e=mu.c=matrix(NA,n.sims,2)

# Fixed costs
# Cost of GP visit to issue NIs prescription
c.gp=19
# Cost of course of treatment with NIs
```

[1]While this is not ideal, it will not be too complicated to find estimates of the utility associated with having influenza

```
c.ni=2.40*6*7*1.175

# Extracts simulations from the object 'flu' (for simplicity in the code)
p1=flu$BUGSoutput$sims.list$p1
p2=flu$BUGSoutput$sims.list$p2
c.inf=flu$BUGSoutput$sims.list$c.inf
l=flu$BUGSoutput$sims.list$l

# Population average costs
mu.c[,1]=(1-p1)*c.gp + p1*(c.gp+c.inf)
mu.c[,2]=(1-p2)*(c.gp+c.ni) + p2*(c.gp+c.ni+c.inf)

# Population average effects
mu.e[,1]=-l*p1
mu.e[,2]=-l*p2

# Now uses 'BCEA' to make the economic analysis
m=bcea(mu.e,mu.c,interventions=c("Status quo","NIs prophylaxis"),ref=2)
# Economic analysis
summary(m,wtp=1000)
```

```
Cost-effectiveness analysis summary

Reference intervention:  NIs prophylaxis
Comparator intervention: Status quo

Optimal decision: choose Status quo for k < 300 and NIs prophylaxis for k >= 300


Analysis for willingness to pay parameter k = 1000

                Expected net benefit
Status quo                   -525.90
NIs prophylaxis              -249.73

                                EIB    CEAC   ICER
NIs prophylaxis vs Status quo 276.18 0.99675 298.71

Optimal intervention (max expected net benefit) for k = 1000: NIs prophylaxis

EVPI 0.063297
```

As is possible to see from the BCEA output, the ICER is very small – around £299 and thus prophylaxis is a very cost-effective strategy, even for very small willingness to pay. We can also use the simulations from our model to summarise directly the differential costs and benefits.

Interestingly, the benefits in terms of number of days with influenza avoided are concentrated to a relatively small number – Figure 6.18 shows a histogram for the posterior distribution of the population average difference $\Delta_e = (\mu_{e2} - \mu_{e1})$, as well as the empirical cumulative distribution function (ecdf).

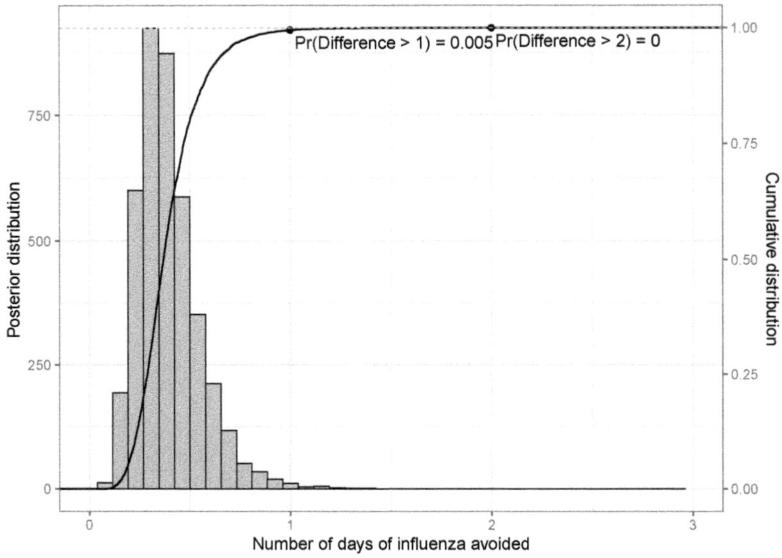

Figure 6.18: Posterior distribution for $\Delta_e = (\mu_{e2} - \mu_{e1})$, i.e. the number of days of influenza avoided. The graph also depicts the empirical cumulative distribution function F_{Δ_e} – the right-hand side y–axis shows the values of this function.

We can read the probability that the benefits exceed a given threshold along the $x-$axis directly off the ecdf; for instance, the chance of more than 1 day of influenza avoided is only around 0% – this can be computed as $\Pr(\Delta_e > 1) = 1 - F_{\Delta_e}(1)$, i.e. the difference between 1 and the ecdf computed for 1.

6.4 Conclusions

This chapter has presented the principles of hierarchical modelling as a compromise between the extreme situations: one in which the data are distinctly heterogenous and therefore should not be pulled together and another in which, on the contrary, we can reasonably assume a single data-generating process, characterised by a single common (set of) parameters, which are then estimated with larger precision because all the information can be pulled together.

These models and a deeper understanding of when each may be appropriate, are the cornerstone of the almost ubiquitous process of "evidence synthesis", which is very prevalent in HTA applications, especially when individual-level data are not directly available (e.g. for reasons due to confidentiality in clinical experimentation) and therefore the analysis is based on connecting various summary statistics.

The next chapter expands on these concepts to consider multiparameter evidence synthesis as well as situations in which the complex nature of the available data include the necessity of "filling the gaps" in a network of evidence for which specific pairwise comparisons are not directly observed.

7

Indirect treatment comparisons

7.1 Introduction

Evidence synthesis and meta-analysis (as presented in Chapter 6) are particularly efficient when we need to pool estimates of a common parameter across different studies. This is typical in much of clinical research, where often there is a number of studies on a common comparison of interest, e.g. treatment $t = 2$ against placebo $t = 1$.

In HTA, this setup is not ideal, however; this is because the actual comparison of interest for the economic model is almost invariably never against a null treatment (as instead happens in clinical studies), but rather against one or more interventions that are already established and available on the market.

This latter consideration is quite important in the context of HTA, because while we may need to consider a number T of treatment of interest, it is fairly unlikely that we have data on all possible pairwise comparisons, or even on all the comparisons between the new interventions (for which we want to the determine the cost-effectiveness) and all the other $T - 1$ existing alternatives.

For this reason, it is useful to expand the framework of Chapter 6 to what is sometimes referred to "multiparameter" (or generalised) evidence synthesis – where the idea is to learn about more than one quantity from combination of *direct* and *indirect* evidence. One such example is given by *Network Meta Analysis* (NMA), a very popular and prevalent methodology in the HTA context (see, among many others, Welton et al., 2012; Dias et al., 2018; Grant and Di Tanna, 2025, chap. 9).

NMA differs from standard pairwise evidence synthesis because it explicitly allows the simultaneous pooling of information across multiple interventions. Thus, instead of restricting the data to the subset of studies that share a specific head-to-head comparison, NMA leverages the whole network of available data (studies), allowing the combination of both direct- (from head-to-head comparisons) and indirect-evidence (i.e. that coming from studies using a common comparator). This makes it possible to estimate relative treatment effects even for pairs of interventions that have never been directly compared in a trial.

In addition, models such as those described in Chapter 6 typically assume that each pairwise comparison is independent, while NMA explicitly models the relationships between multiple treatment comparisons within a connected network. This enables the estimation of a full set of relative effects among all interventions simultaneously, while accounting for correlations induced by shared comparators and study designs.

We expand these ideas in the more comprehensive (and realistically complex) situation of population adjustment, which we consider in Chapter 11.

DOI: 10.1201/9781003771050-7

7.2 Indirect comparisons

In the simplest case, the idea of NMA can be laid out as follows. Imagine that a new treatment C has been recently approved for market authorisation (i.e. it has cleared safety and efficacy tests). Typically, this happens on the back of extensive experimental studies against placebo, A. However, for the same indication for which C has been approved, there is currently another treatment B, which is used as the standard of care. This treatment has also been tested extensively against A.

What we do not have, which is actually what we would need to perform an economic evaluation, is a direct comparison between the two active treatments, B and C. The basic idea of NMA is to use the direct evidence on B vs A and C vs A, to learn, indirectly, about the unobserved contrast B vs C. This process is also known as "mixed treatment comparison" or "multiparameter evidence synthesis", to highlight the fact that we can mix direct and indirect evidence on the same comparison.

Example 7.1. *Smoking cessation (adapted and expanded from Hasselblad, 1998).* We consider the classic example of the "smoking cessation" NMA – this has been originally presented in Hasselblad (1998) and then used in several other tutorials and textbooks (for instance, Welton et al., 2012; Jackson, 2015; Baio et al., 2025a). While this is old and the data may have some limitations, it is also very helpful in showing some of the features and complications of NMA and thus we, once again, use it to showcase the problem.

A total of $S = 24$ studies investigating the effectiveness of different measures to aid smoking cessation are considered. There are $T = 4$ interventions: A (No intervention) can be considered as a "status quo", or "placebo", where people are left to their own device and try to quit smoking by 6-12 months from the enrolment in the study. B (self-help) consists in sending information material (e.g. leaflet) so that people can self-motivate into quitting. C involves individual counselling, where a professional has 1:1 sessions with the individuals enrolled in the study, while D (group counselling) is a different version in which the sessions are held on a 1:many basis.

The full data are presented in Table 7.1; each row identifies one of the S studies; for each the observed number of people successfully quitting smoking out of the sample size in that particular study are reported. So, for instance, in the first study, there are $r_1 = 79$ people who quit smoking out of the $n_1 = 702$ enrolled in the No intervention arm.

Interestingly, although not all the studies involve the full comparison of all the interventions under investigation, all pairwise comparisons have been observed at least once. We can visualise the overall network in Figure 7.1.

The comparison C vs A is very prevalent and there are 15 trials for it, with an overall sample size of over 12 800 individuals. In contrast, there is only one trial comparison B to C, with only 255 people in total.

In addition, because the measure of "success" for a given intervention is defined as "quit smoking within 6-12 months", we may expect some heterogeneity in the outcomes – studies associated with a shorter follow-up may over-estimate the probability of success, as it is perhaps harder to maintain smoking cessation in the long-run; or perhaps it is possible that once a certain amount of time has passed without smoking, then perhaps individuals have effectively quit smoking for good and thus the studies with shorter follow-up may actual under-estimate the relevant success rates. We return to this point in Example 7.2.

Table 7.1: The observed data for the smoking cessation example. Each row indicates one of the 24 selected studies. For each treatment arm, the data represent the number of quitters / the number of participants

ID	A: No intervention	B: Self-help	C: Individual counselling	D: Group counselling
1	79 / 702	77 / 694		
2	18 / 671	21 / 535		
3	8 / 116	19 / 149		
4	75 / 731		363 / 714	
5	2 / 106		9 / 205	
6	58 / 549		237 / 1561	
7	0 / 33		9 / 48	
8	3 / 100		31 / 98	
9	1 / 31		26 / 95	
10	6 / 39		17 / 77	
11	64 / 642		107 / 761	
12	5 / 62		8 / 90	
13	20 / 234		34 / 237	
14	95 / 1107		143 / 1031	
15	15 / 187		36 / 504	
16	78 / 584		73 / 675	
17	69 / 1177		54 / 888	
18	9 / 140		23 / 140	10 / 138
19	0 / 20			9 / 20
20		20 / 49	16 / 43	
21		11 / 78	12 / 85	29 / 170
22		7 / 66		32 / 127
23			12 / 76	20 / 74
24			9 / 55	3 / 26

7.2.1 Fixed effect NMA

We start by considering a "fixed effect" NMA – this is an extension to the "complete pooling" model discussed in Section 6.2.2. In particular, the log odds of the response in each arm is modelled as a function of the effect of study s plus the incremental effect of treatment t, for $s = 1, \ldots, S$, different values of t in each s.

$$\begin{aligned}
r_{st} &\sim \text{Binomial}(\pi_{st}, n_{st}) \\
\text{logit}(\pi_{st}) &= \alpha_s + \delta_{st} \\
\delta_{st} &= d_t - d_{b_s}.
\end{aligned}$$

Here, b_s is a variable that describes the treatment arm chosen as reference in each study s – see Note 20 below for more description of the indexing of the relevant variables in the

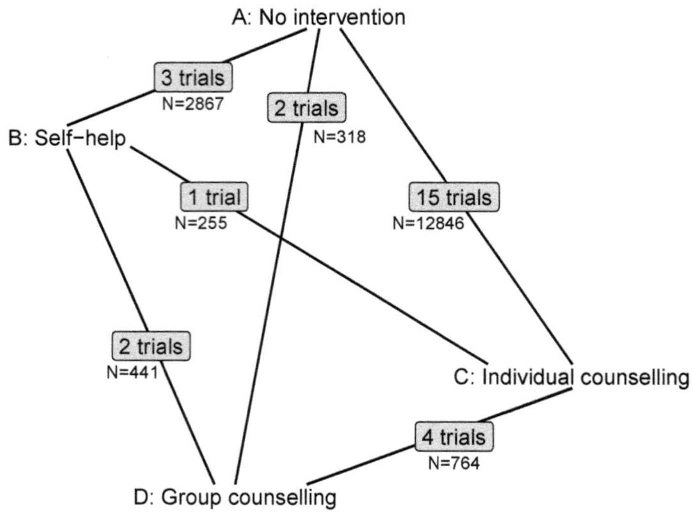

Figure 7.1: The smoking cessation evidence network. The nodes indicate the interventions being considered and edges connecting them indicate the relevant head-to-head studies, with labels reporting the number of trials and the overall sample size.

model. We artificially order the interventions so that whenever the "No intervention" ($t = 1$) option is available, then it is considered as the reference category. If it is not (e.g. in study 23, where $t = 3, 4$: Group and Individual counselling are compared), then we assume the one with the lower index (in that case $t = 3 =$ Individual counselling) to be the reference – see the discussion in Note 16 in Example 6.1.

We complete the model by placing suitable prior distributions on the parameters. The quantities α_s are defined as the study-specific baseline probability for smoking cessation in the treatment arm that is the reference for that particular study, on the logit scale. We model them as $\alpha_s \sim \text{Normal}(0, \text{sd} = 10)$, which implies a large enough variance – when rescaled to $[0; 1]$, this means that, in the prior, 95% of the mass is effectively included in the whole range.

As for the log ORs, we first set $d_1 = 0$ and then model $d_t \sim \text{Normal}(0, \text{sd} = 1)$, for $t = 2, \ldots, T$. This construction amounts to fixing the "No intervention" arm as having no incremental effect over the "untreated population" chances of quitting smoking (as seems reasonable), while allowing the other interventions to have an incremental effect. The choice of the relatively informative standard deviation is again perhaps a red herring: in fact, we can use Monte Carlo simulations to check what the prior range is on the natural scale (i.e. for the ORs), using the following code.

```
rnorm(100000,0,1) |> exp() |> bmhe::stats()
```

```
     mean        sd      2.5%    median     97.5%
1.6473483 2.2039560 0.1392235 0.9959318 7.0881310
```

As is possible to see, even with this seemingly tight prior, we are allowing for most of the mass in the OR distributions to be in a very wide range, i.e. ORs as large as over 7!

Viva Jacob Bernoulli!

Notice that while it is obviously possible that a different distribution is more suitable to model sampling variability for the observed data, in the case of NMAs, it is often the case that the reported summary statistics available from the SLR come in the form of counts for cases over a number of individuals and thus the Binomial model (originally developed by the Swiss mathematician Jacob Bernoulli, in work published posthumously, in 1713) applies naturally.

Extensions are obviously possible, for instance using a Normal model to describe the data and a linear predictor for their mean (see for instance the model for the data presented in Table 9.1), or a Poisson distribution to model sampling variability and a log linear predictor for the mean or the rates. The basic modelling principles described here, however, also apply virtually unchanged.

Example 7.2. *Smoking cessation (continued): fixed effect NMA.* In order to map the modelling assumptions into suitable `JAGS` code, we can efficiently restructure the dataset from the format presented in Table 7.1. In particular, we turn it into a "long-format", i.e. we wrangle the data so that there are multiple rows for each study, one for each intervention involved in it. Table 7.2 shows the resulting dataset, which we save in an object named `smoking_data`, in our `R` workspace.

The variable s indicates the study: for instance, study 1 is indexed in the first two rows. The variables r and n give the number of quitters and participants associated with the treatment arm described in variable t; thus, in the first row, we collect $r = 79$ and $n = 702$, for treatment arm 1 (No intervention), while in the second one, the numbers are those for treatment arm 2 (Self-help), which is the other intervention considered in study 1. Finally, the variable b is the baseline treatment arm for that particular study, as described above.

We then code up a complete pooling/fixed effect model, to estimate the relative effects (in terms of log-odds ratios, `d[t]`).

Table 7.2: An excerpt of the "long-format" dataset. The 24 original studies get expanded into 50 rows, because there are at least two rows for each study (one per comparator). The two three-armed studies contribute three rows each

ID i	Study s	Quitters r	Participants n	Intervention t	Baseline b
1	1	79	702	1	1
2	1	77	694	2	1
3	2	18	671	1	1
4	2	21	535	2	1
...	...	...	...	...	...
47	23	12	76	3	3
48	23	20	74	4	3
49	24	9	55	3	3
50	24	3	26	4	3

```
smoking_fe=function(){
  for (i in 1:N) {
    r[i] ~ dbin(pi[i],n[i])
    logit(pi[i]) <- alpha[s[i]] + delta[s[i],t[i]]
    delta[s[i],t[i]] <- d[t[i]] - d[b[i]]
  }

# Prior for baseline log-odds
  for (s in 1:S){
    alpha[s] ~ dnorm(0,0.01)
  }
# Prior for the incremental effects (log-OR)
  d[1] <- 0  # log odds ratio compared to treatment 1 (e.g. placebo)
  for (t in 2:T) {
    d[t] ~ dnorm(0,1)
  }

# Maps odds ratios for *all* treatment comparisons
  for (A in 1:(T-1)) {
    for (B in (A+1):T)  {
      or[A,B] <- exp(d[A] - d[B])
      or[B,A] <- 1/or[A,B]
    }
  }
# Log odds of quitting successfully under no intervention (from published data)
  rho ~ dnorm(-2.6, 6.925208) # = SD 0.38
# Absolute probability of quitting successfully under each intervention
  for (t in 1:T) {
    logit(p[t]) <- rho + d[t]
  }
}
```

Note 20: Nested indices and long-format datasets

If a dataset is "rectangular", i.e. it has the form of a matrix, where all the variables have the same number of observations, then it is easy to map the mathematical expressions (e.g. d_{st}) in matrix format, using multi-dimensional arrays. In the simplest case, these are just two-dimensional matrices.

However, not uncommonly, the available data do not quite follow this simple pattern and it is possible that there are different sizes – for instance, in the dataset shown in Table 7.1, the number of arms is not always equal to 2 and, in addition, the arms considered in a given study are not always the same.

For this reason, it is helpful to work with "nested indices" and long-format datasets, as in Table 7.2 so that for each row (or value of the main index `i`), we can use the ancillary indexing variables `t` or `b` to correctly specify the data. For instance, for `i=4`, the notation

```
logit(pi[i]) <- alpha[s[i]] + delta[s[i],t[i]]
delta[s[i],t[i]] <- d[t[i]] - d[b[i]]
```

translates into

```
logit(pi[4]) <- alpha[2] + delta[2,2]
delta[2,2] <- d[2] - d[1]
```

correctly indicating that the incremental effect $\delta_{2\,2}$ is modelled for intervention $t = 2$ over the baseline considered in study $s = 2$, i.e. the first intervention and therefore the log OR is $d_2 - d_1$.

We also construct the ORs for all the pairwise comparisons of interest – we do this by rescaling the log ORs. We use two loops and compute the ORs in both directions, e.g. $\text{OR}_{\text{A,B}}$ as well as $\text{OR}_{\text{B,A}}$.

Finally, we also estimate the absolute probability of quitting smoking under each intervention. To do so, we first use evidence from the published literature to estimate this probability in the "No intervention" scenario. This suggests a probability of around 7% with an upper limit of 14% for the probability of quitting without any other intervention being put in place.

We elicit this in the variable

$$\rho \sim \text{Normal}\left(\text{logit}(0.07), \text{sd} = \frac{\text{logit}(0.14) - \text{logit}(0.07)}{2} \approx 0.38\right), \tag{7.1}$$

cfr. Section 1.2.5. This allows us to construct an estimate of the absolute probability of quitting

$$p_t = \frac{\exp(\rho + d_t)}{1 + \exp(\rho + d_t)},$$

for each $t = 1, \ldots, T$ – recall that $d_1 = 0$ and so $p_1 = \exp(\rho)/\left[1 + \exp(\rho)\right]$.

Modelling baseline outcomes

The choice for the baseline logit-scale probability of quitting smoking (i.e. when no intervention is active and people are left to their own devices) selected in Equation 7.1 is obviously not unique. For instance, Baio et al. (2025a) use some sort of average of the "No intervention" arm treatment effect, computed as

$$\rho = \frac{1}{\sum_{s=1}^{S} \mathbb{I}(b_s = 1)} \sum_{s \in \mathbb{I}(b_s = 1)} \alpha_s,$$

where $\mathbb{I}(b_s = 1)$ is the set of studies in which the "No intervention" arm is observed (i.e. studies 1 to 19, in Table 7.1).

Another alternative, perhaps more model-based, would be to distinguish the effect for the "No intervention" arm by modelling the relevant parameter using some partial pooling model, so as to automatically derive a pooled estimate for the baseline probability of quitting smoking.

Equation 7.1 has the advantage of producing an estimate that is, potentially, based on consistent evidence from external data, thus providing a prior distribution that may be more robust against potential selection bias issues present in the S studies.

We finally define the data list with the relevant variables and then run the model using `JAGS`. We select a relatively long burn-in phase of 5000 iterations and also run the MCMC for 25 000 iterations, with thinning of 10, which means we use 4000 simulations for our MC analysis.

```
# Data list
data.list=list(
  t=smoking_data$t,              # Treatment indicator
  s=smoking_data$s,              # Study indicator
  r=smoking_data$r,              # Observed number of quitters
  n=smoking_data$n,              # Total sample size in study s
  b=smoking_data$b,              # Baseline intervention in study s
  N=smoking_data |> nrow(),      # Number of rows in the data
  T=smoking_data$t |> max(),     # Total number of treatment arms
  S=smoking_data$s |> max()      # Total number of studies
)
# Runs model
m_fe=jags(
  data=data.list,parameters.to.save=c("d","or","p"),n.thin=10,
  inits=NULL,n.chains=2,n.burnin=5000,n.iter=25000,model.file=smoking_fe
)
```

We can check convergence and autocorrelation, as usual (for example, as detailed in Section 3.2). In this case, all is in order, with all the relevant nodes having a value of the PSR statistic well below 1.1 and with reasonably large effective sample size, although some parameters do present a non-zero level of autocorrelation.

In this particular case, we have the advantage that we can check the consistency of *all* the indirect comparisons we obtain by pooling together all the data, with the estimates we could obtain from a version of the model in which each pairwise comparison is only informed by the studies in which it is observed (and not indirectly from all the others).

We can do this by modifying the `JAGS` code used for the general fixed effects model to the following

```
d[1] <- 0  # log odds ratio compared to treatment 1 (e.g. placebo)
for (t in 2:T) {
  d[t] ~ dnorm(0,1)
}
or <- exp(d[Active] - d[Baseline])
```

– note that we pass `Active` and `Baseline` as numerical indices for the "active" or "baseline" intervention respectively, in the modified data list; for example, to compare C vs B, we would select `Active=3` and `Baseline=2`. For each combination of `Active` and `Baseline`, we restrict the dataset to only those studies that compare these two options directly.

Figure 7.2 compares the no-pooling model ("direct evidence") with the fixed effect one ("indirect evidence"). As is possible to see, some of the pairwise comparisons are very much aligned; for instance, the estimates for the comparison between C and A are basically identical. This is not surprising, as there are a large number of aggregated observations (over 12 800), to directly obtain them.

In the case of comparisons directly informed by fewer data, the differences between direct and indirect estimates are more striking: the precision for the comparison between D and A is improved by the indirect data for C vs A and C vs D, which pool together a large sample size.

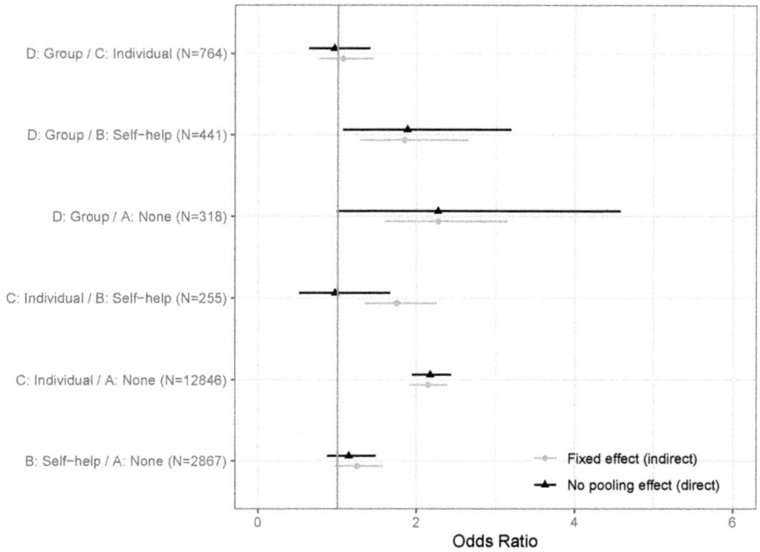

Figure 7.2: Summary of the posterior distributions for the pairwise comparisons, using the no pooling model (to only consider direct evidence) and the complete pooling ("fixed effect"), which uses all the evidence, including indirect.

As for the case of C vs B, the direct effect is substantially different than the indirect one. This is because the direct evidence is only from two relatively small studies ($s = 20, 21$) and therefore the indirect estimate is pulled towards the much bigger indirect C vs A and B vs A data. This suggests some evidence of heterogeneity.

We can also get a better sense of the underlying differences in the individual studies, by running a "no-pooling" model (see Section 6.2.1). In this case, we modify the code for the fixed effect model as in the following `JAGS` code.

```
# Model code for no-pooling individual studies
heterogeneity=function() {
  for (i in 1:N) {
    r[i] ~ dbin(pi[i],n[i])
    logit(pi[i]) <- alpha[s[i]] + delta[s[i],t[i]]
    delta[s[i],t[i]] <- d[s[i],t[i]] - d[s[i],b[i]]
  }
  for (s in 1:S) {
    alpha[s] ~ dnorm(0,0.01)
    d[s,1] <- 0
    for (j in 2:4) {
      d[s,j] ~ dnorm(0,1)
    }
    or[s] <- exp(d[s,Active] - d[s,Baseline])
  }
}
```

In this model, we now consider study- and treatment-specific differential effects d_{st}, to be able to estimate an OR for each combination. Notice that some of the studies are informed by very little data (e.g. $s = 19$), which contributes to large variance, especially in the face

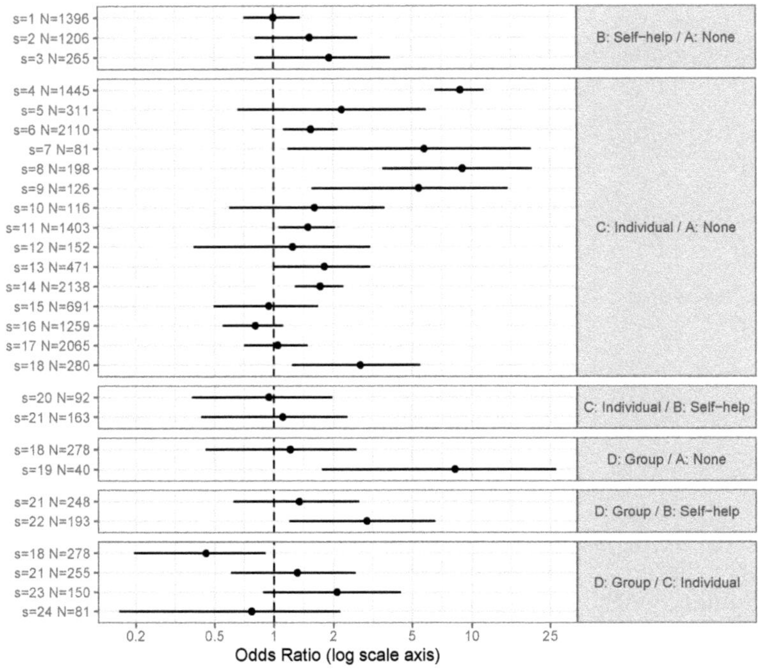

Figure 7.3: Summaries for the posterior distribution of the ORs for all the relevant pairwise comparisons, using direct evidence only and for a no-pooling model. The x–axis is on a log scale; on the y–axis, the study index s and overall sample size N are also reported.

of rather vague priors – we could probably do a better job by regularising the prior range for the ORs, e.g. by increasing the precision for d_{st}. As we are not really using this model for inference, but rather just to gauge the underlying heterogeneity, we just consider the "basic" model, which is consistent with the rest of our analysis.

Figure 7.3 shows the result of this no-pooling model. As is possible to see, there is very large heterogeneity even within studies characterised by the same comparison. In particular, there are quite a few estimates that return a very large OR and uncertainty around the central estimate that is larger still (notice that the x–axis is expressed on a log scale). As is obvious, heterogeneity as well as the precision for the estimates (measured by how tight the intervals around the mean estimates are) depends inversely on the total sample size; so, for instance, smaller studies will be associated with larger variance.

This strongly suggests that we should consider very seriously a partial-pooling version (see Section 6.2.3) of the NMA, to better account for the underlying heterogeneity in the data.

7.2.2 Random effects NMA

To expand to a random effect structure, in line with Section 6.2.3, we need to model the log ORs as exchangeable, which we can do by assuming

$$\begin{aligned} \delta_{st} &\sim \text{Normal}(\mu_{st}, \sigma_{st}) \\ \mu_{st} &= d_t - d_{b_s} \\ \sigma_{st} &\sim p(\sigma_{st}). \end{aligned} \tag{7.2}$$

In contrast to the simplest case of meta-analysis/evidence synthesis discussed in Chapter 6, in a NMA there are T different treatments and $(T-1)$ different pooled effects, relative to treatment 1 (the baseline / reference). We can, in principle, assume that there are $(T-1)$ different random effects distributions to estimate – but often this will not be feasible, unless a large enough number of studies for every single treatment is available.

This means that we generally need to add some identifiability constraints, e.g. by making assumptions such as that the random effects standard deviation is the same for each treatment comparison: $\sigma_{st} = \sigma$. Of course, if we had strong prior knowledge or expectation of differing amounts of heterogeneity for different treatment effects, we should not make this assumption and suitable extensions to this model have been proposed in the literature (Lu and Ades, 2004, 2006) – see also Dias et al. (2018, pp. 35–50) for more details and code suggestions.

Example 7.3. *Smoking cessation (continued): random effect NMA.* To complete the random effect NMA specified in Equation 7.2, we need to define a prior distribution for the random effect standard deviation on the log ORs. We could use one of the models shown previously, e.g. an Exponential PC prior (with the parameter λ defined to elicit a suitable tail-area probability for σ).

In this case, we consider the Half-Cauchy prior suggested by Gelman (2006). In particular, while the Cauchy distribution is not directly implemented in JAGS, we can use its mathematical properties to prove that

$$y \sim \text{Half Cauchy}(\mu = 0, \lambda) = \text{t}(\mu = 0, \tau, \nu = 1)\mathbb{I}(0, \infty)$$

where λ is a scale parameter and $\tau = \lambda^{-2}$ is the precision (cfr. Equations 1.5 and 6.9). Consequently, "truncating" a t distribution with mean $\mu = 0$, precision τ and $\nu = 1$ degree of freedom to only take on $\mathbb{R}^+$ provides the required prior.

Truncated distributions

In a nutshell, a variable y defined in a full range $\mathcal{Y}$ (e.g. $\mathbb{R}$) is "truncated" in a given interval $\mathcal{I} \subset \mathcal{Y}$ (e.g. $\mathbb{R}^+$) if

$$y \sim \begin{cases} p(y \mid \boldsymbol\theta) & \text{if } y \in \mathcal{I} \\ 0 & \text{if } y \notin \mathcal{I}, \end{cases}$$

i.e., for some reason, y is only observed in a subset of its full theoretical range.

Because of this quirk, the distribution $p(y \mid \boldsymbol\theta)$ needs to be re-normalised dividing by $\Pr(Y \in \mathcal{I})$, in order to retrieve the correct contribution to the likelihood – in other words, if (a, b) are the lower and upper bounds of the interval $\mathcal{I}$, then

$$y \sim \frac{p(y \mid \boldsymbol\theta)}{\Pr(Y \in \mathcal{I})} = \frac{p(y \mid \boldsymbol\theta)}{F(b \mid \boldsymbol\theta) - F(a \mid \boldsymbol\theta)}.$$

In JAGS, this is achieved through the `T(,)` operator – for instance, the code

```
sigma ~ dt(0,0.04,1)T(0,)
```

implies a Half Cauchy$(0, 5)$ model for a variable `sigma` – in line with the parameterisation used in Equation 1.5, in JAGS the t distribution is indexed by the precision. Thus a value of 0.04 for the precision τ of the t distribution implies a scale $\lambda = \tau^{-0.5} = 5$ for the resulting Half Cauchy.

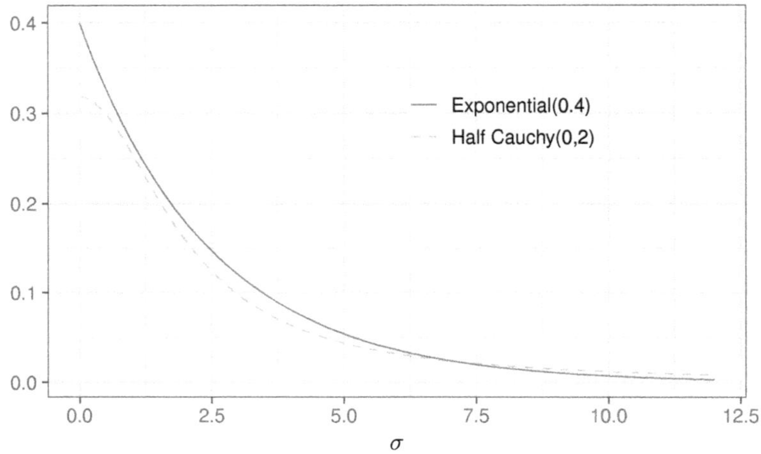

Figure 7.4: Comparison of a Half Cauchy(0,2) and an Exponential(0.4) prior distributions for σ.

In particular, we specify $\sigma \sim \text{Half Cauchy}(0,2) = \text{t}(0,0.25,1)\mathbb{I}(0,\infty)$. This prior can be visualised in Figure 7.4, where we have also overlaid an Exponential(0.4) – this would amount to a PC prior for which $\Pr(\sigma > 6) \approx 0.1$.

The two priors are reasonably aligned – this means that by assuming the Half Cauchy(0,2), we are also implying a very small chance that the random effects standard deviation would exceed a rather large value such as 6; we can use forward sampling (see Section 1.2.6) to estimate that in fact $\Pr(\sigma > 6) \approx 0.102$ for the Half Cauchy prior.

Mean-precision t distribution in R

In R, the built-in commands to compute the density and cumulative distribution for, or to sample from a t distribution (respectively, `dt`, `pt` and `rt`) are based on a different parameterisation, in comparison to the one we use here (see Equation 1.5). More specifically, R implicitly fixes $\mu \equiv 0$ and $\tau \equiv 1$, while BUGS/JAGS allow different values for the parameters – basically, if $y \sim \text{t}(\mu,\tau,\nu)$ and $z \sim \text{t}(\mu \equiv 0, \tau \equiv 1, \nu)$ then $z = (y-\mu)\sqrt{\tau}$.

Consequently, the mean-precision version of the t density and cumulative density can be obtained from the R parameterisations, which we indicate respectively as $p^*(\cdot \mid \nu)$ and $F^*(\cdot \mid \nu)$, applying the rule for change of variable. This yields the following transformations

$$p(y \mid \mu,\tau,\nu) = \sqrt{\tau}p^*\big(\sqrt{\tau}(y-\mu) \mid \nu\big) \quad \text{and} \quad F(y \mid \mu,\tau,\nu) = F^*\big(\sqrt{\tau}(y-\mu) \mid \nu\big),$$

which, in R are obtained using the following commands.

```
density=sqrt(tau)*dt(sqrt(tau)*(y-mu),nu)
cum_dist=pt(sqrt(tau)*(y-mu),nu)
```

We can code up the full random effect NMA model specified above using the following.

```
smoking_re=function(){
  for (i in 1:N) {
```

```
    r[i] ~ dbin(pi[i],n[i])
    logit(pi[i]) <- alpha[s[i]] + delta[s[i],t[i]]
    delta[s[i],t[i]] ~ dnorm(mu[s[i],t[i]],tau)
    mu[s[i],t[i]] <- d[t[i]] - d[b[i]]
  }

# Prior for baseline log-odds
  for (s in 1:S){
    alpha[s] ~ dnorm(0,0.01)
  }
# Prior for the incremental effects (log-OR)
  d[1] <- 0  # log odds ratio compared to treatment 1 (e.g. placebo)
  for (t in 2:T) {
    d[t] ~ dnorm(0,1)
  }
# Half-Cauchy prior for common sd for the random effects. NB: in JAGS, the
# t distribution is indexed in terms of the *precision* (=1/variance)!
  sigma ~ dt(0,0.25,1)%_%T(0,)
  tau <- pow(sigma,-2)

# Maps odds ratios for all treatment comparisons
  for (A in 1:(T-1)) {
    for (B in (A+1):T)  {
      or[A,B] <- exp(d[A] - d[B])
      or[B,A] <- 1/or[A,B]
    }
  }
# Log odds of quitting successfully under no intervention (from published data)
  rho ~ dnorm(-2.6,6.925208) # = SD 0.38
# Absolute probability of quitting successfully under each intervention
  for (t in 1:T) {
    logit(p[t]) <- rho + d[t]
  }
}
```

Note 21: Using truncation in JAGS model code (passed as a function)

Throughout the examples in the book, we have constructed the JAGS model code as an R function. In the case of the model above, we must include the “truncation” operator T(0,), which instructs JAGS to only simulate values for the underlying $t(\mu, \tau, \nu)$ distribution from $\mathbb{R}^+$ and applies the suitable rescaling of the density.

However, the use of the string

```
sigma.delta ~ dt(...)T(0,)
```

within a function is incompatible with R syntax and thus it would break the code, throwing an R error such as the following.

```
Error: unexpected symbol in:
"# Half-Cauchy prior for common sd for the random effects
  sigma.delta ~ dt(0,0.25,1)T"
```

To avoid this issue, when defining the function containing the model code, e.g. `smoking_re()` above, we use a dummy operator `%_%` before the truncation code. This gets automatically parsed out when running `R2jags::jags()`, through the function `R2WinBUGS::write.model()`, which is called in the background to write the model code to a temporary file.

The model can be run using the following `R` code. We again use a burn-in phase of 5000 iterations and run the MCMC for 25 000 iterations, with thinning of 10.

```
# Runs model
m_re=jags(
  data=data.list,parameters.to.save=c("d","or","p","sigma"),n.thin=10,
  inits=NULL,n.chains=2,n.burnin=5000,n.iter=25000,model.file=smoking_re
)
```

Figure 7.5 depicts diagnostics for the model, in terms of the PSR and effective sample size. Generally speaking, we can be satisfied with convergence and the level of autocorrelation does not appear too much of a concern.

Convergence is not an issue in this model and all the main parameters are associated with sufficiently large effective sample size.

We can compare the fixed and random effects NMA, using for instance the DIC. In this case, the complete pooling model is associated with a DIC of 521.62, while the corresponding value for the partial pooling model is 332.7. This large difference, confirms the presence of large heterogeneity in the underlying studies and thus justifies the use of the random effect NMA. More specifically, the amount of shrinkage in the partial pooling model can be computed as a reduction of 43.01% in the number of model parameters (from a nominal 79 to the effective 45.02 parameters, as measured by p_D) – see the discussion in Section 6.2.7.

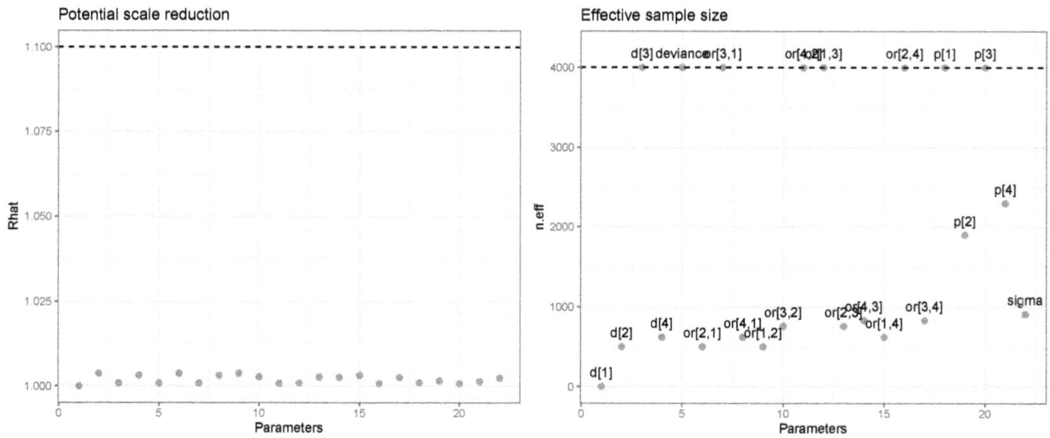

(a) $\hat{R}$. (b) n_{eff}.

Figure 7.5: Diagnostic plots for the random effects NMA.

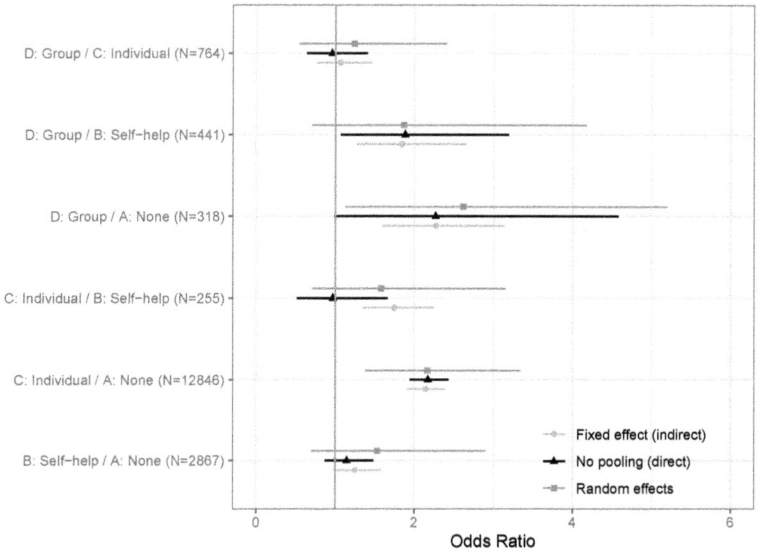

Figure 7.6: Comparison of the three versions of the NMA. The partial pooling ("random effects") generally acts as a compromise between the two extremes of the no- and complete-pooling models. Generally speaking, the uncertainty is higher in the partial pooling model, because of the underlying large heterogeneity inherent in the S studies, which is artificially discarded in the two other models.

Figure 7.6 shows a full comparison of the direct and indirect evidence, using both a fixed and a random effects NMA. Generally speaking, the random effects model is associated with wider intervals, after accounting for heterogeneity. While this may sound as a "disappointing" result, perhaps a more appropriate phrasing would be that, in fact, it is the fixed effects model that tends to give artificially tight interval estimates, which do not fully reflect the underlying variability in the studies.

The comparison between C and B shows that the random effect model is a "compromise" between the direct and indirect evidence, while for D vs A, as it is based on the smallest trials, there is still substantial uncertainty.

7.3 Economic evaluation based on NMA

Generally speaking, the NMA process will be specifically designed to obtain pooled estimates for some relevant *relative* effects and we will want to propagate the inherent uncertainty through some suitable economic model, to obtain estimates for suitable population average benefits and costs and then perform the usual economic analysis.

The power of the Bayesian machinery is that, once the statistical model is fitted, then the remaining steps are more or less repeated in a similar fashion – the propagation of the uncertainty and the PSA come almost for free (see the discussion in Chapter 4).

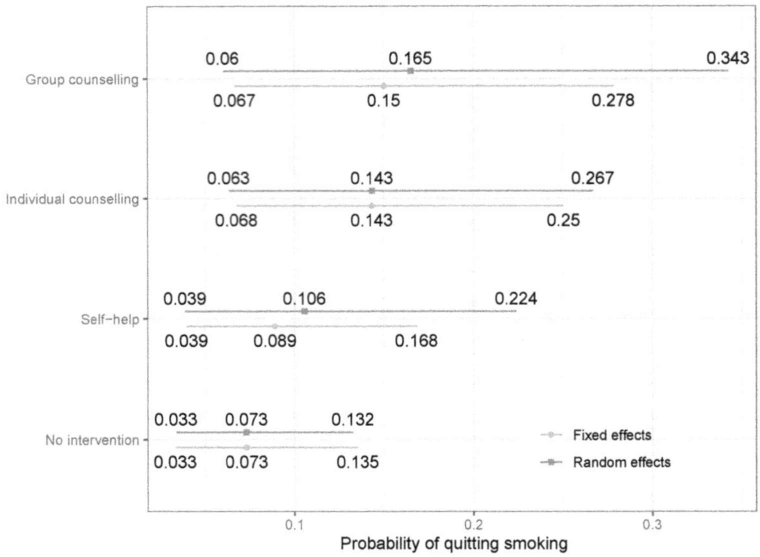

Figure 7.7: Estimates for the absolute probability of quitting smoking for the $T = 4$ competing interventions and under the "fixed" and "random" effect models.

Example 7.4. *Smoking cessation (continued): economic evaluation.* We first turn the estimates for the relative effects obtained in the NMA into suitable *absolute* effects (see the discussion in Note 16 in Chapter 6).

Considering the fixed and random effect models to pool all the available evidence (both direct and indirect), we can automatically consider the nodes `p[t]` defined both in the `smoking_fe()` and `smoking_re()` model code functions. These represent estimates of the absolute probability of quitting smoking, under each of the $T = 4$ interventions considered.

Figure 7.7 compares the posterior distributions under the two models. The numbers indicate the estimates for the 95% interval and the posterior mean – note that the estimates for the "No intervention" arm are essentially identical (up to Monte Carlo simulation error). This is correct, because in both the fixed and random effect models, this baseline probability is modelled using the informative prior on the parameter ρ.

In Figure 7.7, the random effect model produces generally larger intervals, which again reflects the higher uncertainty due to the proper accounting of the underlying heterogeneity in the S studies.

We can use these results and complement them with external data to obtain a measure of clinical benefit from quitting smoking, in terms of life years gained. Specifically, this will vary depending on the age of individuals, with larger benefits encountered for quitters of younger age.

Just to fix ideas, we can consider the results by Mamun et al. (2004), who using the long-running Framingham Heart Study cohort, report increased survival in years of 8.66 (95% interval [7.61; 9.63]) and 7.59 (95% interval [6.33; 8.92]), for men and women, respectively. In addition, using official statistics (e.g. from the UK Office for National Statistics), we can derive the gender distribution of smokers – for instance, ONS (2024) suggest that, in 2023, smokers in the UK were distributed as 3.4 million men and 2.6 million women, which implies a proportional split of 56.67:43.33.

If we model the uncertainty in the life years gained using suitable Normal distributions centred on the point estimates and with standard deviations computed as in Section 1.2.5, we can derive an estimate for the extra life years gained by not smoking (i.e. for quitters) as $l_m \sim \text{Normal}(\text{mean} = 8.66, \text{sd} = 0.495)$ for men and $l_f \sim \text{Normal}(\text{mean} = 7.59, \text{sd} = 0.679)$ for women, respectively. It is easy to check through Monte Carlo simulations that these distributions match closely the interval estimates provided by Mamun et al. (2004).

We can combine these two distributions with weights $w_m = 0.567$ and $w_f = 0.433$ into our final estimate for the overall life years gained as $l = w_m l_m + w_f l_f$ and then derive an intervention-specific measure of clinical benefit as $e_t = p_t l$. We can use the output from our models (and in fact, we consider here only the random effect one) and Monte Carlo simulations, as demonstrated in the following R code.

```
# First computes the life years gained
lm=rnorm(m_re$BUGSoutput$n.sims,8.66,0.495)
lf=rnorm(m_re$BUGSoutput$n.sims,7.59,0.679)
l=0.567*lm + 0.433*lf

# Then weighs these with the probability of quitting for each intervention
e=m_re$BUGSoutput$sims.list$p * l
labs=c(
  "No intervention","Self-help","Individual counselling","Group counselling"
)
# And shows some summary statistics of the resulting distribution
e |> bmhe::stats() |> (\(x) {rownames(x)=labs; x})()
```

```
                            mean        sd      2.5%    median    97.5%
No intervention        0.5990069 0.2135718 0.2741542 0.5649678 1.094705
Self-help              0.8657321 0.4035487 0.3169203 0.7922804 1.855956
Individual counselling 1.1760152 0.4399877 0.5171232 1.1063813 2.190791
Group counselling      1.3543306 0.6097724 0.4906249 1.2504617 2.838233
```

Note 22: Piping functions

Notice that, in R, the code `(\(x) ...)()` can be used as a shortcut for defining a function `func(x){...}`. Here we first consider the object `e`, then we apply the function `bmhe::stats()` to it, to compute the summary statistics from the posterior distributions and then we "pipe" a function to define the names of the four rows of the resulting matrix.

As for the costs, we consider the analysis in Baio et al. (2025a), based on the data provided in Table 7.3, which can be used to determine a central estimate for the overall cost of implementation of each of the interventions. Note that, in a more comprehensive evaluation, we would perhaps need to consider more resources that directly impact on the individuals' quality of life, such as complications (e.g. acute and chronic treatment of cardiovascular disease and events). Here, we keep the modelling relatively simple and only use the direct cost of implementation of the four interventions.

In addition, to account for variance in compliance and potential side treatments, we associate each of the costs with a probability distribution, for the three "active" interventions. In particular, we consider Gamma distributions where the mean is set to the observed total cost and the standard deviation is fixed at 30% of that amount. This is a relatively common

Table 7.3: Point estimates (in £) for the costs associated with the $T = 4$ interventions considered in the smoking cessation example

Intervention	Item cost (in £)	Total cost (£)
No intervention	—	0.0
Self-help	Nicotine replacement therapy (NRT) for five weeks (35 patches at 1.30 each)	45.5
Individual counselling	NRT for five weeks (35 patches at 1.30 each) + five clinic visits (10 each)	95.5
Group counselling	NRT for five weeks (35 patches at 1.30 each) + five clinic visits (19.46 each)	142.8

practice in HTA, where, in the absence of genuine information, the central estimate is perturbed assuming some fixed value for the underlying coefficient of variation $\text{CV} = \mu/\sigma$ – this effectively implies that the standard deviation σ is set to a fraction of the estimated mean μ.

We can use the function `bmhe::gammaPar()` to return the shape and rate parameters for a Gamma distribution to match given values for the underlying mean and standard deviation – other examples for this kind of strategy are presented in Example 9.3. For example, the code

```
bmhe::gammaPar(45.5,.3*45.5)
```

```
$shape
[1] 11.11111

$rate
[1] 0.2442002
```

```
bmhe::gammaPar(45.5,.3*45.5) |>
  (\(x) rgamma(100000,shape=x$shape,rate=x$rate))() |> bmhe::stats()
```

```
    mean       sd     2.5%   median    97.5%
45.56265 13.66428 22.85922 44.20653 75.86524
```

suggests that modelling $c_2 \sim \text{Gamma}(\text{shape} = 11.111, \text{rate} = 0.244)$ would have, at least approximately the required properties. Similar reasoning allows us to model the costs for the individual and group counselling using $c_3 \sim \text{Gamma}(\text{shape} = 11.111, \text{rate} = 0.116)$ and $c_4 \sim \text{Gamma}(\text{shape} = 11.111, \text{rate} = 0.078)$, respectively.

As for the "No intervention" arm, if we do not consider relevant outcomes (such as hospitalisations for major cardiovascular events), we keep the cost of implementation to £0, with no variance. In reality, as mentioned above, we would include costs borne by the health-care provider for resource use related to the underlying condition, e.g. to treat acute heart conditions, which would also impact on the benefit side.

We can then bring all these elements together and perform the cost-effectiveness analysis, for instance using the following `R` code – notice that we could include these calculations inside the `JAGS` object, but since these are pure forward sampling, it would have no effect on the actual estimates based on the computing the posterior distributions for the actual model parameters.

```
# Defines the matrix of cost simulations
c=matrix(
  c(
    rep(0,m_re$BUGSoutput$n.sims),
    rgamma(m_re$BUGSoutput$n.sims,shape=11.111,rate=0.244),
    rgamma(m_re$BUGSoutput$n.sims,shape=11.111,rate=0.116),
    rgamma(m_re$BUGSoutput$n.sims,shape=11.111,rate=0.078)
  ),
  nrow=m_re$BUGSoutput$n.sims,ncol=4
)

# Runs BCEA to perform the economic evaluation
library(BCEA)
m=bcea(e,c,ref=4,Kmax=4000,interventions=labs)
summary(m)
```

```
NB: k (wtp) is defined in the interval [0 - 4000]

Cost-effectiveness analysis summary

Reference intervention:  Group counselling
Comparator intervention(s): No intervention
                          : Self-help
                          : Individual counselling

Optimal decision: choose No intervention for k < 168
                         Individual counselling for 168 <= k < 264
                         Group counselling for k >= 264


Analysis for willingness to pay parameter k = 4000

                       Expected net benefit
No intervention                      2396.0
Self-help                            3417.4
Individual counselling               4608.0
Group counselling                    5274.5


                                             EIB    CEAC   ICER
Group counselling vs No intervention     2878.44 0.98125 189.13
Group counselling vs Self-help           1857.06 0.86525 199.21
Group counselling vs Individual counselling  666.45 0.63550 262.51

Optimal intervention (max expected net benefit) for k = 4000: Group counselling

EVPI 393.8
```

As is clear from the summary, depending on the willingness to pay threshold selected, the optimal intervention does change: when k is less than £168, then do-nothing is the most cost-effective option; Individual counselling becomes the optimal strategy for $k \in$ £[168; 264]; and then Group counselling is the most cost-effective intervention for $k >$ £264.

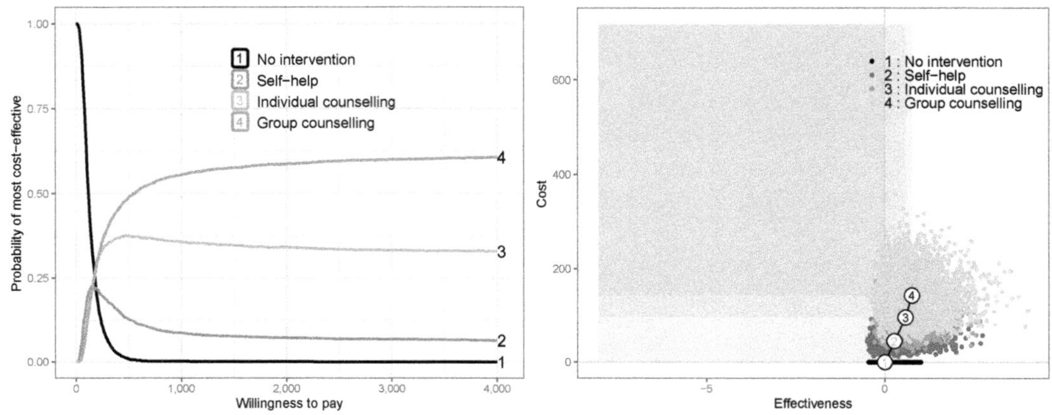

(a) Pr(t is the most cost-effective).

(b) Cost-effectiveness efficiency frontier.

Figure 7.8: Multiple intervention cost-effectiveness analysis for the smoking example.

We can also use the tools described in Section 4.3.3 and produce a more thorough analysis for each intervention. We can do this using BCEA specific functions, as demonstrated in the code below.

```
# Multi-intervention cost-effectiveness analysis
mce=multi.ce(m)
```

The function `multi.ce()` computes and plots the probability that each of the interventions being analysed is the most cost-effective and can be then used to produce the cost-effectiveness acceptability frontier (see Section 4.3.3). The resulting object `mce` can be further processed, e.g. to apply the `ceac.plot` method to draw the CEAC for each intervention – and the `ggplot2` facilities can be used to further customise the resulting graph as shown in Figure 7.8a. This shows the probability that each of the options is the most cost-effective, upon varying the willingness to pay threshold.

Figure 7.8b shows the cost-effectiveness efficiency frontier and, in line with the discussion above, it shows that "Self-help" is inside the frontier, indicating that, for different threshold values, the other three interventions are optimal.

7.4 Conclusions

In this chapter we have introduced the concept of indirect comparison (which will be reprised in Chapter 11) and expanded on the models developed in Chapter 6 to pool together (summary) data obtained from a number of sources. We have showcased the subtle complexity of NMA through the smoking cessation example, which allowed us to explore the potential implications of the underlying heterogeneity in the data. This has also been expanded into a full economic evaluation, by combining the effectiveness measures obtained through the indirect comparison and suitable information on the cost component.

In the next chapter we concentrate on another extremely popular modelling problem in HTA analyses: the use of time-to-event data (which are the most important outcome for e.g. cancer studies) and survival analysis.

8

Survival analysis in HTA

8.1 Introduction

Survival modelling is a cornerstone of biostatistical analysis, specifically designed to model *time-to-event* outcomes, such as the overall time between the beginning of an observation or exposure (e.g. diagnosis of cancer) until a relevant event (typically death, or progression to a different health state). This represents a powerful analytic framework that provides much more granular information than cruder binary (event vs no-event) analyses, thus enabling the estimation of richer output, including instantaneous and cumulative risks, over time.

In typical biostatistics applications, survival modelling is used to understand the magnitude of treatment effects and identify prognostic factors, accounting for the data-generating mechanism. In the context of HTA, it also plays a pivotal role, because decisions are made at the population level and often require extrapolation beyond the follow-up observed in clinical studies. Accurate survival estimates are therefore essential not only for quantifying treatment effectiveness but also for projecting downstream costs, quality-adjusted life years and overall cost-effectiveness.

Whenever possible, modelling at the individual-level allows the incorporation of patient heterogeneity, adjusting for covariates and the propagation of uncertainty that can then inform robust evidence-based policy decisions. This makes survival analysis both a statistical and an economic tool, bridging clinical evidence with the long-term evaluations required for health system decision-making.

While the overall methodology is well established, its application in HTA does have some specific quirks, which are deeply related to the nature of the available data, as well as the fundamental focus on decision-making, rather than simple inference. For these reasons, which we explore in details below, survival methods applied in HTA are often "non-standard", in comparison to those used in "biostatistical" modelling. Despite the underlying complexity, survival analysis is extremely prevalent in HTA, because it is the natural modelling framework for cancer studies, which represent a large proportion of all the HTA appraisals (Latimer, 2011).

In this chapter, we provide a general framework for survival analysis, specifically for HTA and focus on a number of "typical" distributional assumptions, as well as on computational methods that are particularly efficient for this type of outcome. Jackson et al. (2025) provide a wider introduction (with larger focus on non-Bayesian modelling), while aspects of HTA modelling related to survival analysis are also presented in Dias et al. (2018, chap. 10) and in Sharples and Demiris (2020).

DOI: 10.1201/9781003771050-8

Notation for survival modelling

As suggested in Note 9 in Section 4.2, throughout this chapter we slightly modify our general notation, in which we have used the symbol t to index the treatments under consideration.

In order to align with the general survival analysis literature (and because, hopefully, there is no major confusion with the rest of the book), *in this chapter*, we indicate with t_i the main outcome of the analysis, i.e. the time until a relevant event happens for individual i.

We also use throughout this chapter the index $k = 1, \ldots, K$ to indicate relevant parts of the models, as in Equation 8.8, or in Equation 8.13.

8.2 General framework for survival analysis

The general modelling framework for time-to-event, can be described as follows. The main outcome is the observed time at which the event under study is recorded for the i–th individual, t_i. We can describe the sampling variability in the observed times using a density $f(t_i \mid \boldsymbol{\theta})$, as a function of a set of relevant parameters.

In addition, we can consider a number of helpful quantities to describe the survival mechanism: the first and, perhaps, most important is the *survival function*

$$S(t \mid \boldsymbol{\theta}) = \Pr(T > t) = 1 - F(t \mid \boldsymbol{\theta}) = 1 - \int_0^t f(u \mid \boldsymbol{\theta}) du,$$

where $F(t \mid \boldsymbol{\theta})$ is the cumulative density of the variable T. The survival function describes the probability of an individual surviving beyond time t.

Other important quantities are the *hazard function*

$$h(t \mid \boldsymbol{\theta}) = \lim_{dt \to 0} \frac{\Pr(t \leq T < t + dt \mid T \geq t)}{dt}, \tag{8.1}$$

which quantifies the instantaneous risk of experiencing the event, as well as the related *cumulative hazard function*

$$H(t \mid \boldsymbol{\theta}) = \int_0^t h(u \mid \boldsymbol{\theta}) du.$$

Brothers and sisters

By their mathematical properties, we can retrieve a set of useful relationships that allow us to connect $F(\cdot)$, $S(\cdot)$. $f(\cdot)$, $h(\cdot)$ and $H(\cdot)$. Thus, specifying one of them is sufficient to fully characterise the survival model.

1. By definition, the density function is the derivative of the cumulative function, with respect to the time variable

$$f(t \mid \boldsymbol{\theta}) = \frac{d}{dt} F(t \mid \boldsymbol{\theta}) = F'(t \mid \boldsymbol{\theta}). \tag{8.2}$$

2. As the numerator of Equation 8.1 is a conditional probability, it can be factorised into the ratio of the joint to the marginal probabilities (see Section 5.2.2) and thus

$$\begin{aligned} h(t \mid \boldsymbol{\theta}) &= \lim_{dt \to 0} \frac{\Pr(t \leq T < t + dt, T \geq t)}{\Pr(T \geq t) dt} = \lim_{dt \to 0} \frac{\Pr(t \leq T < t + dt)}{S(t \mid \boldsymbol{\theta}) dt} \\ &= \frac{f(t \mid \boldsymbol{\theta}) dt}{S(t \mid \boldsymbol{\theta}) dt} = \frac{f(t \mid \boldsymbol{\theta})}{S(t \mid \boldsymbol{\theta})}, \end{aligned} \tag{8.3}$$

because, obviously, the probability that T is in the interval $[t; t + dt)$ and, at the same time, $T \geq t$ is just $\Pr(t \leq T < t + dt)$; and, by definition, $f(\cdot)dt$ is the probability that the variable T is in a small interval of width dt.

3. Combining the definition of the survival function and Equation 8.2, its derivative with respect to the time variable is the negative of the density function

$$S'(t \mid \boldsymbol{\theta}) = \frac{d}{dt} S(t \mid \boldsymbol{\theta}) = \frac{d}{dt} [1 - F(t \mid \boldsymbol{\theta})] = -f(t \mid \boldsymbol{\theta}). \tag{8.4}$$

4. Combining Equations 8.3 and 8.4, the hazard function can be represented as the ratio of the derivative to the actual survival function

$$h(t \mid \boldsymbol{\theta}) = -\frac{S'(t \mid \boldsymbol{\theta})}{S(t \mid \boldsymbol{\theta})}. \tag{8.5}$$

5. Given Equations 8.1 and 8.5, as well as the basic properties of differential calculus, the cumulative hazard function can also be expressed also as the negative log-survival

$$H(t \mid \boldsymbol{\theta}) = \int_0^t -\frac{S'(u \mid \boldsymbol{\theta})}{S(u \mid \boldsymbol{\theta})} du = -\log(S(t \mid \boldsymbol{\theta})). \tag{8.6}$$

8.2.1 Censoring

Another important defining feature of time-to-event data is the fact that, almost invariably, the evidence in the observed data is limited. This is because, most often, the length of the follow-up is not enough for us to be able to observe the event under study on all the individuals involved – a phenomenon typically referred to as *censoring*[1].

Thus, in addition to the observed times t_i, we usually consider an event indicator d_i (for "dummy" variable), taking value 1 if the event actually happens within the time horizon during which the data are observed, or 0 when the i–th individual is "censored".

If $d_i = 1$, then t_i is fully observed; conversely, if $d_i = 0$, we do not know whether the event actually occurs – it may in the future, but we just do not have this information. Consequently, when $d_i = 0$, then the observed t_i does not represent the true "survival time". Figure 8.1 depicts this by showing that for some individuals the entire history is known, while for others, key information (e.g. whether the event is actually occurred) is not available.

[1]Technically, this is only one of the possible forms of "censoring", indicated in the literature as "right censoring". As this is the most common for applications in HTA, we limit our attention to it, here.

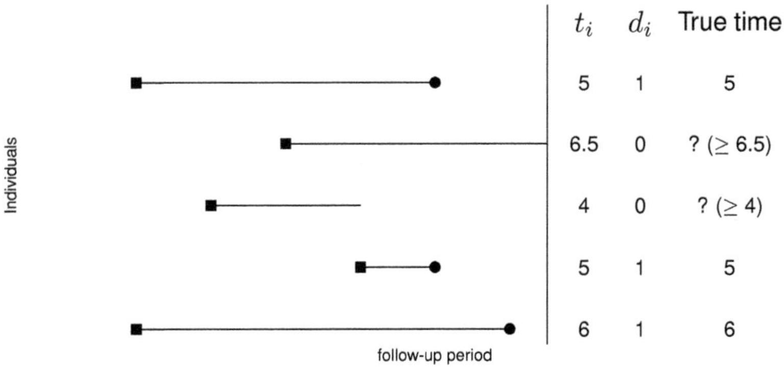

Figure 8.1: A graphical representation of the concept of (right) censoring. For some individuals, we know the full history, i.e. the point in time when they enter (the black square) and exit the observation because the event under study has occurred (the black dot). In other cases, this information is not available: we only know that, at some point, the individual has ceased to be observed and therefore the actual time-to-event is only known partially.

Censoring is important, because just like missing data (see Chapter 10), it implies that the information present in the data is not complete. Consequently, in the presence of censoring, the individual contribution to the likelihood function is expressed as

$$\mathcal{L}(\boldsymbol{\theta} \mid t_i, d_i) = h(t_i \mid \boldsymbol{\theta})^{d_i} S(t_i \mid \boldsymbol{\theta}). \tag{8.7}$$

Basically, if the individual is not censored (i.e. they have survived up to t and hence $d_i = 1$), their risk of experiencing the event is simply described by the full density function, expressed as $h(t_i \mid \boldsymbol{\theta})S(t_i \mid \boldsymbol{\theta})$ – see Equation 8.3; if, on the other hand, they are censored (i.e. $d_i = 0$), then their risk is measured by the survival function as the probability that they will experience it in the future (after time t).

Equation 8.7 can be used (typically taking the log, for computational stability) to perform calculations on the density $f(\cdot)$ – we return to this point in Section 8.3.4.

8.3 Survival analysis in HTA

In typical applications of survival analysis, e.g. in the context of randomised clinical trial, the main objective of the statistical analysis is to estimate the impact of a number of covariates (including the treatment arm) on the survival time. This sort of structure is applied specifically for cancer drug trials. In these cases, typically, the analysis is focused on a head-to-head comparison between a new intervention (e.g. a new cancer drug) and some sort of standard of care (e.g. chemotherapy).

In the case of survival modelling in HTA, there are at least two added complications that must be carefully taken into account.

8.3.1 Extrapolation

Almost invariably, the nature of these studies implies a time horizon that does not allow to follow-up all the individuals enrolled until they experience the event of interest (usu-

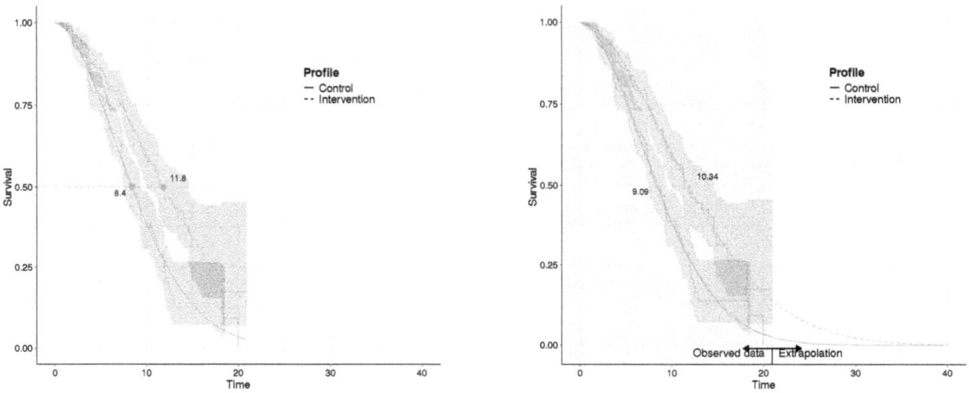

(a) Typical trial data.

(b) Extrapolation.

Figure 8.2: Survival analysis in HTA. Panel (a) shows the observed data over the available time-horizon (e.g. from a trial), while panel (b) shows the extrapolation over a longer time-horizon, highlighting how median and mean survival times may differ substantially.

ally, sadly, death), through the effect of censoring and other considerations (e.g. treatment switching for lack of efficacy – see for instance Latimer et al., 2016).

Figure 8.2a shows the typical representation of trial data in the form of Kaplan-Meier (KM) curves (Kaplan and Meier, 1958) – see Note 23 below for more technical details. These are non-parametric estimators for the probability of survival at any given time point over the duration of the follow-up in a study and are shown as the step curves (surrounded by a non-parametric 95% interval estimate). KM estimates are ubiquitous in survival analysis, as they are a very efficient way of summarising the observed data.

Alongside the KM curves for the two treatment arms (generically labelled as "Control" and "Intervention"), we have included two smooth curves, fitted to the observed data to estimate survival over the observed study period. The two dots on the smooth curves indicate the estimated *median* survival time, i.e. the point along the x–axis in correspondence of the value of 50% along the y–axis.

In typical survival studies, the median time is one of the quantities of interest because, as shown in Figure 8.2a, we do not have enough observations to be able to estimate the survival curves *all the way down to 0*, i.e. at the point when all the observed individuals actually experience the event. Notice that in the case depicted in Figure 8.2a, censoring is actually not too extreme, as indicated by the fact that both curves are reasonably close to 0 (especially for the controls). Nonetheless, for the intervention arm, there is about 15% of individuals for whom we do not know the time at which the event (death) occurs and hence both the KM and the smooth curve end abruptly at the end of the follow-up time.

This is in contrast with the needs of the HTA analysis: we cannot just rely on the difference we measure in the study period, e.g. in this case a treatment effect of $11.8 - 8.4 = 3.4$ units of time, say months, in terms of median survival. That is because the economic analysis must take a "life-time horizon": if a treatment is approved for reimbursement, it will be provided to individuals for as long as they need it and the effects must then be measured in terms of *mean*, rather than median survival time.

Figure 8.2b shows this by expanding the smooth curve beyond the duration of the observed times – this is typically referred to as *extrapolation*. By expanding the time horizon to, in this particular case, over 40 units of time, we ensure that the survival curves go down to 0, to the point where *all* the individuals will have experienced the event under study. This is necessary because, integrating by part and using Equation 8.4, we can prove that the mean survival time is equivalent to the full area under the survival curve:

$$\mathrm{E}[T] := \int_0^\infty t f(t \mid \boldsymbol{\theta}) dt = \int_0^\infty S(t \mid \boldsymbol{\theta}) dt.$$

Importantly, if we are able to extrapolate the survival curve over a longer time horizon, the treatment effect may vary even substantially: in the case of Figure 8.2b, it is $10.34 - 9.09 = 1.25$ units of time, in terms of mean survival – that is basically half the median treatment effect that we get from the trial data with no extrapolation.

There are two main obvious implications of this issue. Firstly, in HTA it is harder to apply standard modelling for survival analysis, such as Cox Proportional Hazard models (Cox, 1972). This is because, while they have the great advantage of not committing to a fully parametric specification for the time-to-event variable, their semi-parametric nature makes it harder to produce time-quantile predictions, e.g. extrapolate the survival curves.

For this reason, in HTA we tend to rely more heavily on parametric models for survival analysis, which do require more explicit assumptions. Therefore, the way in which we produce this extrapolation beyond the observed trial data becomes crucial and may exert notable sensitivity to the overall economic results (Latimer, 2011).

Note 23: Kaplan-Meier estimates

Imagine we have a fictional dataset recording the time-to-event for $n = 10$ individuals, as $\boldsymbol{t} = (0.03, 0.03, 0.92, 1.48, 1.64, 1.64, 1.7, 1.7, 1.74, 1.77)$. The data can be aggregated by listing the unique times at which events happen and counting the progression of individuals from being "at risk" (i.e. exposed to the risk of the event) to having actually experiencing it. Table 8.1 shows this aggregation.

Table 8.1: The Kaplan-Meier representation for the fictional data presented above. The "survivors" are computed as the difference between the number of individual at risk and the total number of events occurred at a certain time

Time	At risk	Events	Survivors
0.00	10	0	10
0.03	10	2	8
0.92	8	1	7
1.48	7	1	6
1.64	6	2	4
1.70	4	2	2
1.74	2	1	1
1.77	1	1	0

The KM estimator for the survival curve is formally defined as

$$S^{\text{KM}}(t) = \prod_{i:t_i \leq t} \left(1 - \frac{m_i}{r_i}\right),$$

where: $\mathcal{R}_t = \{i : t_i \leq t\}$ indicates the *risk set*, i.e. the set of observed times below the index value t; m_i is the total number of events observed in each of the times in the risk set; and r_i is the number of individuals at risk in each of the times included in the risk set.

In the example of Table 8.1, the survival curve for the third time ($t = 0.92$) can be computed as

$$\begin{aligned} S^{\text{KM}}(0.92) &= \left(1 - \frac{0}{10}\right)\left(1 - \frac{2}{10}\right)\left(1 - \frac{1}{8}\right) \\ &= 1 \times \frac{8}{10} \times \frac{7}{8} = \frac{7}{10}. \end{aligned}$$

This estimate holds until the next observed unique time – thus, in this case, we would estimate $S^{\text{KM}}(t) = 0.7$ for $t \in [0.92; 1.48)$. This gives KM estimates the typical "step-function" shape displayed in Figure 8.2a. Note that censoring is automatically accounted for in this computation, because the denominator is represented by the risk set, which excludes censored individuals.

8.3.2 Digitised data

One further problem with survival modelling in HTA is that, while it may be possible to access individual-level data for a specific study comparing an active (and typically innovative) treatment against some standard of care (placebo, or existing technologies, such as chemotherapy), it is very unlikely that we have available all individual-level data for all the relevant treatments, for which we may only have access to aggregated level data (cfr. Chapter 6).

Interestingly, graphical representations of the data are typically produced in the literature, in the form of Kaplan-Meier estimates, as shown in Figure 8.2a. Suitable algorithms exist that are able to process the image depicting the KM curves from a given study and recreate a synthetic dataset that resembles the original one, in the sense that if a KM estimated is produced using the synthetic data, the images would be very close. Zhang et al. (2024) have recently produced an `R` package (and a corresponding `R` Shiny web-application) to perform this operation, while other proprietary software, e.g. `DigitizeIT` or `Enguage`, is also available for the same purpose.

The use of digitised survival data has become increasingly popular, especially in HTA, because it allows to recreate a set of individual-level datasets that can be used to expand the full survival modelling to all the relevant comparators in an economic evaluation, effectively expanding the analysis of aggregated data. One (but not the only – we return to this point in Section 9.3.2) key limitation of digitised data is that the KM estimates are typically presented conditionally only on the treatment arm, as in Figure 8.2a. Every other covariate that may be of interest (e.g. sex, age, comorbidities or cancer stage at diagnosis) is averaged out in the KM curves that can be digitised. Nonetheless, this form of synthetic information is very often the only one available to modeller and thus it can be helpful, if used wisely.

In addition (and perhaps even more importantly), landmark trials upon which the evaluation of the time-to-event is based report outcomes both in terms of *overall survival* (OS; i.e. the time from enrolment to death) and using a surrogate *progression-free survival* (PFS, indicating the time from enrolment until "progression" to a worse status of prognosis). While the focus of the economic evaluation is on OS, often data from clinical experimentation are not mature enough to observe many deaths during the course of the follow-up; conversely, progression data tend to have lower amount of censoring and thus are often used as a proxy for OS – see also Green et al. (2025b), who develop a model based on a Bayesian hierarchical structure similar to those discussed in Chapter 6, to "borrow" strength from the more mature PSF curves and estimate OS with increased precision.

In the case of digitised data, because the curves are presented separately, in the absence of further information, it is impossible to embed the underlying correlation in the two outcomes. In other words, in the actual dataset, there may be individuals who first progress and then die and these will contribute to both the PFS and OS curves. However, simple digitisation process will not allow us to determine who they are and effectively only generate two separate, independent datasets: one with synthetic data on the time to progression and one with synthetic data on the time to death.

Using suitable algorithms (such as the one described in Guyot et al., 2012), it is possible to correctly estimate the number of individuals at risk at different points on a time-grid, thus properly accounting for censoring. Nonetheless, the overall limitation of using digitised over fully individual-level survival data remains.

Example 8.1. *NICE Technical Appraisal 174 (adapted from Williams et al., 2017a).* We focus here as a running example on one of NICE's technical appraisals (TAs), specifically TA174 (NICE, 2009). This considers a full economic evaluation of rituximab in combination with fludarabine and cyclophosphamide (RFC) against fludarabine and cyclophosphamide alone (FC) for the first-line treatment of chronic lymphocytic leukaemia (CLL-8).

Although the original data used in NICE (2009), mainly based on Hallek et al. (2010), are not publicly accessible, in their tutorial on using `R` to model survival analysis for economic evaluation, Williams et al. (2017a) make available a digitised version of the dataset, which we use as our motivating example. This version of the original dataset is also included in the `R` package `survHE` (Baio, 2020) – see Section 8.4.

Note 24: Digitising well is hard work...

The data presented by Williams et al. (2017a) benefit from a further layer of substantive post-processing, which allowed the research team to reconstruct (a very good approximation of) the full trajectory of each individual patients.

First, the KM curves for OS, PFS and Post-Progression Survival (PPS), available from Hallek et al. (2010) have been digitised, accounting for censoring, so that there were as many times points as there were patients.

Secondly, an iterative process was performed, to keep calculating KM estimates with the generated data, until all the event and censored times were reconstructed "in the right place", i.e. so that they matched the survival probabilities from the curves at each time to within an arbitrary margin of error of 0.005, in most cases.

The event times from the PFS and OS curves that most closely matched were assumed to be deaths without progression. This left the other PFS events as progressions and the other OS events as deaths after progression. This process is fairly straightforward in this particular study, because there are not too many deaths. The progression and death time for each individual were finally recreated by matching a progression time from the PFS curve with a time from the PPS curve that gave a death after progression time from the OS curve.

Obviously, this procedure does not retrieve the original data for all the individual trajectories with absolute certainty and therefore the digitised and post-processed dataset is merely an approximation to the "truth".

The data contain much information – for each individual (labelled in the ID column, in Table 8.2), we observe a treatment indicator, along two further indicators for whether progression and/or death have been observed (`1`) or not (`0`). The time (in months) at which these occur is also recorded – if either progression or death do not occur, the time is the point at which the individual is censored, i.e. they exit the observation. Because of the approximation in the digitisation and post-processing, there are some (relatively minor) discrepancies with the original data: for instance, Hallek et al. (2010) report 106 progressions in the RFC arm, while the synthetic data only count 104.

In the rest of this chapter, we consider a version of the overall dataset (which we, creatively, name `data`), which focuses on progression. In other words, if an individual either dies or is not observed to progress within the follow-up of the study, they are considered as censored (and the variable `status` is set to 0 – see Example 9.5 for more details on how to retrieve this dataset).

Figure 8.3 shows the KM curves for the two treatment arms. In the beginning and at the end of the follow-up period, there does not seem to be much separation among the two curves, when we also consider the interval estimates. In the middle of the observation period, however, the RFC arm seem to have better survival, as the KM curve is higher.

Table 8.3 shows the estimated numbers behind the KM curves. We report here, for simplicity, the first and last three times at which the estimates are produced, for both the treatment arms. In each row, we include the number of observed events (individuals who have a progression within the period defined by the two consecutive times), the overall number of individual at risk and the number of individuals censored, in that period.

Table 8.2: A snippet of the NICE TA174 digitised data. The progression and death time are shown in months since enrolment

ID	Progression?	Death?	Progression time	Death time	Treatment
1	1	0	31.991	32	RFC
2	1	0	30.552	30.6	RFC
3	1	0	27.906	28	RFC
4	1	0	2.877	3	FC
5	1	0	0.978	1.11	FC
6	1	0	1.611	1.77	FC

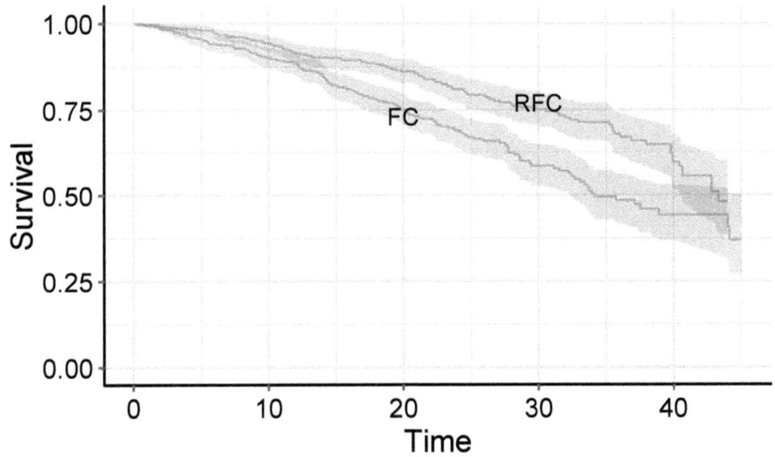

Figure 8.3: The Kaplan-Meier curves for the two treatment arms in the digitised TA174 data.

8.3.3 Modelling

Generally speaking, assuming the data include a vector of covariates $\boldsymbol{x}$, (e.g. age, sex, comorbidities, clinical history, trial arm, etc.), we can describe the vector of relevant parameters as $\boldsymbol{\theta} = (\mu(\boldsymbol{x}), \alpha(\boldsymbol{x}))$, where $\mu(\boldsymbol{x})$ is a *location* parameter, which indicates the mean or the scale of the probability distribution used to model the sampling variability in the time-to-event data, described by the density $f(t \mid \boldsymbol{\theta})$. As for $\alpha(\boldsymbol{x})$, this is a (set of) *ancillary* parameters, characterising the shape or variance of the underlying distribution.

Even though we may assume that the observed covariates modulate both the location and the ancillary parameters, most often, we simply limit the dependence for $\mu(\boldsymbol{x})$ and model α independently on $\boldsymbol{x}$ – Latimer (2011) suggests ways in which we can still incorporate the dependence on the covariates in shape parameters too (see Section 8.4.5 for more discussion).

Table 8.3: The estimated numbers underlying the KM curves for the two treatment arms. For each time point, we report the estimated number of events, the number at risk before that time point and the number of individuals censored at that time

RFC				FC			
Time	Events	At risk	Censored	Time	Events	At risk	Censored
0.058	0	407	1	0.058	0	403	1
0.748	1	406	0	0.173	1	402	0
0.806	0	405	1	1.266	1	401	0
...	...	...	...	...	...	...	...
44.016	1	12	0	43	0	22	4
44.131	1	11	0	43.326	1	18	0
45	0	10	10	44	0	17	17

Table 8.4: Some distributions commonly used in parametric survival modelling in HTA. The linear predictor η_i is defined as in Equation 8.8 throughout. The function $\gamma(a, x) = \int_0^x t^{a-1}\exp(-t)dt$ is the incomplete lower gamma function, while $\Phi(\cdot)$ is the cumulative distribution function of a Normal(0, 1) random variable.

Distribution	Density $f(t_i \mid \mu_i, \alpha)$	Location μ_i	Survival $S(t_i \mid \mu_i, \alpha)$
Exponential	$\mu_i \exp\left(-\mu_i t_i\right)$	$\exp(\eta_i)$	$\exp\left(-\mu_i t_i\right)$
Weibull	$\frac{\alpha}{\mu_i}\left(\frac{t_i}{\mu_i}\right)^{\alpha-1}\exp\left(-\left(\frac{t_i}{\mu_i}\right)^{\alpha}\right)$	$\exp(\eta_i)$	$\exp\left(-\left(\frac{t_i}{\mu_i}\right)^{\alpha}\right)$
Gamma	$\frac{\mu_i^{\alpha}}{\Gamma(\alpha)} t_i^{\alpha-1}\exp(-\mu_i t_i)$	$\exp(\eta_i)$	$1 - \frac{1}{\Gamma(\alpha)}\gamma(\alpha, \mu_i t_i)$
Gompertz	$\mu_i e^{\alpha t_i}\exp\left(-\frac{\mu_i}{\alpha\left(e^{\alpha t_i} - 1\right)}\right)$	$\exp(\eta_i)$	$\exp\left(\frac{-\mu_i}{\alpha(e^{\alpha t_i} - 1)}\right)$
log-logistic	$\frac{(\alpha/\mu_i)(t_i/\mu_i)^{\alpha-1}}{1 + (t_i/\mu_i)^{\alpha}}$	$\exp(\eta_i)$	$\left(1 + \left(\frac{t_i}{\mu_i}\right)^{\alpha}\right)^{-1}$
log-Normal	$\frac{1}{t_i\alpha\sqrt{2\pi}}\exp\left(-\frac{(\log t_i - \mu_i)^2}{2\alpha^2}\right)$	η_i	$1 - \Phi\left(\frac{\log t_i - \mu_i}{\alpha}\right)$

Notice also that in a parametric formulation such as this, the main quantities of interest, $S(t \mid \boldsymbol{\theta})$ and $h(t \mid \boldsymbol{\theta})$ can be written down as functions of $(\mu(\boldsymbol{x}), \alpha(\boldsymbol{x}))$ and thus, once we can produce suitable estimates for them, we can simply plug in any value for t in that functional form to extrapolate the survival or hazard.

We typically use a generalised linear formulation

$$g(\mu_i) = \eta_i = \beta_0 + \sum_{k=1}^{K} \beta_k x_{ik}[+\ldots] \tag{8.8}$$

Here, the function $g(\cdot)$ is usually the logarithm – and, in line with Baio (2020), we slightly abuse the notation and omit the dependence of μ_i on $\boldsymbol{x}$, for simplicity. As discussed in Section 5.2, the notation $[+\ldots]$ indicates that Equation 8.8 can be extended to additional terms, e.g. random effects to account for repeated measurements or clustering. This may be relevant, for instance, in the case of multi-site trials, or for "tumour-agnostic" experimentation, in which the same treatment is used across different cancer types, if they share the same underlying molecular abnormality.

Table 8.4 presents some selected choices to model the sampling variability for the observed and censored times, as well as the mathematical expression for the resulting density, the relationship linking the location parameter μ_i to the linear predictor η_i, as defined in Equation 8.8 and the functional form of the survival function, depending on the model parameters $\boldsymbol{\theta} = (\mu_i, \alpha)$. More detailed accounts for parametric survival models are presented, for example, in Latimer (2011), Cox (2008), or Jackson et al. (2025).

Note 25: Weibull parameterisations

Table 8.4 shows one specific parameterisation for the Weibull distribution, in terms of a *scale* μ_i and a *shape* α. This particular parameterisation gives rise to an *accelerated failure time* (AFT) interpretation, which amounts to assuming that the effect of a covariate is to accelerate or decelerate the life course of a disease by some constant.

To give a general intuition, we may consider the old cliché that every year in a dog's life is equivalent to about seven human years. Indicating the survival functions for humans and dogs as $S_H(t \mid \boldsymbol{\theta})$ and $S_D(t \mid \boldsymbol{\theta})$ respectively, we can summarise this by assuming that

$$S_D(t \mid \boldsymbol{\theta}) = S_H(7t \mid \boldsymbol{\theta}),$$

which essentially implies that the chances of a dog surviving past t years are identical to those of a human surviving past $7t$ years – in other words, dogs go through life seven times faster than humans.

Generally speaking, in an AFT model, we compare survival across two different "profiles" (e.g. covariates specifications) through an acceleration factor (e.g. the multiplier set at the value 7, in the dogs' life example). If this acceleration factor is greater than 1, then "exposure" benefits survival, while if it is less than 1, then it is detrimental.

The Weibull distribution also has a different parameterisation, which allows the *proportional hazard* (PH) interpretation. If we model

$$t \sim \text{Weibull}(\mu_i^*, \alpha) \qquad \text{with} \qquad p(t \mid \mu_i^*, \alpha) = \mu_i^* \alpha t_i^{\alpha-1} \exp\left(-\mu_i^* t_i^\alpha\right),$$

then we can prove that $S(t \mid \mu_i^*, \alpha) = \exp\left(-\mu_i^* t_i^\alpha\right)$. Using Equation 8.3, the hazard function is computed as

$$\begin{aligned} h(t \mid \mu_i^*, \alpha) &= \mu_i^* \alpha t_i^{\alpha-1} \\ &= \exp(\eta_i^*) \alpha t_i^{\alpha-1} \\ &= \exp\left(\beta_0^* + \sum_{k=1}^{K} \beta_k^* x_{ik}\right) \alpha t_i^{\alpha-1}. \end{aligned}$$

This implies that if we compare two profiles differing only in the value of one covariate in the linear predictor by taking the ratio of their respective hazard functions, then all the other terms cancel out and the coefficient of that covariate, β_k^*, is the (log-)hazard ratio.

Some simple algebra shows that, interestingly, we can retrieve the PH parameterisation from the AFT one, by setting

$$\mu_i = \exp\left(-\frac{\eta_i}{\alpha}\right) = \exp\left(-\frac{\beta_0 + \sum_{k=1}^{K} \beta_k x_{ik}}{\alpha}\right). \tag{8.9}$$

We return to this point in Section 8.3.5.

More generally, of the models described in Table 8.4, in the basic format: the Weibull and Exponential have both a PH and AFT interpretation, the Gompertz is PH only and the Gamma, log-Normal and log-logistic are AFT only.

NICE Decision Support Unit document (Latimer, 2011) presents an even larger set of potential distributional assumptions for the density $f(\cdot)$ than these in Table 8.4; while this was never intended to be prescriptive, but rather to serve as guidance for practitioners, many applications of survival modelling in HTA have taken this literally, with the consequence that, often, practitioners feel like they must test all the models described in the NICE guidance document.

8.3.4 Bayesian modelling

In a Bayesian setting, in addition to identifying a parametric model to describe the sampling variability in the observed (and censored) data, we need to include a suitable prior distribution for the model parameters $\boldsymbol{\theta}$. Baio (2020) summarises the main features of the various parametric models mentioned in Latimer (2011), alongside some default minimally vague specification for the prior distributions for the relevant specification of $\boldsymbol{\theta}$.

In the context of Equation 8.8, this amounts at least to the set of regression coefficients $\boldsymbol{\beta} = (\beta_0, \ldots, \beta_K)$, for which we can typically use a prior of the form $\boldsymbol{\beta} \stackrel{iid}{\sim} \text{Normal}(0, s)$ for some suitable standard deviation s, depending on the scale of the linear predictor.

The vast majority of the distributions suggested by Latimer (2011) is also indexed by a number of ancillary parameters $\boldsymbol{\alpha}$. The actual number of elements in $\boldsymbol{\alpha}$ varies with the mathematical function. For instance, as is clear in Table 8.4, one extreme case is the Exponential distribution, which is only indexed by a *rate* parameter, modelled as in Equation 8.8 with $g(\cdot) = \log(\cdot)$ and thus does not include any ancillary parameters. Using again Equation 8.3, we can see that the resulting hazard function for an Exponential distribution is

$$h(t \mid \mu_i) = \frac{\mu_i \exp(-\mu_i t_i)}{\exp(-\mu_i t_i)} = \mu_i,$$

which means that, for each individual profile i, the hazard is constant over time (and identical with the rate μ_i) – cfr. the discussion in Section 2.2.3.

Similarly, when considering the Weibull, Gamma, Gompertz or log-logistic distributions, the linear predictor is still defined on the log scale, but there is also an additional *shape* parameter, whose presence makes these distributions much more flexible than the often too simplistic Exponential. In these cases, because the shape parameter is $\alpha > 0$, a suitable prior may be a relatively vague Gamma(ϵ, ϵ) for some small constant ϵ, say $\epsilon = 0.1$. The log-Normal distribution is also characterised by two parameters, but it is already defined on the log scale and thus the function $g(\cdot)$ transforming the linear predictor is just the identity.

Note 26: The importance of being Bayesian (in survival modelling in HTA)

Latimer (2011) also mentions the Generalised Gamma and Generalised F as even more flexible options (the actual details of the mathematical definitions are not important, here – we also refer the reader to Jackson et al., 2010; and Jackson, 2016 and for more information).

These two distributions have, respectively, 2 and 3 ancillary parameters, which indeed contribute to making the shape of the resulting survival curve more "wiggly". On the other hand, because of the larger number of free parameters, they tend to be "data-hungry" and it is generally harder to estimate all the parameters precisely.

In the case of the Generalised F, the ancillary parameters are $\boldsymbol{\alpha} = (\sigma, p, q)$, representing a scale and two shape parameters, with $\sigma, p > 0$ and $q \in \mathbb{R}$ – see Cox (2008) for more details.

Consider for instance the fictional data presented in Figure 8.2a. If we try to fit a Generalised F to the underlying data using MLE, we obtain the results presented in Table 8.5.

Table 8.5: The parameter estimates for the Generalised F model fitting, using maximum likelihood estimates

Parameter	Mean	2.5%	97.5%
μ	2.291	2.135	2.448
σ	0.5873	0.4611	0.7481
q	0.8487	0.3575	1.34
p	0.002683	6.305505e-32	1.141320e+26
Treatment	0.3465	0.1744	0.5185

While running the model using MLE is very quick (the running time is only 0.118 seconds), there is an interesting finding in Table 8.5. The estimate for the parameter p has a 95% interval estimates that effectively spans over the entire $\mathbb{R}^+$ range – the lower limit is effectively 0, while the upper limit is, for all intents and purposes, ∞.

The reason for this quirky result is that there is not enough information in the data to be able to estimate properly all the model parameters – this is essentially a problem of "identifiability".

Conversely, in the absence of substantial information coming from the data (which is often the case with censoring), we could use a Bayesian approach and set the priors to "nudge" the posterior in the right direction. For instance, we could set up the following relatively vague (and yet not totally clueless) priors: $\sigma \sim \text{Gamma}(0.1, 0.1)$, $\log p \sim \text{Normal}(0, 0.5)$ and $q \sim \text{Normal}(0, 2.5)$. Using this model structure, the results are pretty comparable with the MLE estimate for all the model parameters – except for p, which this time has a rather different and most sensible estimate, both for the point and the interval values.

Table 8.6: The parameter estimates for the Generalised F model fitting, using Bayesian modelling

Parameter	Mean	2.5%	97.5%
μ	2.2571	2.0824	2.4227
σ	0.5085	0.3715	0.6517
q	0.7079	0.1104	1.3498
p	1.1023	0.378	2.6053
Treatment	0.3474	0.1851	0.5196

The priors have the important effect of regularising the inference, by complementing the limited information contained in the data and placing suitably finite ranges for the parameters that are harder to identify, thus leading to a 95% estimate for p that is much more sensible. Notice, however, that similarly to our discussion in Example 6.3, none of these priors are extreme: using simple Normal theory or Monte Carlo simulations, we can see that the prior for $\log p$ implies that $\Pr(p < 2.65) \approx 0.975$.

We may relax this assumption and increase the standard deviation for $\log p$ and perhaps we should run a few versions of the model to assess the sensitivity of the results to changes in the priors; for instance, if we set $\log p \sim \text{Normal}(0, 1)$, then the posterior point estimate would change to 1.53 and the 95% posterior interval for p would expand up to 6.36. This does show some sensitivity to the prior, which is consistent with the failure of convergence in the MLE – but essentially, we need to do something, because pretending that the only information we have is sufficient, will simply return ridiculous (and potentially dangerous!) estimates, as in Table 8.5.

The advantages in the Bayesian approach come at a computational cost: the model now runs in 16.678 seconds – still not unbearable, but substantially higher than for the MLE equivalent. On this occasion[2], clearly time well spent...

8.3.5 Bayesian computation for survival modelling in HTA

In theory, coding up a survival model in standard Bayesian software (e.g. BUGS or JAGS) is not that complicated, although this is one of the few places in which the syntax used by BUGS differ from that used by JAGS in dealing with censoring and thus care is needed when using either of these two pieces of software for survival modelling – see Lunn et al. (2013, sec. 12.6.2) for details in the syntax differences, as well as Alvares et al. (2021) for a detailed description of how JAGS can handle various types of survival models.

In addition, Gibbs sampling can struggle with survival models: compilation and running time can be rather long, mainly because the main outcome t has missing values in the data (the censored times). To combat this problem, it is generally useful to set initial values for t in a clever way to avoid problems in running the MCMC. In addition, convergence may be difficult to reach even with relatively simple models (e.g. Weibull Proportional Hazard).

For these reasons, survival modelling is one of the arguably limited number of applications in HTA in which the use alternative modes of Bayesian inference can be helpful to overcome or at least limit these issues. One option is to consider Integrated Nested Laplace Approximation (INLA – see Section 3.1.2). This is typically very fast and accurate, although, at present, it can only run a limited number of survival models (e.g. Weibull, Exponential, Gompertz, log-Normal and log-logistic).

Another important alternative is Hamiltonian Monte Carlo (HMC – see Section 3.1.2 and Section 2.3.3). HMC is typically very efficient and flexible for survival modelling and we can implement virtually any distributional assumption – the software Stan and the relevant R package rstan allow the user to build different blocks in which custom sampling distributions can be defined (which is helpful for instance to account for censoring – typically expressing the individual likelihood as in Equation 8.7). More details on Stan and rstan are given in Carpenter et al. (2017) and the comprehensive online user's guide (Stan development team, 2024).

The code below shows an example, in which we construct a PH parameterisation for the Weibull distribution, starting from the AFT model described in Table 8.4, making use of Equation 8.9.

```
// Stan code for Weibull survival model (with PH parameterisation)

functions {
  // Defines the log hazard (using the AFT parameterisation)
  vector log_h (vector t, real shape, vector scale) {
```

[2]Actually, in the author's considered opinion, being Bayesian is *always* time well spent...

```
    vector[num_elements(t)] log_hvec;
    // NB: The './' operator is the element-wise division
    log_hvec = log(shape)+(shape-1)*log(t ./ scale)-log(scale);
    return log_hvec;
  }

  // Defines the log survival (using the AFT parameterisation)
  vector log_S (vector t, real shape, vector scale) {
    vector[num_elements(t)] log_Svec;
    for (i in 1:num_elements(t)) {
      log_Svec[i] = -pow((t[i]/scale[i]),shape);
    }
    return log_Svec;
  }

  // Defines the sampling distribution (using the AFT parameterisation)
  real surv_weibullPH_lpdf (vector t, vector d, real shape, vector scale) {
    vector[num_elements(t)] log_lik;
    real prob;
    // NB: And the '.*' operator is the element-wise multiplication
    log_lik = d .* log_h(t,shape,scale) + log_S(t,shape,scale);
    prob = sum(log_lik);
    return prob;
  }
}

data {
  int n;                            // number of observations
  vector[n] t;                      // observed times
  vector[n] d;                      // censoring (1=observed, 0=censored)
  int K;                            // number of covariates
  matrix[n,K] X;                    // matrix of covariates (n rows, K columns)
  vector[K] mu_beta;                // mean of the covariates coefficients
  vector<lower=0> [K] sigma_beta; // sd of the covariates coefficients
  real<lower=0> a_alpha;            // parameters for the shape
  real<lower=0> b_alpha;
}

parameters {
  vector[K] beta;           // Coefficients in linear predictor (with intercept)
  real<lower=0> alpha;      // shape parameter
}

transformed parameters {
  vector[n] eta;
  vector[n] mu;
  eta = -(X*beta)/alpha;    // rescales the linear predictor to get PH
  for (i in 1:n) {
    mu[i] = exp(eta[i]);
  }
```

```
}

model {
  alpha ~ gamma(a_alpha,b_alpha);
  beta ~ normal(mu_beta,sigma_beta);
  t ~ surv_weibullPH(d,alpha,mu);
}

generated quantities {
  real scale;                    // scale parameter
  scale = exp(beta[1]);
}
```

A Stan programme is made by a number of "blocks", each of which defines specific elements of the probabilistic model. Blocks are labelled by keywords (for instance functions, or data) and enclosed in curly brackets. Unlike in R, comments are indicated using the C++ syntax of double slash //.

In the example above, we start the code with a functions block, in which we define customised functions to be used in the sampling process. Here, we define the log hazard log_h() and the log survival log_S() functions. Unlike R, Stan requires the user to specify the type associated with each variable – for instance, the block

```
vector log_h (vector t, real shape, vector scale) {
...
```

tells the compiler that inputs t, shape and scale are, respectively a vector, a real number and another vector; in addition we specify that the output value for the function log_h is also a vector.

In the functions block, we combine the log hazard and log survival functions to determine the individual likelihood contributions log_lik (again, in line with Equation 8.7). The function surv_weibullPH_lpdf() returns the sum of all the individual likelihood contributions into the real number prob, containing the overall log-likelihood – this effectively creates a new, custom-made distribution surv_weibullPH() that can be used to model sampling variability.

The next block defines the data. Here, we mostly need to explicitly specify the type (and length) of each data variable. The notation vector<lower=0> [K] sigma_beta instructs the compiler that the variable sigma_beta is a positive vector of length K.

Next, in the block parameters, we specify the type and dimension for all the core parameters, i.e. those that are directly modelled using a probability distributions. The parameters that are defined as deterministic functions of other (possibly random) quantities are all defined in the transformed parameters block. Here, for instance, we define the linear predictor (indicated as η_i in Equation 8.8 and as eta in the model code) using the relationship described in Equation 8.9.

The model block is where we specify the distributional assumptions: in this case, we set the prior distributions for the shape $\alpha \sim \text{Gamma}(a_\alpha, b_\alpha)$ for set constants a_α and b_α, as well as the coefficients for the linear predictor $\beta_1, \ldots, \beta_K \stackrel{iid}{\sim} \text{Normal}(\mu_\beta, \sigma_\beta)$. Because the parameter beta is defined as a vector of size H in the model code, Stan understands the vectorised definition of the prior, which gives the same Normal with set mean μ_β and *standard deviation* σ_β – notice that, unlike BUGS or JAGS, Stan indexes the Normal distribution more naturally in terms of mean and standard deviation. The variable t, representing the observed times is modelled using the custom-made surv_weibullPH distribution, which takes as inputs the vector of censoring indicators d, the shape alpha and the location parameter mu.

Finally, we can specify other generated quantities, which are typically functions of basic parameters, which are simply forward sampled – in this case we create a variable scale, which is the rescaled intercept in the linear predictor.

The code described above can be run from R using the package rstan. However, the vast majority of the relevant computational facilities for the specific objective of performing Bayesian modelling in HTA have been coded up into the package survHE, which we use in the rest of the chapter and introduce in Section 8.4.

8.4 Using the R package survHE

survHE (Baio, 2020) is an R package designed with the specific objective to perform survival analysis for HTA. In a nutshell, survHE is designed as a modular package, with a basic component (the actual survHE package), which is essentially a "wrapper" to one of the most popular survival packages, flexsurv (Jackson, 2016), which is a general-purpose tool for performing several types of survival analysis using maximum likelihood estimates. The core survHE package also defines several facilities that are helpful when performing the analysis in an HTA context, including standardised post-processing of the estimates, both in tabular and graphical format, as well as for the purposes of PSA (Section 4.3).

There are also two "add-on" packages, called survHEinla and survHEhmc, which code specific functions to run Bayesian survival modelling, using either INLA or HMC through Stan and rstan.

Installing survHE

The core code for survHE can be installed directly from the main R repository, the Comprehensive R Archive Network (CRAN), which is hosted at https://cran.r-project.org/. In a R terminal, we can use the standard command

```
install.packages("survHE")
```

to install the package. This creates the backbone for the whole survHE infrastructure to work. All the basic MLE estimation routines are installed, as well as the basic functions that perform plotting, printing, data pre- and post-processing, including for PSA.

The two Bayesian modules can be installed from their GitHub repositories, using R commands such as the following.

```
# Installs the package 'remotes', that can be used to download packages
# off a GitHub repository (only need to run this command once)
install.packages(remotes)

# Uses 'remotes' to install the package from GitHub
remotes::install_github("giabaio/survHEhmc")
remotes::install_github("giabaio/survHEinla")

# Or via the alternative repository at at https://giabaio.r-universe.dev/
install.packages(
  c("survHEhmc","survHEinla"),
  repos=c("https://giabaio.r-universe.dev","https://cloud.r-project.org")
)
```

– again, the latter method is perhaps more user-friendly and we thus recommend it. It is not necessary to install both the Bayesian add ons, or even one of them (although, obviously, in case neither `survHEinla` nor `survHEhmc` are present in the user's system, they will not be able to run the Bayesian versions of the models...).

Depending on the user's specification, `survHE` maps internally to different code, which calls either `flexsurv`, `rstan` or `INLA` in the background to produce the relevant estimates. The resulting output is also standardised and presented in a form that is common, irrespective on the underlying inferential engine. Further post-processing can happen directly in `R`.

We use NICE TA174 as a running example to demonstrate the use of `survHE` to perform Bayesian modelling in the context of survival analysis in HTA. Of course, the use of `survHE` is absolutely not a necessity and the user could write bespoke code to run the MCMC analysis (either in `BUGS`/`JAGS` or in `Stan`).

Nonetheless, we do take advantage of the fact that `survHE` is somehow tailor-made for this specific context and thus use it throughout. We also refer the user to Baio (2020), as well as the package website (`https://gianluca.statistica.it/software/survhe/`) and GitHub repository (`https://github.com/giabaio/survHEhmc`) for further information.

Example 8.2. *NICE TA174 (continued): running the models using* `survHE`**.** We use `survHE` to fit a Bayesian model using different distributional assumptions to the NICE TA174 data described in Example 8.1. To fix ideas, we consider three options. The first one is a Weibull (AFT) model, specified as in Equation 8.10.

$$
\begin{aligned}
t_i &\sim \text{Weibull}(\mu_i, \alpha) \\
\log(\mu_i) &= \beta_0 + \beta_1 \text{Treatment}_i \\
\beta_0, \beta_1 &\overset{iid}{\sim} \text{Normal}(0, 5) \\
\alpha &\sim \text{Gamma}(0.1, 0.1).
\end{aligned}
\tag{8.10}
$$

For the second model, we use a similar specification, but choose a Gompertz sampling distribution, as in Equation 8.11.

$$\begin{aligned} t_i &\sim \text{Gompertz}(\mu_i, \alpha) \\ \log(\mu_i) &= \beta_0 + \beta_1 \text{Treatment}_i \\ \beta_0, \beta_1 &\overset{iid}{\sim} \text{Normal}(0, 5) \\ \alpha &\sim \text{Gamma}(0.1, 0.1). \end{aligned} \tag{8.11}$$

Finally, we specify a log-Normal model, as in Equation 8.12.

$$\begin{aligned} t_i &\sim \text{log-Normal}(\mu_i, \alpha) \\ \mu_i &= \beta_0 + \beta_1 \text{Treatment}_i \\ \beta_0, \beta_1 &\overset{iid}{\sim} \text{Normal}(0, 100) \\ \log(\alpha) &\sim \text{Uniform}(0, 5). \end{aligned} \tag{8.12}$$

Notice that the prior distributions set out for the model parameters in the three specifications are the ones used by default by `survHE` – see Baio (2020) and Section 8.4.1 for more details.

We can use the function `fit.models()` in the package `survHE` to run the three models using `Stan` and `rstan` in the background, for instance using code such as the following.

```
# Runs the Bayesian analysis using 'survHE'
m=fit.models(
  Surv(time,status)~treatment,
  data=data,
  distr=c("wei","gom","lno"),
  method="hmc"
)
```

`fit.models()` takes as input:

- a model "formula", in which we specify the outcome `Surv(time,status)`, indicating the observed times and the censoring indicator, as a function of the linear predictor. In this case, we only include the treatment arm as a covariate (technically, this is a "factor", i.e. a categorical variable, taking values `RFC` and `FC`) and, in line with standard `R` notation, we can omit the intercept, which we could explicitly add or remove by writing `Surv(time,status)~1+treatment` or `Surv(time,status)~treatment-1`, respectively, as it is included by default.
- A named dataset (in this case, we assume that the subset for the TA174 data shown in Figure 8.3 is stored in an object named `data`).
- A vector of named distributions. `survHE` has a set of built-in abbreviations[3] – the string vector `c("wei","gom","lno")` instructs `R` to run the models for the three sampling distributions specified in Equations 8.10–8.12. It is not essential to store multiple models in the same object (`m`, in this case). We could have run three separate instances of `fit.models()` giving as input a different distribution, in each.
- The inferential method, in this case `hmc`. The default considers the MLE.

[3]It is possible to run the "hidden" function `survHE:::load_availables()` to see all the available distribution names and the relevant abbreviation for each inferential engine.

A potentially helpful optional argument is `save.stan`; if set to `TRUE`, when `method="hmc"`, then `survHE` will save the pre-compiled `Stan` model code on the user's working directory. This can then be used to customise the model further, starting from the working template that is built-in the `survHE` package.

The object `m` contains the output generated for the three models considered; in particular, it contains four components, as can be seen by typing the `R` command `names(m)`. The first one (`models`) is the object in which `survHE` stores the output produced by the underlying inferential engine (in this case, `rstan`). `survHE` has a number of methods that can be applied to this object, in order to print and plot the outcome in suitable formats.

The second element of `m` is the object `model.fitting`, which contains a set of model fitting statistics, i.e. the AIC and BIC, as well as the DIC, if the model has been fitted using a Bayesian method – see Section 5.3.1 for more details on information criteria.

The other two objects, which can be accessed using the notation `m$method` and `m$misc` are really just for `survHE` internal consumption and contain a string with the inferential method used (`hmc`, in this case) and a set of "miscellanea", including the actual data object, the running time (in seconds) and the formula specified to fit the model. As mentioned above, the user does not really need to use this information, but other functions in `survHE` do, in order to create plots and relevant summaries.

We can summarise the models using the `print()` method, for instance using the following code.

```
# Prints the summary stats for the first model (Weibul AFT)
print(m,mod=1)
```

```
Model fit for the Weibull AF model, obtained using Stan (Bayesian inference via
Hamiltonian Monte Carlo). Running time: 2.928 seconds

                   mean        se       L95%      U95%
shape          1.501199 0.0861131   1.338545  1.680990
scale         45.813915 2.8580690  40.948629 52.102713
treatmentRFC   0.360521 0.0881215   0.195345  0.532749

Model fitting summaries
Akaike Information Criterion (AIC)....: 2594.718
Bayesian Information Criterion (BIC)..: 2613.506
Deviance Information Criterion (DIC)..: 2592.803
```

```
# Prints the summary stats for the second model (Gompertz)
print(m,mod=2)
```

```
Model fit for the Gompertz model, obtained using Stan (Bayesian inference via
Hamiltonian Monte Carlo). Running time: 3.480 seconds

                    mean          se        L95%       U95%
shape         0.04151302 0.00609955  0.02962516  0.0529226
rate          0.00873628 0.00121314  0.00661164  0.0111927
treatmentRFC -0.55315606 0.12988454 -0.81820588 -0.3011726

Model fitting summaries
Akaike Information Criterion (AIC)....: 2591.911
```

```
Bayesian Information Criterion (BIC)..: 2610.700
Deviance Information Criterion (DIC)..: 2590.088
```

```
# Prints the summary stats for the third model (log-Normal)
print(m,mod=3)
```

```
Model fit for the log-Normal model, obtained using Stan (Bayesian inference via
Hamiltonian Monte Carlo). Running time: 4.407 seconds

                  mean        se      L95%      U95%
meanlog       3.730758 0.0847732 3.562578 3.896071
sdlog         1.218969 0.0612683 1.106838 1.343186
treatmentRFC 0.432944 0.1086174 0.230513 0.651142

Model fitting summaries
Akaike Information Criterion (AIC)....: 2626.819
Bayesian Information Criterion (BIC)..: 2645.607
Deviance Information Criterion (DIC)..: 2624.965
```

As is possible to see, the `print()` method in `survHE` returns a standardised table (this is independent on the inferential method chosen) and reports some key information. First, it specifies what model has been fitted and with which inferential method, as well as the running time (extracted from the object `m$misc$time2run`). Then, the table shows the point estimate for the model parameters, as well as a measure of standard error and a 95% interval. As we are using a Bayesian model, here, these are obtained by summarising the HMC simulations from the posterior distributions. Finally, the `print()` method provides some model fitting statistics – as this is a Bayesian model, AIC, BIC and DIC are all computed and reported.

One interesting aspect from the summary tables above is that the coefficients of the models are estimated to substantially different values. This is not surprising for the core parameters: for instance, the parameter `scale` in the Weibull AFT model is the intercept β_0 of the linear predictor $\eta_i = \beta_0 + \beta_1 \text{Treatment}_i$. In the Gompertz model, β_0 is still the intercept of η_i, but in this model it represents a *rate*, instead of a scale – effectively, it is defined on an inverse scale as rate = 1/scale. In the log-Normal model, β_0 is simply the mean survival time, on the log scale, for individuals over which there is no treatment effect (i.e. the controls) and thus the interpretation is also different, which explains the difference in the estimated value.

Similarly, the nuisance parameters α represents a shape for the Weibull and Gompertz (albeit in regard to a scale and a rate, respectively), while it is a log standard deviation for the log-Normal model, which again justifies the different values shown in the summary tables above.

As for the treatment effect, the Weibull and the log-Normal models described above are both characterised by an AFT interpretation. This explains why the resulting coefficient for the treatment effect (indicated as `treatmentRFC` in the summary tables and equivalent to β_1 in the models of Equations 8.10 – 8.12) are reasonably similar, at least in the point estimate. The Gompertz model, conversely, has a PH interpretation, whereby $\exp(\beta_1)$ is the hazard ratio, i.e. a measure of how much more likely a random individual from the target population is to experience the event under study if they are in the treatment arm, as opposed to the control. In this case, we can see that $\exp(\beta_1) = \exp(-0.5531561) = 0.575$ indicates that the intervention arm (RFC) is beneficial as it decreases the hazard of experiencing the event (progression) – this is because the hazard ratio is less than 1.

Consistently with this finding and the discussion in Note 25 in Section 8.3.3, the acceleration factor for both the Weibull and the log-Normal models is positive, to indicate a beneficial treatment effect.

8.4.1 Setting prior distributions

One of the main advantages of `survHE` is that, similarly to other packages that use `rstan` in the background (e.g. the very popular `brms` – see Bürkner, 2017), the user does not have to code up a full Bayesian model using `Stan` code. Rather, for a set of defined models, the package "pre-compiles" the code (which makes the running time shorter, overall) and the user needs to specify commands similar to the `R` built-in function `lm()` to define the distributional assumptions and data, in order to run the analysis.

On the one hand, this is a very attractive feature, because it removes a potential barrier for the user, thus possibly improving uptake of the Bayesian machinery in complex cases. On the other hand, however, this somehow constrains the modelling to a more or less pre-defined setup, which may limit the generalisability and use of the tool.

Fortunately, neither these potential issues are insurmountable: for `survHE`, the average user can probably use the default setup (with the usual caveat that extensive post-processing and sensitivity analysis are essential to any statistical modelling, perhaps even more so in a Bayesian context). In addition, the package has some built-in facilities that allow to modify the default code as well as the default prior distributions.

Example 8.3. *NICE TA174 (continued): setting non-default priors.* If we are happy with the distributional assumptions specified in the default models encoded in `survHE` (e.g. considering a Normal distribution for the linear predictor coefficients $\boldsymbol\beta$, or a Gamma prior for the shape α of the Weibull distribution), we can use the optional argument `priors` to instruct `fit.models()` to use customised values *for the parameters* of these distributions (see Baio, 2020 for more details on how to define this argument).

For instance, suppose we want to model the shape parameter for the Weibull model using an Exponential(3) distribution. By the properties of the Gamma distribution, this is equivalent to modelling $\alpha \sim \text{Gamma}(1, 3)$. In addition, we want to change the prior for the regression coefficients to $\beta_0, \beta_1 \stackrel{iid}{\sim} \text{Normal}(0, 10)$, to double the standard deviation from the default choice. We can specify this version of the model using the following command – see again Baio (2020, sect. 5.2) specifically on how to structure the list `priors` in the presence of multiple distributions specified in the input `distr`, in the call to `fit.models()`.

```
m1=fit.models(
  Surv(time,status)~treatment, data=data, distr="wei", method="hmc",
  priors=list(
    wei=list(
      a_alpha=1,b_alpha=3,
      sigma_beta=rep(10,2)
    )
  )
)
```

Here, we need to specify `sigma_beta=rep(10,2)` because the vector of regression coefficients $\boldsymbol{\beta}$ has two values (β_0, β_1). We do not have to assume the same standard deviation for all the elements of $\boldsymbol{\beta}$ and we could have set a vector of different values, e.g. `sigma_beta=c(1,4)`.

In this particular instance, the output of the model does not vary dramatically, as we can check by comparing the summary tables (cfr. the results in Example 8.2).

```
# Prints the results with the revised priors
print(m1)
```

```
Model fit for the Weibull AF model, obtained using Stan (Bayesian inference via
Hamiltonian Monte Carlo). Running time: 3.443 seconds

                    mean        se      L95%      U95%
shape           1.492758 0.0856485  1.328224  1.673059
scale          46.010411 2.9410947 40.734988 52.213182
treatmentRFC    0.361651 0.0931622  0.182556  0.559986

Model fitting summaries
Akaike Information Criterion (AIC)....: 2594.755
Bayesian Information Criterion (BIC)..: 2613.543
Deviance Information Criterion (DIC)..: 2593.055
```

If we wanted to completely change the distributional assumptions for the priors, then we would need to set the `save.stan` option to `TRUE` in a dummy call to the `fit.models()` function and save the model template to a `.stan` file. The resulting object, say `x`, would also include an element `x$misc$data.stan`, which is a list with the relevant data formatted in a way that `rstan` would accept. At that point, we can modify the `Stan` code directly – for instance we could replace the code

```
model {
  alpha ~ gamma(a_alpha,b_alpha);
  ...
}
```

with the code

```
model {
  alpha ~ normal(0,3);
  ...
}
```

to encode the assumption that the shape parameter for the Weibull AFT model has a Half-Normal distribution, i.e. a Normal truncated to be positive – because we have specified in the `parameters` block

```
  real<lower=0> alpha;
```

then `Stan` knows that `alpha` must be positive and thus can automatically rescale the set distribution to fit the range for the parameter. Notice however that, in this case, we cannot run the model using `survHE`, but we would need to use pure `rstan` to specify data and model code see the `rstan` manual (Stan development team, 2024), for details on how to do so.

8.4.2 Assessing model convergence

Much as for any Bayesian model, before we can use the output of a call to `fit.models()` that specifies `method="hmc"`, we need to perform extensive model diagnostics to check convergence and autocorrelation, as discussed in Section 2.3.2. This is fundamental, because of course we need to make sure that the estimates are representative of the target posterior distribution, before we can use them to derive the important quantities for the HTA analysis, e.g. the survival curves.

We can use a combination of `survHE` and `rstan` (and, possibly, `bmhe`) facilities to streamline this process, as demonstrated in the next example.

Example 8.4. *NICE TA174 (continued): assessing model convergence.* Outputs obtained running `survHE` are saved onto the `R` workspace as objects in the `survHE` class. As mentioned above, these are effectively lists with several elements, one of which, `model`, in fact contains all the output generated by the underlying inferential engine. Because in the object `m` described in Example 8.2 is created running `rstan` in the background, we can use all the `rstan` features to assess convergence, much as we have discussed in Section 2.3.2.

Firstly, the `print()` method in `survHE` has an option that allows to show the original, "unstandardised" results obtained by the package that has been called in the background to perform the analyses (this would be `flexsurv` for MLE, or `Stan/INLA` for a Bayesian model). We can do this by using the option `original=TRUE`, as in the following code.

```
print(m,mod=2,original=TRUE,digits=2,print_priors=TRUE)
```

```
Inference for Stan model: Gompertz.
2 chains, each with iter=2000; warmup=1000; thin=1;
post-warmup draws per chain=1000, total post-warmup draws=2000.

              mean se_mean   sd     2.5%      25%      50%      75%    97.5% n_eff Rhat
beta[1]      -4.75    0.01 0.14    -5.02    -4.85    -4.75    -4.65    -4.49   684 1.00
beta[2]      -0.55    0.00 0.13    -0.82    -0.64    -0.55    -0.46    -0.30  1113 1.01
alpha         0.04    0.00 0.01     0.03     0.04     0.04     0.05     0.05   683 1.00
rate          0.01    0.00 0.00     0.01     0.01     0.01     0.01     0.01   708 1.00
lp__      -1294.28    0.05 1.29 -1297.62 -1294.77 -1293.96 -1293.37 -1292.84   799 1.00

Samples were drawn using NUTS(diag_e) at Tue May 26 14:30:02 2026.
For each parameter, n_eff is a crude measure of effective sample size,
and Rhat is the potential scale reduction factor on split chains (at
convergence, Rhat=1).

Prior modelling assumptions
alpha ~ gamma(0.1, 0.1)
(Intercept): beta[1] ~ normal(0, 5)
treatmentRFC: beta[2] ~ normal(0, 5)
t ~ surv_gompertz(d,alpha,mu)
```

The output is a summary table where the parameters are named using the convention defined in the `Stan` code that is automatically used by `survHE` when calling `rstan` in the background. In this case, the coefficients are presented on the log scale, which is how the linear predictor is defined in the `Stan` code. The parameter `beta[1]` maps onto the log of the parameter `rate`, while `beta[2]` maps onto the parameter `treatmentRFC` presented in the

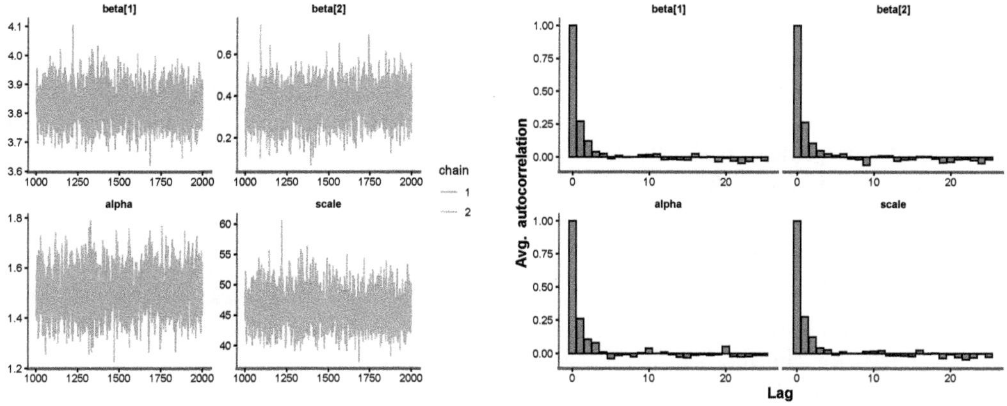

(a) Traceplot for a Stan object. (b) Autocorrelation plot for a Stan object.

Figure 8.4: Convergence diagnostics for the model.

summary table shown in Example 8.2. The parameter `alpha` is the `shape` in Example 8.2. In the `Stan` code, the `rate` is also directly computed (in fact, in the `generated quantities` block – cfr. the code discussed in Section 8.3.5).

The original table also shows familiar quantities such as `n_eff` and `Rhat` that can be used to check convergence and autocorrelation (see Section 2.3.2). In this case, we have also used the option `print_priors=TRUE`, which, in combination with `original=TRUE`, instructs `survHE` to append a summary of the distributional assumptions used in the prior distributions to the table. This option can be omitted and obviously has no effect when the model is run using `flexsurv`.

In addition, as mentioned above, we can use `rstan` built-in functions to visualise and assess convergence, for example as in the following code and the resulting output in Figure 8.4.

```
# Generates traceplots for the Weibull model's parameters
rstan::traceplot(m$models[[1]])

# Generates autocorrelation plots for the Weibull model's parameters
rstan::stan_ac(m$models[[1]])
```

This sort of diagnostic checks should *always* be performed when running Bayesian modelling, but, again, there is no overheads in carrying them out following a `survHE` run, because the resulting object is, fundamentally, a `rstan` output and thus all "standard" Bayesian procedures for post-processing directly apply.

8.4.3 Visualisation and assessment of the survival curves

Once a model has been fitted to observed data and the estimates for the model parameters obtained (e.g. in terms of simulations from the joint posterior distribution, in a Bayesian context), we need to move our analysis to a slightly different level, in which we try and get a sense of the treatment effect, in terms of improvement in survival.

As mentioned in Section 8.3, the main reason why we focus on parametric modelling is because we can use the posterior for the model parameters $\boldsymbol{\theta}$ to induce a posterior on the survival curve $S(t \mid \boldsymbol{\theta}) = g(\boldsymbol{\theta})$, where the function $g(\cdot)$ depends on the specific model chosen, as shown in Table 8.4.

Especially as the general guideline is to try a number of parametric models to then produce the "base-case" evaluation using the one that "fits the data best" (we clarify the actual meaning of this phrase in the next few sections), it is vital to visualise the results and be able to argue for a specific choice of model, on a combination of numerical and clinical evidence.

Example 8.5. *NICE TA174 (continued): estimating the survival curves.* survHE has a built-in plot() method, which is based on ggplot2 and can be used to visualise the resulting survival curve for the models fitted using the function fit.models(). For instance, in the NICE TA174 example, we can simply use the following code – notice that we take advantage of the ggplot2 processing facilities and overwrite survHE colouring scheme to ensure that the three models are most distinguishable both when visualised in colour and in grey-scale. We do this by adding the ggplot2 function scale_color_manual() and specifying colours with significant differences in luminance, which are then markedly separated in grey-scale.

```
# Plots the survival curves for all models and adds some customisation
plot(
  m,
  # Adds the KM estimates (optional)
  add.km=TRUE,
  # Customises the treatment labels (optional)
  lab.profile=c("RFC","FC")
) +
# Customises the position of the legend (optional)
theme(
  legend.position.inside=c(.2,.2)
) + scale_color_manual(values=c("#000000","#1F77B4","#FF7F0E"))
```

Figure 8.5 shows the KM curves for the two treatment arms with the survival curves estimated from the models in Equations 8.10 – 8.12. Typically, we seek the model that tends to approximate the trajectory in the KM best: for instance, in Figure 8.5 the log-Normal model seems relatively badly calibrated, particularly in the FC arm, where it under-estimates the survival pattern, especially at the beginning of the observation (when the curve is outside the interval around the KM estimates). It also seem to slightly over-estimate survival towards the end of the trial, although in this case the curve is within the KM interval.

As for the other models, the Gompertz does reasonably well for the RFC arm, seemingly capturing the dip in survival at the end of the follow-up. In the FC arm, it perhaps tends to under-estimate survival at the end of the follow-up, perhaps due to some sort of "plateau", probably due to censoring.

The Weibull model seems perhaps to adapt best to the FC arm, especially at the end of the follow-up, but it is maybe a bit over-optimistic in the last part of the observed data, for the RFC arm.

While perhaps the main objective of the survival analysis in HTA is to produce an estimate of the survival curves, it is generally very helpful to also look at the resulting hazards, to get a sense of the clinical plausibility of the results.

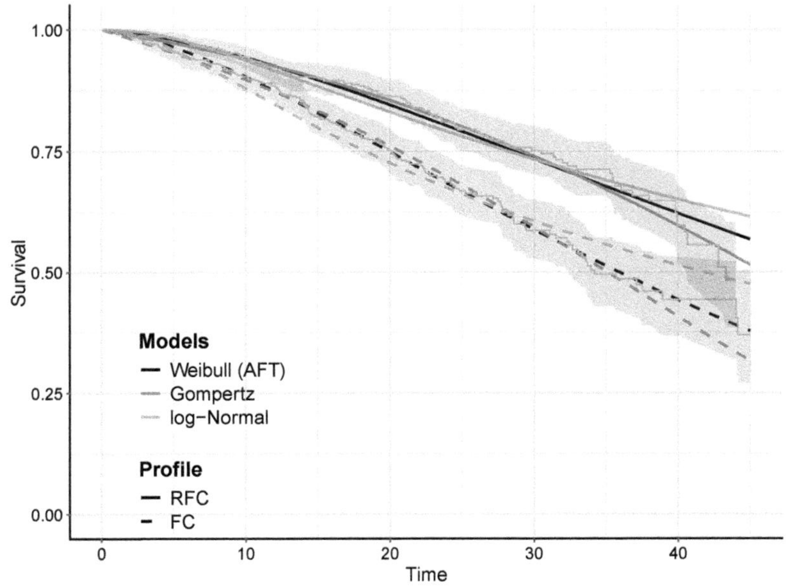

Figure 8.5: The survival curve estimates for the three models fitted to the TA174 data on progression.

The hazard functions tell us about the instantaneous (and cumulative) risk of experience the event – for instance, it is possible that the risk of dying is very high immediately after a given surgery, but then stabilises or even decreases, over time. Or: it may be completely unrealistic that, with time passing, the risk of a given clinical event becomes lower. These considerations should be used to assess the meaningfulness of alternative model specifications.

In `survHE`, we can also plot the hazard and cumulative hazard functions adding the option `what="hazard"` or `what="cumhazard"` to the call to the `plot()` method. The latter (Figure 8.6b) is simply computed using Equation 8.6. The former (Figure 8.6a) is computed as the *numerical* derivative of $-\log S(t \mid \boldsymbol{\theta})$.

Example 8.6. *NICE TA174 (continued): estimating the hazard curves.* Figure 8.6 shows the hazard functions derived from the models in Equations 8.10 – 8.12. In Figure 8.6a it is possible to see how the hazard function has a big increase towards the end of the observation period, while it actually decreases for the log-Normal model. While these are related to the mathematical functions describing these two distributions, it is also helpful to compare the trajectories with clinical knowledge about the underlying disease.

Very often, studies based on survival analysis in HTA tend to report graphs such as that in Figure 8.5; these are arguably very important and useful and should be used as the basis for comparison and assessment of model fit and plausibility. However, as they are the output of a statistical modelling, we know that they are subject to inherent uncertainty, because the underlying model parameters are. Thus, it is also important to report a measure of implied uncertainty on the average survival curves.

This is naturally embedded in `survHE`, which simply needs to add the option `nsim` to the call for the `plot()` method. This instructs `R` to not just take into account the point estimates

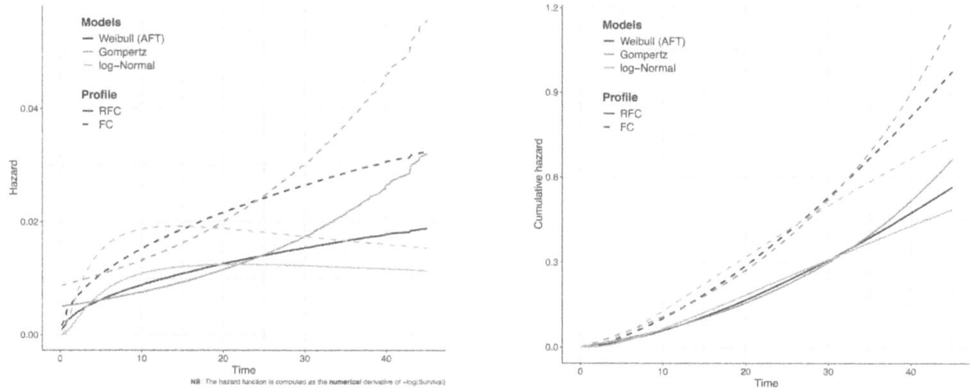

(a) Hazard functions. (b) Cumulative hazard functions.

Figure 8.6: Hazard and cumulative hazard plots for the models fitted to the TA174 data.

and plug the relevant values to compute the survival curves; rather, in a full Bayesian approach (particularly when using HMC), we can use the simulations from the joint posterior distribution of all the model parameters $\boldsymbol{\theta}$ and propagate the uncertainty to the implied distribution of the survival curve $S(t \mid \boldsymbol{\theta})$.

If the input `nsim` is set to a value greater than 1, then `survHE` will automatically construct simulations for the entire distribution of the underlying survival curves. Technically, this automatically calls in the background another `survHE` function, `make.surv()`, which produces the required number of simulations.

The importance of being Bayesian (in survival modelling in HTA) – again

While, strictly speaking, assessing fully the uncertainty in model outputs is not a Bayesian feature only, arguably, the Bayesian philosophy and machinery make this perhaps their key aspect – as discussed in Chapters 1, 2 and 4, the main object of the inference, within a Bayesian approach, is directly the joint posterior distribution, which we can summarise using point estimates, but that, fundamentally, we want to assess and evaluate in its entirety.

As mentioned in Section 5.2.1, this is particularly relevant when there is potential correlation among the model parameters, which we need to reflect appropriately in reporting inference for any function thereof, as is the case in the survival analysis, when we are not just interest in $\boldsymbol{\theta}$, as much as we are in $g(\boldsymbol{\theta}) = S(t \mid \boldsymbol{\theta})$.

Frequentist procedures (such as those used by `flexsurv` in the background) achieve this through bootstrapping, which, *numerically*, can be thought of as a (sometimes, but not universally) precise approximation to the full posterior distribution – but again, as the model complexity increases to mimic more closely the complex reality we are trying to understand and estimate, the computational complexity in moving to the Bayesian approach becomes marginally lower and thus potentially much more efficient.

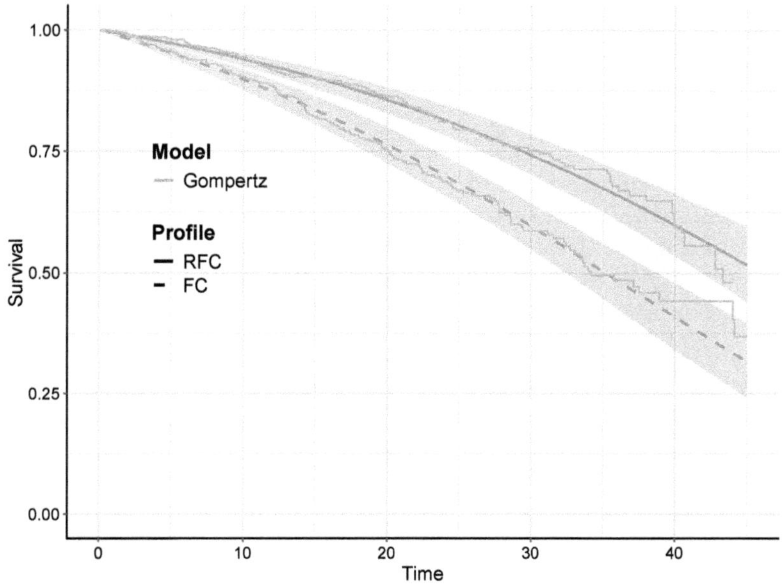

Figure 8.7: The estimated survival curve for the Gompertz model, alongside the 95% interval around the point estimate. This is computed using the simulations from the joint posterior distribution of the parameters, which induces a whole distribution for the survival curve. The plot also retains the point estimate from the Kaplan-Meier curves.

Example 8.7. *NICE TA174 (continued): probabilistic sensitivity analysis.* The code `plot(m,nsim=1000)` is sufficient to extend the plot shown in Figure 8.5 and add a 95% interval band around the point estimate for $S(t \mid \boldsymbol{\theta})$.

Looking at multiple survival curves, with the uncertainty around them, within the same plot becomes however quite confusing; for this reason, we can also use the optional argument `mods`, which allows us to select only one of a few of the distributions fitted in the object `m`.

For instance, as we have specified in the call to the function `fit.models()` the option `distr=c("wei","gom","lno")` to fit the three distributions in the same object, we can simply use the `plot()` method with the option `mods=2` to instruct R to only show the survival curve for the second model (i.e. the Gompertz), as shown in Figure 8.7.

The R code below takes advantage of the fact that the `plot()` function in `survHE` generates a `ggplot` object and, as such, can manipulate it for further customisation. First, we save the plot onto an object `p` – this makes it easier to modify its components. Here we choose to add both the KM estimates (with the interval around the step curve), as well as the point and interval estimates for the survival curve for the Gompertz model.

```
# Saves the plot to a 'ggplot' object, named p, for further customisation
p=plot(
  m,
  # Selects only the Gompertz model (the 2nd in the argument 'distr' when
  # calling the function fit.models() to obtain the object 'm')
  mods=2,
  # Adds the KM curves
  add.km=TRUE,
  # Customises the treatment labels
```

```
  lab.profile=c("RFC","FC"),
  # Uses 'nsim=1000' simulations from the posterior to do the PSA
  nsim=1000
)
```

If we just show the resulting plot (by just calling `p` in the `R` terminal), we see that the picture is very busy, with multiple uncertainty bands overlaid on top of each other, which makes it very confusing and hard to process. We can still post-process this object to remove the bands around the KM estimate, while including the step function so that we can assess how closely the point and interval around the survival curve matches the KM.

In fact, the newly created object `p` contains several elements, including one named `layers`, which describes the features of the various parts that make up the plot. We can visualise what these are using the command `p$layers` – in this case, there are four parts. A little trial and error (or deeper knowledge of the `ggplot` machinery...), allows us to identify that the fourth one:

```
p$layers[[4]]
```

```
mapping: x = ~time, y = ~S, ymin = ~lower, ymax = ~upper, group =
            ~as.factor(strata:object_name)
geom_ribbon: na.rm = FALSE, orientation = NA, lineend = butt, linejoin = round,
            linemitre = 10, outline.type = both
stat_identity: na.rm = FALSE position_identity
```

is actually the one we want to remove, i.e. the interval bands around the KM estimates. We can do this by setting that layer to `NULL` and then show the revised object `p`.

```
# Removes the 'ggplot' layer showing the interval estimate around the KM curves
p$layers[[4]]=NULL

# Shows the revised plot and customise the position of the legend
p + theme(legend.position.inside=c(.2,.6))
```

The resulting graph in Figure 8.7 becomes much more readable and helpful – with a clear measure of how well the Gompertz survival curve matches the observed data. For the most part, the KM estimates are all enclosed within the interval band around the point estimate for $S(t \mid \boldsymbol{\theta})$ – with the only exception of the FC arm, at the very end of the observation period. Throughout most of the follow-up, the solid curves do a reasonable job at approximating the trajectory shown in the observed data – this is one of the key feature we seek when visualising the estimated survival curves.

8.4.4 Model selection

As we have hinted at earlier, given that the advice is to try several distributional assumptions on a given dataset, it obviously becomes important to be able to select one of the options as "the best" – of course, what this qualifier actually means, remains a bit vague. We know that whatever our choice, we will most likely not be in a position of characterising perfectly to true underlying data-generating process.

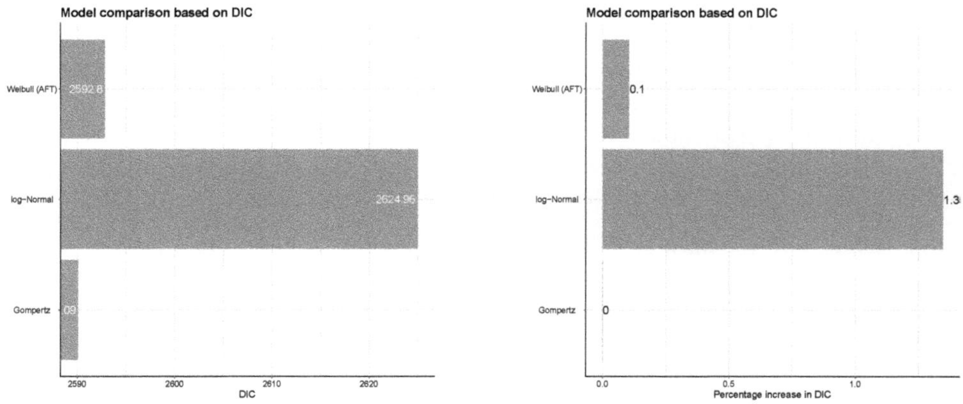

(a) Absolute values for the DIC. (b) Relative values for the DIC.

Figure 8.8: Visualisation of the model fitting statistics, based on DIC. Panel (a) shows the absolute value of the DIC for the models being compared, while panel (b) shows the percentage increase in the DIC in comparison to the model associated with the lowest DIC value, overall.

In line with the discussion of Section 5.3 and Section 6.2.6, it is helpful to consider some model-fitting criteria (e.g. DIC, in a Bayesian context), to say something on "how well does a single model fit the observed data" – we return to this idea in Section 8.4.6.

Example 8.8. *NICE TA174 (continued): model selection.* Figure 8.8 illustrates how we can use survHE to visualise and compare the model fitting performance for the competing models. Figure 8.8a uses the function model.fit.plot() with the only argument type="DIC" to display a bar-chart with the absolute value of the DIC for the three models.

```
# Model fitting plot (specifies the DIC)
model.fit.plot(m,type="DIC")

# Model fitting plot (on a relative scale, wrt the best fitting model)
model.fit.plot(m,type="DIC",scale="relative")
```

The graph seems to indicate that there is little difference, in the model fit, between the Weibull and the Gompertz model, but that the log-Normal is substantially worse, based on the DIC.

Figure 8.8b also adds the optional argument scale="relative" to display the bar-chart using the best-fitting model as reference and showing the percentage incremental in the DIC from the other two. Again, this highlights that the log-Normal does have a relatively higher value for the DIC, while the Weibull only contributes an increase in DIC (i.e. worse performance) of 0.1%. Displaying the results on a relative scale is sometimes useful to appreciate the magnitude of how much better one of the model seems to be doing, in comparison to the others.

8.4.5 Separate modelling by treatment arm

While Example 8.8 indicates that the Gompertz model may be the best fitting, albeit marginally over the Weibull, the analysis of Example 8.5 seems to indicate that, actually, there may not be a single model fitting the observed data best, in both the treatment arms. This is not uncommon, particularly when we are not able to account for more potential covariates of interest and can only control for the treatment arm.

In these situations, we may stipulate that instead of modelling the linear predictors as functions of the treatment indicator, as we have specified in Equations 8.10 – 8.12, we could run separate models by subsetting the data to only include the controls and then the intervention arm, with only an intercept in the expressions for η_i. This approach effectively assumes that both the location and the ancillary parameters depend on the treatment arm (as they are estimated using separate models).

Generally speaking, HTA submissions tend to focus on a main model (as the base-case analysis) and Latimer (2011) comments that:

> *Fitting separate parametric models to each treatment arm involves fewer assumptions, although it does also require the estimation of more parameters. While fitting separate parametric models to individual treatment arms may be justified, it is important to note that fitting different types of parametric model (for example a Weibull for one treatment arm and a log normal for the other) to different treatment arms would require substantial justification, as different models allow very different shaped distribution.*

Example 8.9. *NICE TA174 (continued): separate modelling by treatment arm.* We can use the following code to run the models on the two subsets of the TA174 data, filtering for the treatment arm and thus selecting only the controls or only the intervention arm. In the formula to describe the linear predictor, we only specify the intercept term using the `R` notation `~1`.

```
# Model for the control arm only
m.ctl=fit.models(
  Surv(time,status)~1,
  data=data |> dplyr::filter(treatment=="FC"),
  distr=c("wei","gom","lno"),method="hmc"
)

# Model for the treatment arm only
m.trt=fit.models(
  Surv(time,status)~1,
  data=data |> dplyr::filter(treatment=="RFC"),
  distr=c("wei","gom","lno"),method="hmc"
)
```

The resulting model fit can be summarised again using the `model.fit.plot()` function: the option `stacked=TRUE` instructs `R` to create grouped bar-charts so that it is easier to compare across different objects (`m.ctl` vs `m.trt`, here).

```
# Then assess model fit across the models
model.fit.plot(FC=m.ctl,RFC=m.trt,type="DIC",stacked=TRUE)
```

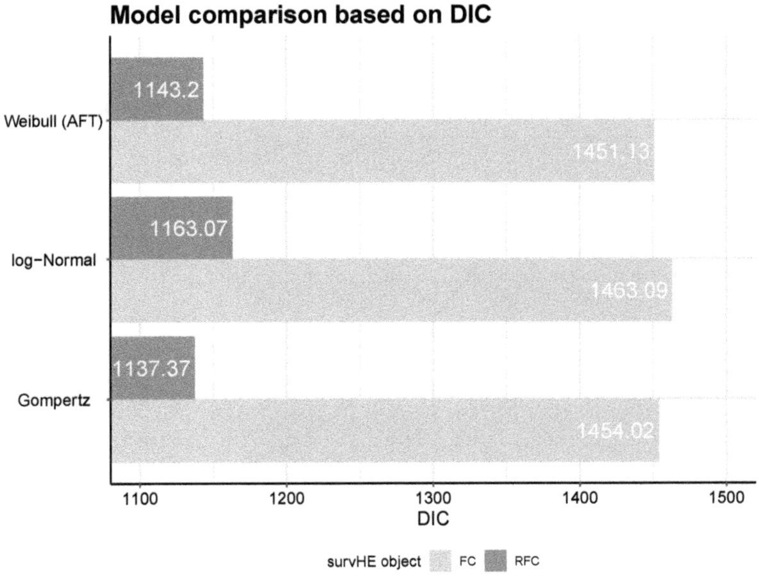

Figure 8.9: Visualisation of the model fitting statistics, based on DIC, when fitting the models to subset of the data by treatment arm. This confirms that the best fitting model varies depending on the treatment arm.

As is possible to see, this confirms the fact that the Gompertz does (marginally) better than the Weibull for the controls (FC), but the reverse is true for the treatment arm (RFC).

8.4.6 Extrapolation

As mentioned in Section 8.3, in "standard" biostatistical analysis of time-to-event data, the main objective is to estimate the effect of a set of covariates (including, most importantly the treatment arm) on the survival time, as well as an estimate of the median survival – this is because most often, trial data at least cover the situation in which at least half of the sample experience the event of interest.

In HTA, the main focus is not so much on either of these objectives, but rather in determining the long-term benefits of a given treatment (see Figure 8.2). We then face a complicated assessment process, which by necessity needs to mix statistical and clinical considerations, together with unavoidable uncertainty about the extrapolation into the future.

On the one hand, we want to ensure that the model we select is able to represent the observed data (within the trial follow-up) as well as possible – as in the discussion on model fitting in Example 8.8. This is perhaps the more "statistical" side of the assessment.

On the other hand, we also want to select a model that has clinical plausibility in the long-term extrapolation, i.e. for which the resulting survival at a time reasonably far in the future is generally justifiable and defensible, given the clinical expertise. Interestingly, because extrapolation, by nature, has to do with data that have not yet occurred, there is very little that we can do to assess how reasonable it is, simply based on model fitting statistics.

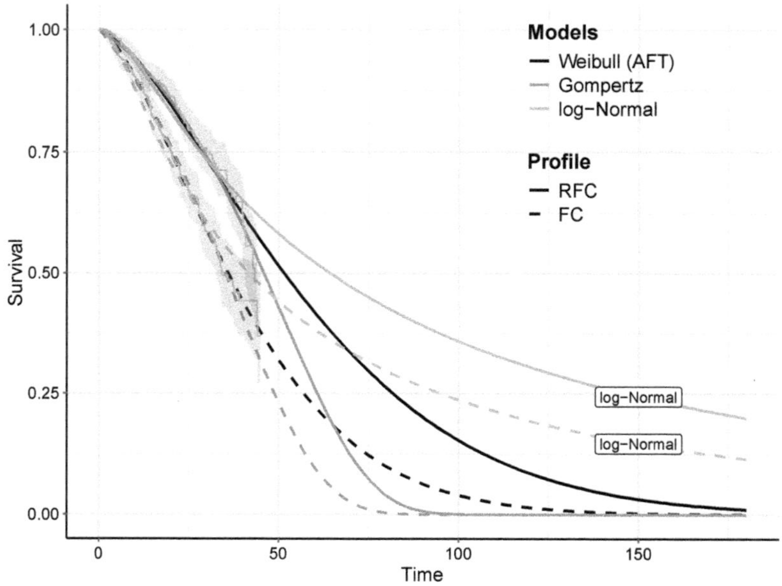

Figure 8.10: Extrapolation up to 180 months (=15 years) for the survival curves for the TA174 subset of data.

Consequently, model fitting cannot be an overarching guiding principle to selecting one of the models, because it can only tell us about how well a given distributional assumptions setup does *with respect to the observed data* – but can say nothing at all about the extrapolation period. Mathematically, this is evident if we consider model fitting criteria based on the deviance, which in turn is a function of the (log)likelihood, i.e. given observed data (and a situation not too dissimilar to the one discussed in Chapter 10).

One important implication of this discussion is that it is crucial to visualise the extrapolated curves and, even more importantly, to accept the inherent and unavoidable uncertainty that is associated with this process.

Example 8.10. *NICE TA174 (continued): extrapolation.* Figure 8.10 shows the extrapolated curves for the models in Equations 8.10 – 8.12, over a time horizon spanning up to $t = 180$ months (i.e. 15 years).

It is possible to directly add this to the `plot()` function in `survHE` by simply adding the optional argument `t`. In this case, we can use code such as `t=seq(0,180)`, to extrapolate the underlying survival curves up to $t = 180$, as required.

As is possible to see, although it does have a decent fit to the observed time period (e.g. around 45 months), the log-Normal model does extrapolate in a rather peculiar way, with curves that, even at $t = 180$ would suggest a rather high probability of not having experienced the event (progression) – the two curves labelled as "log-Normal" are well above 10%, for both treatment arms. This may be considered as unrealistic, drawing on clinical experience and thus the log-Normal model would be considered as unrealistic and discarded on that basis.

Irrespective of the model fitting statistics, we can continue to consider the clinical plausibility of all the models, from the visualisation of the extrapolated survival curves: if we consider the Gompertz and the Weibull, we may stipulate that the latter tends to give a survival probability that is just too high, at later points in the time horizon. For instance, in the

RFC arm, $S(t \mid \boldsymbol{\theta}) > 0.12$, at around 100 months, which clinicians may deem too optimistic. Similar considerations may apply, perhaps to a lower extent, for the FC arm too where $S(t \mid \boldsymbol{\theta}) \approx 0.04$, at $t = 100$.

On the other hand, the Gompertz model may penalise particularly the FC arm, by dropping the survival curve a bit too abruptly, although the point in the time horizon at which the survival curves for the two arms hit 0 may be deemed reasonable by clinical experts.

In line with the discussion in Section 8.4.5, we may also decide to consider different distributional assumptions for the two treatment arms – we can isolate the Weibull survival for FC and the Gompertz survival for RFC using the following code (this is effectively identical to removing all the other curves from Figure 8.10).

```
plot(
  # Selects and names the 'survHE' objects to plot; automatically creates a
  # list combining 'm.ctl' and 'm.trt' (so 3+3=6 models overall)
  FC=m.ctl,RFC=m.trt,
  # Selects which of the models in two objects to plot:
  #  mods=1 => 1st model in m.ctl => Weibull model for FC
  #  mods=5 => 2nd model in m.int, 5th overall => Gompertz for RFG
  mods=c(1,5),
  # Adds KM and extrapolates to 180 months
  add.km=T, t=seq(0,180)
) + scale_color_manual(values=c("#000000","#1F77B4"))
```

Figure 8.11 highlights that, for this particular analysis, we would be willing to violate the assumption of proportional hazard, as the curves cross just after $t = 50$.

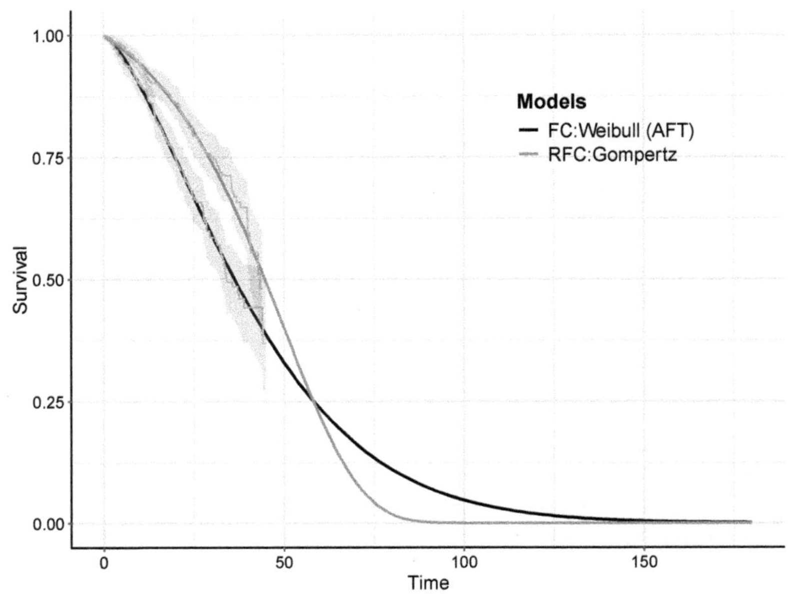

Figure 8.11: Extrapolation up to 180 months (=15 years) for the survival curves for the TA174 subset of data, using the separate best fitting models (Weibull for FC and Gompertz for RFC).

The analysis in Example 8.10 highlights the inherent uncertainty in the extrapolation process – the data *seem* to suggest that in the control arm the Weibull distribution is a very good fit and, perhaps, the extrapolated curve is meaningful clinically. The trajectory of the Gompertz in the intervention arm, as well as the violation of PH, may be real, as dictated by a fast waining treatment effect, or maybe is artificially influenced by small numbers at the end of the trial follow-up when we see a marked number of events, which in turn, perhaps unduly, pulls the extrapolated survival curve towards 0, very quickly.

Note 27: Hazardous ratios

The subtle nature of the PH assumption and the use of HRs as a main measure of inference are a well known issue in the biostatistical (and causal inference) literature. Notably, Hernán (2010) highlights that hazard ratios compare the hazard rates between treatment groups at specific time points, *conditional on survival up to that time*. This implies that the HR reflects the instantaneous risk among individuals who have survived to a particular time, rather than providing an overall measure of treatment effect across the entire study population.

In addition, HRs are *non-collapsible* (see also Example 11.1 in Section 11.2), meaning that HRs calculated for the entire study population may differ from those estimated within subgroups, even in the absence of confounding. This property can lead to discrepancies between *marginal* and *conditional* estimates, complicating the interpretation of HRs as measures of average treatment effect. This is also related to the fact that, as time progresses in a study, the way in which individuals remain at risk can change non-uniformly in different treatment arms. This dynamic can introduce selection bias, as the groups being compared may no longer be comparable due to differential survival, potentially distorting the HR.

This latter feature has the potential of fundamentally generating a violation of the PH assumption; crossing of the underlying survival curves may be generated by a "real" non-PH in the underlying DGP, but may also result as a consequence of selection bias, especially in the presence of large censoring.

Ultimately, it is very possible that with relatively immature data (which are often a feature of HTA modelling based on survival), a single dataset is just not good enough to provide, at the same time, the best characterisation of the observed trial data, as well as a clinically meaningful extrapolation to the long-term effects.

8.5 Advanced survival modelling in HTA

Recent research developments in statistical modelling for survival data in HTA have concentrated on flexible alternative to the "standard" parametric models described above. For example, drawing on methodology originally introduced by Royston and Altman (1994), Jansen (2011) and Jansen et al. (2015) have presented methods based on "*fractional polynomials*". These are flexible functions used to model time-dependent effects by allowing non-linear transformations of time using non-integer powers. One drawback of this method is that they can be quite computationally intensive and hard to interpret, because of the nature of the fundamental parameters.

Another interesting approach to provide more flexibility in the modelling of censored time-to-event data is to use "*poly-hazard*" models. The main idea is to describe survival as arising from multiple independent failure processes, each with its own hazard function – essentially, this amounts to assuming a mixture of a number of terms, each characterised by an independent hazard function. One convenient model is to assume a poly-Weibull structure (Demiris et al., 2015; Benaglia et al., 2015), where a set number of individual Weibull hazard functions combine additively to capture complex, multi-risk survival patterns.

Hardcastle et al. (2025) have recently produced computational advancements to expand on the basic poly-hazard model and allow model- and variable-selections within the MCMC algorithm. In particular, the model allows data-driven selection of the number of components, can switch covariates on and off (by allowing their coefficient to spike at 0) and jump across different distributional assumptions for the hazards.

More recently, much of the research has focused on using splines, which are flexible, piecewise polynomial functions that model complex, non-linear relationships over time by smoothly connecting intervals at predefined knots. While, especially in a Bayesian context, fitting splines can still pose computational challenges, their interpretation and use for extrapolation is much simpler and thus they are currently one of the "good" methods to use in the context of survival analysis in HTA.

8.5.1 M-splines models

M-splines (Ramsay, 1988) are a set of non-negative, piecewise polynomial functions that provide a flexible yet smooth representation of hazard over time, defined over a series of "knots", which are specific time points that partition the time axis. By default, the knot locations are automatically selected based on quantiles of the observed event times, but it is possible to select specific values, depending on the data at hand.

A relevant application in HTA is the model specified by Jackson (2023) and defined as

$$h(t \mid \boldsymbol{\theta}) = \phi \sum_{k=1}^{K} \omega_k b_k(t), \tag{8.13}$$

where $\phi > 0$ is the baseline hazard scale parameter, $\boldsymbol{\omega} = (\omega_1, \ldots, \omega_K)$ is a vector of coefficients for the M-spline basis terms and $b_k(t)$ are deterministic functions of time t, known as "basis functions".

The hazard function is expressed as a linear combination of the basis functions, with coefficients estimated within a Bayesian framework. Beyond the boundary knots, i.e. outside the range of the data, the model assumes that the hazard remains constant, adopting the value at the last knot. This assumption provides a pragmatic approach to extrapolation, acknowledging uncertainty in areas lacking data while avoiding unwarranted complexity.

In general, the baseline hazard scale parameter is modelled by defining a prior on the log scale: $\log\phi \sim \text{Normal}(0, \text{sd} = 20)$, although it is possible to include dependence of the hazard function on a set of C covariates $\boldsymbol{x} = (\boldsymbol{x}_1, \ldots, \boldsymbol{x}_C)$ by assuming a PH model in which $\phi^*(\boldsymbol{x}) = \phi \exp(\boldsymbol{\beta}^\top \boldsymbol{x})$, with a default prior $\beta_1, \ldots, \beta_C \overset{iid}{\sim} \text{Normal}(0, \text{sd} = 2.5)$.

The M-spline coefficients are subject to the constraint that $\sum_{k=1}^{K} \omega_k = 1$ and are modelled using partial pooling to ensure smoothing, with the following specification

$$\gamma_k = \log\left(\frac{\omega_k}{\omega_1}\right) \sim \text{Logistic}(\mu_k, \sigma),$$

where $\gamma_1 = \mu_1 = 0$ and, in general

$$y \mid \mu, \sigma \sim \text{Logistic}(\mu, \sigma) \quad \Rightarrow \quad p(y \mid \mu, \sigma) = \frac{1}{\sigma} \exp\left(-\frac{y-\mu}{\sigma}\right)\left(1 + \exp\left(-\frac{y-\mu}{\sigma}\right)\right)^{-2}.$$

This formulation is useful to prevent overfitting, effectively penalising excessive flexibility and allowing the model to adapt its complexity based on the amount and quality of the available data.

The location parameters $\boldsymbol{\mu} = (0, \mu_2, \ldots, \mu_K)$ are selected using a data-driven procedure based on the location of consecutive knots for the basis functions, so as to ensure that, in the prior, for each μ_k, the corresponding weight ω_k implies a constant hazard.

The scale parameter σ controls the level of smoothness of the fitted hazard curve and it is given a default prior $\sigma \sim \text{Gamma}(2, 1)$ – this amounts to considering $\Pr(\sigma > 4) \approx 0.1$. If $\sigma \to 0$, then the hazard is closer to constant.

Another way to include dependence on the covariates $\boldsymbol{x}$ while also relaxing the PH assumption is to add a term to the location of the Logistic distribution, so that it becomes $\mu + \boldsymbol{\delta}_k^\top \boldsymbol{x}$, where $\boldsymbol{\delta}_k = (\delta_{k1}, \ldots, \delta_{kC})$ and $\boldsymbol{\delta}_1 = \mathbf{0}_C$. For each covariate $\boldsymbol{x}_c$, the resulting coefficient δ_{kc} quantifies the level of departure from the basic PH assumption. In the prior, $\delta_{kc} \sim \text{Normal}(0, \tau_k)$, where $\tau_k \sim \text{Gamma}(2, 1)$, by default.

Jackson (2023) provides more discussion on the modelling framework for Bayesian M-splines, while Phillippo et al. (2024) discuss an application of this family of models in the context of multilevel NMA (see Chapter 11) and, in particular, the use of Random Walk priors to induce smoothness.

Example 8.11. *NICE TA174 (continued): modelling M-splines using* `survextrap`. Similarly to `survHE`, the M-splines model is fully implemented in the `R` package `survextrap` (Jackson, 2023). Detailed tutorials are also included in the software website `https://chjackson.github.io/survextrap/` and in the GitHub repository `https://github.com/chjackson/survextrap/`. We demonstrate the basic use of `survextrap` in the following.

The first task is to set up the basic structure of the M-spline model. The fundamental information, which is coded up in the `survextrap` function `mspline_spec()`, involves: *i)* the model `formula` (which specifies the linear predictor – in this case, we only consider the intercept and model the impact of the covariates later); *ii)* the dataset to be analysed (which is used to construct the knots, based on the quantiles of the observed data); *iii)* the number of basis functions (in this case, 6), which determine the "degrees of freedom" of the M-spline procedure; and *iv)* the additional knots (in this case up to $t = 180$), which are used to extrapolate beyond the observed time-frame.

```
# Loads the package
library(survextrap)

# Spline specification
mspline=mspline_spec(
  formula=Surv(time,status)~1,
  data=data,
  # Defines the number of basis function (=degrees of freedom of the spline)
  df=6,
  # Define additional knots (for the extrapolation part)
```

```
  add_knots=180
)
```

The resulting object mspline stores a set of variables that are instrumental to actually fitting the model in Equation 8.13.

The Bayesian estimation is actually performed by the call to the survextrap function survextrap(), specified as in the following code.

```
# Runs the model
msp=survextrap(
  formula=Surv(time,status)~treatment,
  data=data,
  mspline=mspline,
  chains=2,iter=4000
)
```

Here, we first specify the model formula, which includes the treatment arm as a covariate. In addition, we pass the set up information stored in the object mspline and then select 2 chains, each with 4000 iterations for the HMC run – more options are available and described both in the package vignettes (https://chjackson.github.io/survextrap/articles/) and the R help. The results can be visualised by simply calling the object msp in the R terminal.

```
Individual data: 810 individuals, 248 events
External data: 1 period
M-spline survival model
6 knots, degree 3, 7 basis terms.
Fitted using MCMC
Smoothness SD: full Bayes
Priors:
  Baseline log hazard scale: normal(location=0,scale=20)
  Log hazard ratios:
  treatmentRFC: normal(location=0,scale=2.5)
  Smoothness SD: gamma(shape=2,rate=1)
Sample of 4000 from the posterior
Posterior summary:
# A tibble: 11 x 9
   variable basis_num term            median    lower   upper      sd  rhat ess_bulk
   <chr>        <dbl> <chr>            <dbl>    <dbl>   <dbl>   <dbl> <dbl>    <dbl>
 1 alpha           NA <NA>           0.493    0.120    0.797  0.172   1.00      1696.
 2 coefs            1 <NA>           0.00930  0.00325  0.0174 0.00357 1.00      1241.
 3 coefs            2 <NA>           0.0189   0.00964  0.0330 0.00602 1.00      2252.
 4 coefs            3 <NA>           0.0369   0.0204   0.0634 0.0110  1.00      2128.
 5 coefs            4 <NA>           0.0718   0.0451   0.111  0.0170  1.000     3039.
 6 coefs            5 <NA>           0.110    0.0622   0.194  0.0326  1.00      2370.
 7 coefs            6 <NA>           0.682    0.419    0.813  0.102   1.00      1743.
 8 coefs            7 <NA>           0.0690   0.00243  0.224  0.0592  1.00      1522.
 9 loghr           NA treatmentRFC -0.542    -0.794   -0.289  0.129   1.000     2364.
10 hr              NA treatmentRFC  0.582    0.452    0.749  0.0756  1.000     2364.
11 hsd             NA <NA>           1.21     0.532    2.89   0.622   1.000      610.
```

This returns first detailed information on the prior setup, including the default distributions selected for the model parameters. In the priors block, Baseline log hazard scale is $\log(\phi)$

in Equation 8.13; `treatmentRFC` indicates the coefficient β for the only covariate included in the model, in this case; and `Smoothness SD` indicates σ above.

In the main body of the table, for each model parameter, the summary reports the posterior median, 95% interval estimates and standard deviation, as well as some (`rstan`-based) convergence metrics. The parameter reported as `alpha` is the baseline log-hazard scale, i.e. $\log(\phi)$ in the notation of Equation 8.13. The parameters labelled as `coefs` indicate the elements of the vector $\boldsymbol{\omega}$, i.e. the coefficients for the basis functions. The parameter `loghr` indicates the coefficient β for the covariate included in the linear predictor (the treatment arm), while `hr` is its exponentiated value, i.e. the HR. Because the underlying M-spline model assumes PH, this estimate is comparable with that provided by the Gompertz model in Example 8.2. Finally, the parameter indicated as `hsd` is the smoothing scale σ.

The object `msp` can be further processed using built-in functions from `survextrap` or other `R` packages (including `rstan` or `ggplot2`). For instance, we can reconstruct the estimates survival curves using the following code. Here, for consistency with `survHE`, we use the mean (rather than the median) and the 95% interval estimates and save these in the object `S`.

```
# Extracts the survival curves
S=survextrap::survival(
  # For consistency with survHE, selects the mean (rather than the median)
  msp,summ_fns=list(mean=mean,~quantile(.x, probs=c(0.025, 0.975)))
)
```

This, in turn, can be used to plot the survival curves. Figure 8.12a (generated by the code below) shows the fitted curves using `survHE` and the Weibull and Gompertz models, as well as the M-spline based estimates computed by `survextrap`. Here we can take full advantage of `ggplot2` to combine different objects into the same plot, effectively by customising the `survextrap` object `S` to align with the `survHE` output.

```
# Puts together the data to show plots from survHE and survextrap
plot(
  # Plots the fit for Weibull and Gompertz models
  m,mods=c(1,2),add.km=T,t=seq(0,180),
  lab.profile=c("RFC","FC")
) +
  # Adds the data from the M-spline survival curves
  # (recodes the treatment to strata, to be consistent with survHE)
  geom_line(
    data=S |> mutate(
      model="M-spline",
      strata=case_when(
        treatment=="FC"~"treatmentRFC=0",TRUE~"treatmentRFC=1"
      ) |> factor(level=c("treatmentRFC=1","treatmentRFC=0"))
    ),
    aes(t,mean,col=model,linetype=strata),size=0.9
    ) +
  scale_color_manual(values = c("#000000", "#1F77B4", "#FF7F0E"))
```

While both the parametric models and the M-spline cover well the observed data, the extrapolations are quite different. The M-spline model seems to produce slightly higher curves towards the end of the extrapolation, in comparison to the Weibull and even more

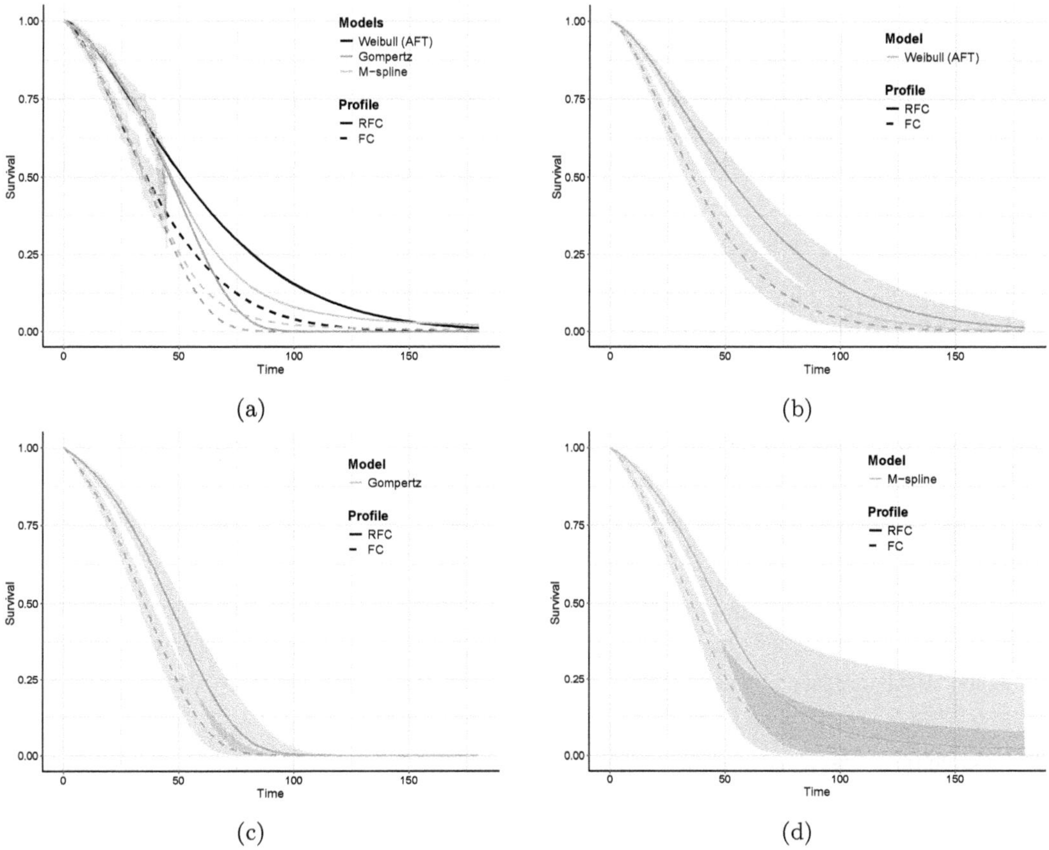

Figure 8.12: Survival extrapolation based on parametric and M-spline models. Panel (a) combines the KM estimates from the observed data with the fit and extrapolation from both the parametric models (Weibull and Gompertz) and the M-splines estimate. The solid curves are for the active treatment (RFC), while the dashed curves are for the controls (FC). Panels (b), (c) and (d) show the uncertainty around the survival curves and over the long-term extrapolation for the Weibull, Gompertz and M-spline models, respectively.

so to the Gompertz models. This latter seems to suggest a steeper decrease towards 0, especially for the treatment arm.

The differences are better appreciated in Figures 8.12b–8.12d, which show the survival curves together with a 95% interval estimates for the Weibull, Gompertz and M-spline models, respectively. Interestingly, the M-spline model shows substantial uncertainty in the extrapolation period, in comparison with the parametric models. This is not surprising: there are no observed data beyond the end of the follow-up and thus the M-spline responds by giving very wide interval estimates for the survival curves. Conversely, the two parametric models are "mathematically forced" to give increasingly narrow uncertainty as time progresses along the x–axis.

In a sense, neither model is necessarily "correct": on the one hand, the parametric models naturally encode in their mathematical formulation the fact that, eventually, survival will go down to 0 – if we wait for long enough. On the other hand, M-splines respond to the lack of observed data by showing large uncertainty around the survival (basically being more naturally agnostic about "how long is *long enough*").

More pragmatically and importantly, this consideration highlights the fact that, in reality, the observed data on a limited follow-up are most often just not informative enough to have a model that fits them as well as possible, while also extrapolating in the most sensible way possible...

8.5.2 Including external information

The Bayesian framework allows naturally the incorporation of different sources of information, which is particularly relevant in the case of survival modelling based on limited/immature data for the follow-up period, but for which we need to extrapolate over a much longer time horizon.

One typical situation is when, alongside the individual-level data for the follow-up, we also have information, perhaps in the form of aggregated or summary data, over the longer term. One common way to deal with this scenario is when aggregated data are available in the form of counts $r_j \sim \text{Binomial}(\pi_j, n_j)$, where, for each of the $j = 1, \ldots, J$ available time intervals $\mathcal{I}_j = (t_j^{\text{start}}, t_j^{\text{stop}})$, we observe n_j, the total number of individuals alive at t_j^{start} and r_j is the total number of people who survive the end of $\mathcal{I}_j$ and thus are still alive at t_j^{stop}.

We can combine these aggregated data with ILD by assuming a single data-generating process characterised by a common hazard function by modelling

$$\pi_j = \frac{S(t_j^{\text{stop}} \mid \boldsymbol{\theta})}{S(t_j^{\text{start}} \mid \boldsymbol{\theta})}$$

i.e. the ratio of the probability to survive beyond t_j^{stop}, given survival at least at t_j^{start}.

This situation applies naturally to M-spline models, where using Equations 8.6 and 8.13, we can estimate the survival probabilities for a generic time t using the following relationships:

$$\begin{aligned}\log S(t \mid \boldsymbol{\theta}) &= -H(t \mid \boldsymbol{\theta}) = -\int_0^t h(u \mid \boldsymbol{\theta}) du \\ &= -\int_0^t \phi \sum_{k=1}^K \omega_k b_k(u) du = -\phi \sum_{k=1}^K \left(\omega_k \int_0^t b_k(u) du\right) \\ &= -\phi \sum_{k=1}^K \omega_k I_k(t), \end{aligned} \tag{8.14}$$

where $I_k(t) = \int_0^t b_k(u)du$ is the k–th *integrated* basis function, which can be computed using a recursion formula (Ramsay, 1988), e.g. as implemented in the R package `splines2` (Wang and Yan, 2021). Thus, the aggregated data can be used to contribute to the overall likelihood through Equation 8.14 – this can act as an "anchoring" factor and thus help stabilise the extrapolation of the survival curves.

We return to this type of data in a different context and using simpler parametric models in Example 9.2, when discussing the issue of treatment effect waning.

Example 8.12. *NICE TA174 (continued): modelling M-splines with external data in* `survextrap`. We start by considering aggregated data made by the expected number of individuals still alive at the end of a given observation period (beyond the end of the ILD follow-up), out of the total number of individuals who had not experienced the event at the beginning of a given interval of that observation period (typically a closed interval). Note that these may come from published summary statistics (e.g. obtained by "real world evidence" or observational dataset), but may also be derived using elicitation of expert opinion, e.g. by asking clinicians what is reasonable to expect, in their opinion. We can collect these in a format suitable for processing in `survextrap` as in the following code.

```
#' Construct a dataset with expected number of people still alive at the end
#' of an observation period, out of a total number of people alive at the
#' beginning (to use for anchoring the survival extrapolation)
extdat=tibble(
  start=c(100,120,150),
  stop=c(120,150,180),
  n=c(100,100,100),
  r=c(8,6,2),
  treatment=as.factor(c("FC","FC","FC"))
)
```

Next, we can re-run the M-spline model by adding the optional argument `external=exdat`, to instruct `survextrap` to use the extended model in Equation 8.14, which we do using the following code.

```
msp_ext=survextrap(
  Surv(time,status)~treatment,data=data,mspline=mspline,chains=2,iter=4000,
  external=extdat
)
```

Finally, we can derive the resulting survival curves, which we plot in Figure 8.13a, alongside the corresponding output of the M-spline models based only on the observed follow-up data, derived in Example 8.11.

```
S_ext=survextrap::survival(
  # For consistency with survHE, selects the mean (rather than the median)
  msp_ext,summ_fns=list(mean=mean,~quantile(.x, probs=c(0.025, 0.975)))
)
```

As is possible to see, the model using external data gets pulled towards 0 at later times (i.e. during the extrapolation part). Interestingly, the extra information also contributes to lower uncertainty (compare for instance Figure 8.13a with Figure 8.12d).

Another recent way of incorporating formally external information into the survival modelling is the "*blended survival model*" of Che et al. (2023), implemented in the `R` package `blendR` (available from `CRAN`, with a development version at the GitHub repository `https://github.com/StatisticsHealthEconomics/blendR`).

The main idea is to consider two separate processes. The first one is a model driven exclusively by the observed data; this is the same as the "standard" HTA analysis described above and is used to estimate $S_{obs}(t \mid \boldsymbol{\theta}_{obs})$, with the aim of producing the best fit possible to the observed information.

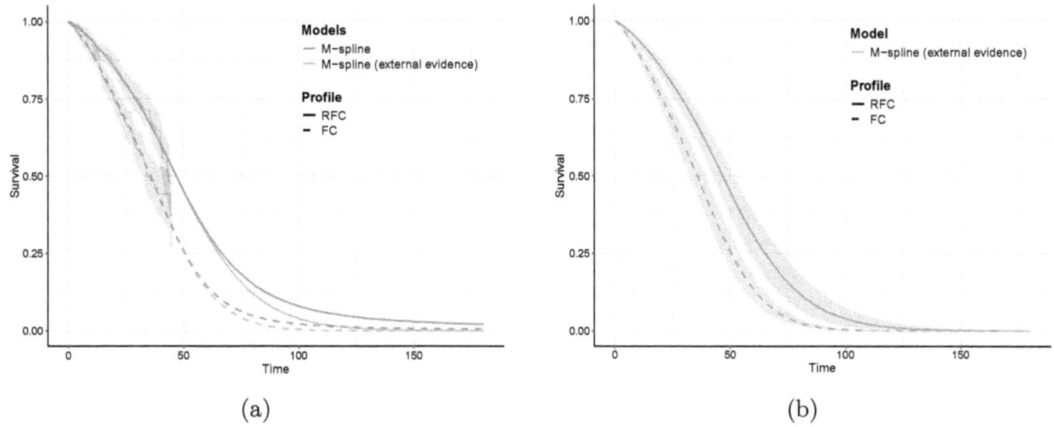

Figure 8.13: Output of the survival analysis using M-splines. Panel (a) shows the comparison between the results produced with and without the external data, while panel (b) shows the uncertainty characterising the latter analysis.

Note that, unlike in standard modelling, we are not (too) concerned with overfitting, because we also consider a second process, which is used to derive a separate survival curve, $S_{ext}(t \mid \boldsymbol\theta_{ext})$ to describe the long-term estimate for the survival probabilities. This may be based on "hard" evidence (e.g. real world evidence, registries, or cohort studies), or purely subjective knowledge elicited from experts (as described in Example 8.12) – or even both.

The two processes are "blended" together as

$$S_{ble}(t \mid \boldsymbol\theta) = S_{obs}(t \mid \boldsymbol\theta_{obs})^{1-\pi(t;\alpha,\beta,a,b)} \times S_{ext}(t \mid \boldsymbol\theta_{ext})^{\pi(t;\alpha,\beta,a,b)},$$

where $\boldsymbol\theta = \{\boldsymbol\theta_{obs}, \boldsymbol\theta_{ext}, \alpha, \beta, a, b\}$ is the vector of model parameters; the weight function

$$\pi(t;\alpha,\beta,a,b) = \Pr\left(T \leq \frac{t-a}{b-a} \mid \alpha,\beta\right) = F_{\text{Beta}}\left(\frac{t-a}{b-a} \mid \alpha,\beta\right)$$

controls the extent to which $S_{obs}(\cdot)$ and $S_{ext}(\cdot)$ are blended together in the *blending period* $[a,b]$; and $t \in [0,T^*]$, is the interval of times over which we want to perform our evaluation.

This is not dissimilar to "*mixture cure model*" (De Angelis et al., 1999; Latimer and Rutherford, 2024), in which we assume that the underlying population is in fact made up by individuals who respond to treatment (and become "cured") and others who do not as much ("uncured"), with a resulting mixed survival curve to model heterogeneity in the population. Conversely, in blended survival short- vs long-term processed are modelled explicitly with smooth transition and the main objective of extrapolation.

8.5.3 Network meta-analysis for survival data

In line with the discussion in Chapters 6 and 7, in HTA we often cannot access individual-level data for all the relevant interventions we need to compare. In the case of survival analysis, aggregated summaries typically consist of reported estimates for the (log)HRs, together with a measure of variability (e.g. a standard deviation).

We can expand the ideas of Chapter 7 to the case of survival outcomes, to make a suitable model that can pool together the "data" on the HRs (see Dias et al., 2018, chap. 10; Jackson et al., 2025). For example, the summary statistics for study $s = 1,\ldots,S$ typically consist an estimated log HR, y_{sa}, defined for treatment arm $a = 1, \ldots, A$ against the reference arm considered in that study, with variance estimated as v_{sa}.

Perhaps the simplest model in this situation is to consider $y_{sa} \sim \text{Normal}(\mu_{sa}, v_{sa})$, where μ_{sa} is the true underlying log HR. Under a random effects specification, we have

$$\mu_{sa} \sim \text{Normal}(\delta_{sa}, \sigma^2_\mu) \qquad \text{and} \qquad \delta_{sa} = d_a - d_{b_s}.$$

Here, d_a is the pooled log HR for treatment a relative to the reference ($d_1 = 0$, by convention) and b_s is the reference arm of study s. The parameter σ^2_μ is the between-study heterogeneity variance. In a Bayesian context, the model is completed by placing suitable priors on the parameters d_a and σ_μ.

This model produces posterior estimates of all pairwise log HRs across the network, which can be used to estimate the underlying survival curves. Assuming we have at least one ILD (possibly based on digitised data – see Section 8.3.2 for more details) to estimate the baseline hazard, one way to do so is to expand the M-spline model of Equation 8.13. Under the PH assumption, we model

$$h_a(t \mid \boldsymbol\theta) = h_0(t \mid \boldsymbol\theta) \exp(d_a).$$

and then use Equation 8.6 to derive an estimate of the resulting survival curves.

When PH is implausible (e.g. for immunotherapies with delayed separation of survival curves), treatment effects can instead be introduced at the level of the spline coefficients $\boldsymbol\omega$, allowing the log HR to vary smoothly over time, as described in Phillippo et al. (2024). The package `multinma` (Phillippo, 2024) can be used to run this sort of NMA.

8.6 Conclusions

This chapter has presented a long account of the intrinsic complexities associated with modelling time-to-event in HTA and the potential advantages produced by using the Bayesian approach. This is specifically related with the nature of the data, which is almost invariably characterised by limited follow-up and large censoring, which implies a lack of real information. This in turn makes the objective of extrapolation over a (much) longer time horizon, which is key to the HTA application, extremely complex and is particularly helped by the Bayesian feature of allowing a principled combination of different sources of information (be it prior knowledge, or additional data).

We have presented more "basic" parametric models and their use in `survHE`, as well as more "advanced" and flexible ones, through the use of `survextrap`. Both packages are based on a different MCMC algorithm (Hamiltonian Monte Carlo, see Section 2.3.3) – another consequence of the underlying complexity of modelling this sort of data, which renders computation more convoluted (and thus best effected using the, in this case, more efficient HMC).

The next chapter concentrates on so-called Markov models, another important tool that is very popular in HTA, which is used to describe the natural history of a specific condition by using a simulation approach for a "virtual" cohort of individuals. This sort of modelling tool is particularly helpful for economic modelling and has close links with survival analysis.

9

Markov models

9.1 Introduction

In the context of HTA, Markov models (sometimes referred to more generically as "Multistate models", in the wider Statistical literature) are tools used to assess the long-term benefits and associated costs of a set of interventions, whose effect materialise on potentially repeating events (see Thom et al., 2025a; Thom et al., 2025b, as well as references therein for more details). The popularity of Markov models in HTA mainly derives from the fact that they are particularly effective at describing the "natural history of the disease" for many chronic conditions, which must be evaluated over a long enough time horizon.

Markov models are characterised by a set of relationships that identify the movement of a cohort of individuals across a number of "states", or hypothetical outcomes that characterise a specific condition or disease. The way in which movements occur over time and across these states is determined by a set of relevant probabilities (or rates, in continuous time). A Bayesian approach can be particularly effective to model these probabilities, either from directly observed data or through evidence synthesis procedures.

In this chapter, we first give an introduction to the general "cohort Markov model in discrete times". We do so by using a combination of data to feed into the estimation of the relevant probabilities and demonstrate the features of the tool in extrapolating the economic outcomes over longer time horizons, which again is a key feature for economic evaluation.

Then, we consider a specific case, the "Three-state cancer Markov model", which is very popular and prevalent in much of the applications of HTA, combining this analysis with the methods described in Chapter 8.

9.2 Cohort Markov models

Generally speaking, we define a Markov model structure by considering a set $\mathcal{S}$ made by S clinically relevant health states. These represent specific conditions or levels of the underlying pathology and are assumed to be *exhaustive* (i.e. they include all the relevant possible stages of the natural history of the disease) and *mutually exclusive*, meaning that if an individual is a state $s = 1, \ldots, S$ at time $j = 0, \ldots, J$, then they cannot also be in a different state $s' \neq s$, at the same time.

DOI: 10.1201/9781003771050-9

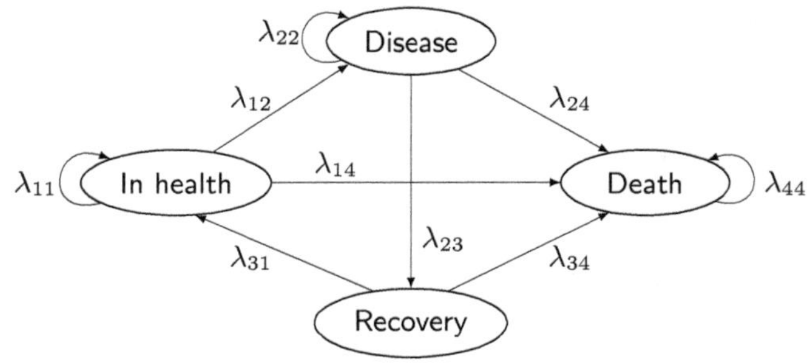

Figure 9.1: A general graphical representation of a Markov model structure.

From one period to the next, subjects can move among the states according to the rules specified by the Markov model's assumptions. The movements occur according to suitable *transition probabilities*

$$\lambda_{ss'} = \Pr(\text{individual is in state } s' \text{ at time } (j+1) \mid \text{individual was in state } s \text{ at time } j).$$

The times j are often referred to as "*Markov cycles*" and a Markov model considers a "virtual follow-up" during which the cohort is free to move across the states.

Figure 9.1 shows a graphical representation of a Markov model structure. Here, arrows indicate the possibility of moving from the state from which the arrow originates to the state in which the arrow ends. The absence of an arrow indicates that the transition between these nodes is not allowed.

For instance, in Figure 9.1, we are assuming that individuals cannot move from the state "Recovery" back to "Disease", without going through the state "In health" first. The state "Death" is an *absorbing* state – once individuals reach it, they cannot abandon it.

The assumption that the states are exhaustive and mutually exclusive implies that

$$\sum_{s'=1}^{S} \lambda_{ss'} = 1. \tag{9.1}$$

We can use some simple matrix algebra to fully characterise the Markov model in terms of the *occupancy probabilities*, describing the proportion of individuals who transition in each of the S states, at any given time. These can be obtained as

$$\boldsymbol{\pi}_{j+1} = \boldsymbol{\pi}_j \boldsymbol{\Lambda}, \tag{9.2}$$

where $\boldsymbol{\pi}_j = (\pi_{j1}, \ldots, \pi_{jS})$ is the vector of probabilities for each state at time j and

$$\boldsymbol{\Lambda} = \begin{pmatrix} \boldsymbol{\lambda}_1 \\ \vdots \\ \boldsymbol{\lambda}_S \end{pmatrix} = \begin{pmatrix} \lambda_{11} & \ldots & \lambda_{1S} \\ \vdots & \ddots & \vdots \\ \lambda_{S1} & \ldots & \lambda_{SS} \end{pmatrix}$$

is a transition matrix, describing the probability of moving from state s to state s' at time j. The vector $\boldsymbol{\lambda}_s$ indicates the s–th row of the matrix $\boldsymbol{\Lambda}$.

In this case, we imply that the transition probabilities do not vary over time – and thus for any Markov cycle j, $\lambda_{ss'}$ always indicate the probability of moving between the two states s and s' over two consecutive time points.

However in many cases the transition matrix should be allowed to vary over time (and would hence be indicated as $\boldsymbol{\Lambda}_j$); for instance, if the movements are affected by an individuals' age, then the transition probabilities may vary in older ages (i.e. for later Markov cycles). Similarly, we may add a further index and write $\boldsymbol{\Lambda}_j^{(t)}$, to indicate that the transition matrix changes for different treatment arms.

In the more general case where the transitions are allowed to vary over time, Equation 9.2 compactly computes the total probability of being in state s at time $j+1$ as

$$\pi_{j+1\,s} = \pi_{j1}\lambda_{j1s} + \pi_{j2}\lambda_{j2s} + \ldots + \pi_{jS}\lambda_{jSs}.$$

If we define m_{js} as the absolute number of individuals in state s at time j, then we can also compute

$$m_{j+1\,s} = m_{j1}\lambda_{j1s} + m_{j2}\lambda_{j2s} + \ldots + m_{jS}\lambda_{jSs},$$

which we can again write in matrix algebra as

$$\begin{aligned} \boldsymbol{m}_{j+1} &= \boldsymbol{m}_j\boldsymbol{\Lambda}_j \qquad (9.3) \\ (m_{j+1\,1},\ldots,m_{j+1\,S}) &= (m_{j1},\ldots,m_{jS}) \begin{pmatrix} \lambda_{j11} & \ldots & \lambda_{j1S} \\ \vdots & \ddots & \vdots \\ \lambda_{jS1} & \ldots & \lambda_{jSS} \end{pmatrix}. \end{aligned}$$

In general, we can simulate a "virtual cohort" of individuals and their movements across the states for a period of time to evaluate the economic performance of a set of relevant interventions.

Example 9.1. *HIV (adapted and expanded from Briggs et al., 2006).* We consider the example originally discussed in Chancellor et al. (1997), also used in the description of the R package hesim (Incerti and Jansen, 2021), which can be used as a general framework for integrating statistical analyses with economic evaluation.

The economic evaluation considers two interventions for the treatment of HIV infection: zidovudine monotherapy (ZDV) and zidovudine + lamivudine in combination therapy (3TC+ZDV). The model includes 4 health states.

We label them as "State A" (HIV positive/non-AIDS with CD4 cells $>$ 200 and $<$ 500 cells/mm3, which we also label as "Compromised CD4"), "State B" (HIV positive/non-AIDS with CD4 $<$ 200 cells/mm3, also labelled as "Low CD4"), "State C" (HIV positive/AIDS diagnosed, or "AIDS") and "State D" ("Death"). This labelling indicates an implied ordering of severity of the underlying condition (so that A is less severe than B, which is less severe than C, etc.) and the model assumes only "forward" transitions, i.e. that patients can transition to any state that is more severe but cannot transition back to a less severe state.

Figure 9.2 shows a graphical representation of the modelling assumptions in terms of a DAG. For simplicity, we do not add a superscript (t) to indicate that the transition probabilities are different in the two treatment options.

The simulation of the trajectories of patients across the S states is considered for $J = 20$ annual cycles, starting from $j = 0$.

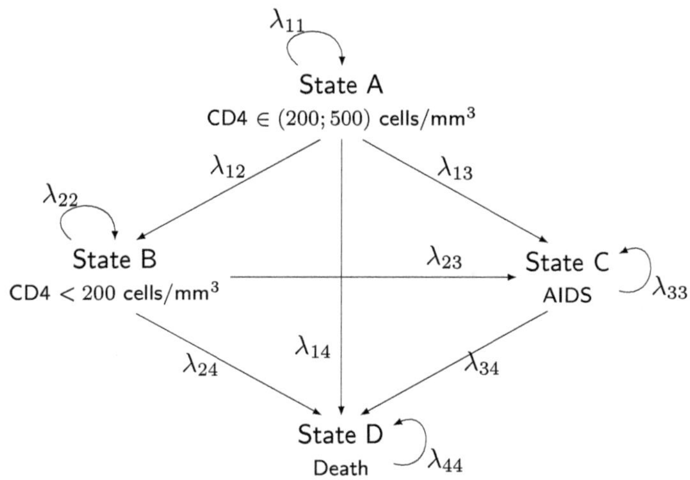

Figure 9.2: A graphical description of the assumptions embedded in the HIV Markov model. Source: Chancellor et al. (1997).

9.2.1 Estimating the transition probabilities

While "running the Markov model" is reasonably simple and amounts to the basic matrix algebra defined by Equation 9.3, from the statistical perspective, the main complexity is in obtaining suitable estimates of the transition probabilities off each state, $\boldsymbol{\lambda}_s$.

The simplest case is when we have observed data informing directly all the transitions. These amount to an $S \times S$ matrix in which the number of movements between s and s' for all $s, s' = 1, \ldots, S$ are recorded over a suitable period of time. We can represent these data as

$$\boldsymbol{y} = \begin{pmatrix} \boldsymbol{y}_1 \\ \boldsymbol{y}_2 \\ \vdots \\ \boldsymbol{y}_S \end{pmatrix} = \begin{pmatrix} y_{11} & y_{12} & \cdots & y_{1S} \\ y_{21} & y_{22} & \cdots & y_{2S} \\ \vdots & \vdots & \cdots & \vdots \\ y_{S1} & y_{S2} & \ddots & y_{SS} \end{pmatrix},$$

where

$$n_s = \sum_{s'=1}^{S} y_{ss'} \qquad \text{and} \qquad \boldsymbol{n} = \begin{pmatrix} n_1 \\ n_2 \\ \vdots \\ n_S \end{pmatrix}$$

is the vector of sample sizes.

We can reasonably describe the sampling variability characterising this particular data-generating process using a Multinomial distribution

$$\boldsymbol{y}_s \sim \text{Multinomial}(\boldsymbol{\lambda}_s, n_s) \quad \Rightarrow \quad p(\boldsymbol{y}_s \mid \boldsymbol{\lambda}_s) = \frac{n_s!}{\prod_{s'=1}^{S} y_{ss'}} \prod_{s'=1}^{S} \lambda_{ss'}^{y_{ss'}}, \tag{9.4}$$

where $\boldsymbol{\lambda}_s = (\lambda_{s1}, \ldots, \lambda_{sS})$. Equation 9.4 can be seen as a multivariate generalisation of a Binomial distribution (cfr. Equation 1.16).

From a Bayesian perspective, we need a suitable probability distribution to model our epistemic uncertainty over $\boldsymbol{\lambda}_s$. In the simplest of cases, we can assume

$$\boldsymbol{\lambda}_s \sim \text{Dirichlet}(\boldsymbol{a}_s) \quad \Rightarrow \quad p(\boldsymbol{\lambda}_s \mid \boldsymbol{a}_s) = \frac{\Gamma\left(\sum_{s'=1}^S \lambda_{ss'}\right)}{\prod_{s'=1}^S \Gamma\left(\lambda_{ss'}\right)} \prod_{s'=1}^S \lambda_{ss'}^{a_{ss'}}. \tag{9.5}$$

The Dirichlet distribution is a multivariate generalisation of the Beta. Specifically, where the Beta(a, b) is a good model for a single parameter ranging between 0 and 1, the Dirichlet can be used to model S parameters $\lambda_{s1}, \ldots, \lambda_{sS}$ that are all constrained in the range $[0; 1]$ and such that $\sum_{s'=1}^{S} \lambda_{ss'} = 1$.

The parameters $\boldsymbol{a}_s$ have a relatively intuitive interpretation, as they are proportional to the expected probability associated with the various outcomes. So if a_s is very large in comparison to the other parameters $a_1, \ldots, a_{s-1}, a_{s+1}, \ldots, a_S$, then we are encoding the fact that outcome s is much more likely to occur than the others.

The scale of the parameters indicates the precision. So for example, in a $S = 3$-dimensional case, a Dirichlet$(1, 1, 1)$ encodes the assumption that the three possible categories are all equally likely (because the underlying parameters a_1, a_2, a_3 are all the same). But in the same way, so would a Dirichlet$(100, 100, 100)$, or for that matter a Dirichlet$(0.01, 0.01, 0.01)$. In all cases the three parameters have the same value. The third distribution implies the lowest level of precision, while the second one implies large precision: intuitively, the larger the value, the more prior knowledge we consider.

Figure 9.3 shows six *simplexes* (which, in three dimension, are just triangles): each side of the triangles represents one of the Dirichlet parameters (in this case we assume an underlying variable with three possible categories).

When $a_1 = a_2 = a_3 = 0.85$ (Figure 9.3a), the mass for the underlying Dirichlet distribution is spread all over the area in the triangle. This is the equivalent of a vague prior where the probability mass is spread all over the range of the variable.

Conversely, when $a_1 = a_2 = a_3 = 50$ (Figure 9.3f), the mass is concentrated in a small, central part of the triangle – intuitively, this means that the three dimensions carry the same weight (because the parameters have the same value); because that value is large, then the variance of the points is relatively low and thus the coloured part of the triangle (which indicates highest probability mass) is concentrated around the barycentre of the triangle.

When one of the dimensions has a much larger value than the others, the probability mass tends to be pulled towards that area, as happens when we consider a Dirichlet$(10, 5, 2)$ in Figure 9.3e, where a_1 is larger than both a_2 and a_3 and thus pulls the mass towards it. The remaining subfigures show different examples of Dirichlet distributions in which one of the three dimensions carries more weight than the others.

Just as the Beta distribution is related to the Binomial sampling distribution, so the Dirichlet is to the multivariate generalisation of the Binomial, i.e. the Multinomial distribution. Modelling a vector $\boldsymbol{\lambda} \sim$ Dirichlet$(a_1, \ldots, a_S)$ is the equivalent of the *conjugated* Beta-Binomial model (see Example 2.3) – i.e. with the added benefit that the posterior distribution given a vector of observed data $\boldsymbol{y}$ is also a Dirichlet:

$$\boldsymbol{\lambda} \mid \boldsymbol{y} \sim \text{Dirichlet}(a_1 + y_1, \ldots, a_S + y_S). \tag{9.6}$$

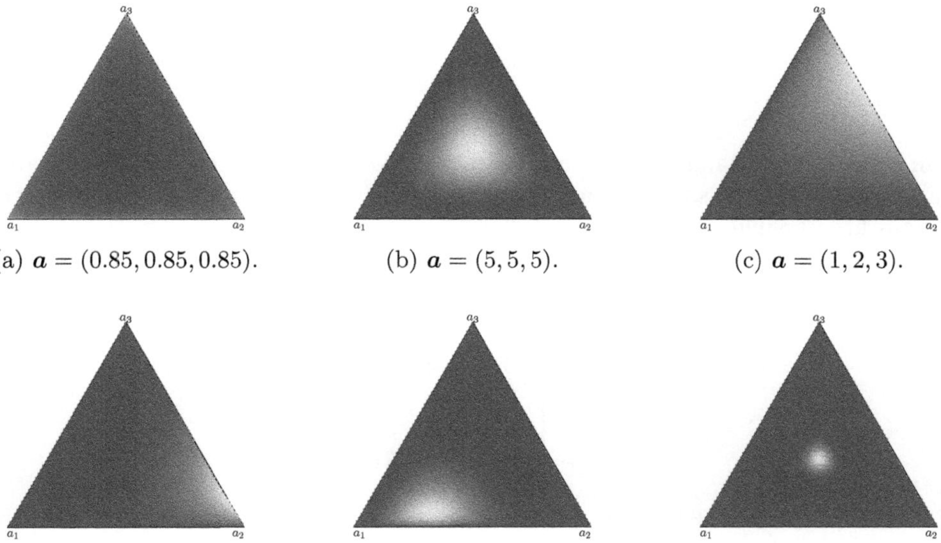

(a) $\boldsymbol{a} = (0.85, 0.85, 0.85)$. (b) $\boldsymbol{a} = (5, 5, 5)$. (c) $\boldsymbol{a} = (1, 2, 3)$.

(d) $\boldsymbol{a} = (1, 7, 2)$. (e) $\boldsymbol{a} = (10, 5, 2)$. (f) $\boldsymbol{a} = (50, 50, 50)$.

Figure 9.3: Examples of a Dirichlet density on a 3d simplex. The lighter colours indicates areas of higher mass in the underlying distribution.

Example 9.2. *HIV (continued): Bayesian modelling.* We can combine a number of data sources to estimate all the model parameters (including the transition probabilities) and then run the Markov model to perform the full economic evaluation.

Transition probabilities in the ZDV arm

We firstly set up the number of states $S = 4$. Also, we load the data, given in the form of matrices with the observed transitions across the states, during the actual follow-up in the trial. These are available for the control intervention (ZDV) The code is relatively straightforward – we use the `R` built-in function `matrix()` to define the data. Notice that the numbers included in the matrix are read by row (as the input `byrow=TRUE` suggests).

```
# Sets up the number of states and the names of the states
S = 4
states=c("Compromised CD4","Low CD4","AIDS","Death")
y=matrix(
  c(
    1251, 350, 116, 17,
    0, 731, 512, 15,
    0, 0, 1312, 437,
    0, 0, 0, 469
  ),ncol = 4, nrow = 4, byrow = TRUE
)
colnames(y)=rownames(y)=states
# Row-wise sample size
n=apply(y,1,sum)
# Visualises the data (observed transitions across states)
y
```

```
                  Compromised CD4 Low CD4 AIDS Death
Compromised CD4              1251     350  116    17
Low CD4                         0     731  512    15
AIDS                            0       0 1312   437
Death                           0       0    0   469
```

We can model the data $\boldsymbol{y}_s$ using the Multinomial-Dirichlet structure described above – notice that, in this case, some of the cells in the transition matrix are fixed to 0 as not all transitions are possible.

In particular, we select a value of 3 for the scale parameter of the Dirichlet prior and define $\boldsymbol{\lambda}_s \sim \text{Dirichlet}(\boldsymbol{a}_s)$, where $\boldsymbol{a}_s$ is the $s-$th row of the matrix

$$\boldsymbol{A} = \begin{pmatrix} 3 & 3 & 3 & 3 \\ 0 & 3 & 3 & 3 \\ 0 & 0 & 3 & 3 \\ 0 & 0 & 0 & 3 \end{pmatrix}.$$

Combining this with the observed data guarantees that the inadmissible transitions (e.g. from "AIDS" back to "Compromised CD4", governed by the parameter λ_{31}) are associated with probabilities identical with 0 (cfr. Equation 9.6). The posterior for the vectors $\boldsymbol{\lambda}_s$ make up the full transition matrix for the ZDV arm, which we indicate as $\boldsymbol{\Lambda}^{(1)}$.

Of course, other choices are possible – we use this a as a reasonably vague prior and explore sensitivity analysis to other configurations (noting that the sample sizes in the data are generally reasonably large). If covariates were available to inform the posterior distribution of $\boldsymbol{\lambda}_s$, we could expand this model to use Multinomial-logistic regression (see for instance Lunn et al., 2013, pp. 129–132).

Relative risk of progression in the 3TC+ZDV arm

In this case, we do not have direct access to similar data for the "active" intervention (3TC+ZDV); however, Chancellor et al. (1997) consider a number $L = 4$ of relevant published studies in which the results of head-to-head comparisons (in terms of progression to fully established AIDS diagnosis) have been reported in the form of relative risks (RRs) and the resulting 95% interval estimates. These are reported in Table 9.1.

We can model these summary statistics to produce a pooled estimate for the RR and then apply it to the ZDV estimates for the transition probabilities, to derive the equivalent values for the 3TC+ZDV group. In particular, for each data point $l = 1, \ldots, L$, we use a partial

Table 9.1: Summary results of the relevant randomised clinical trials of 3TC vs ZDV. Source: Chancellor et al. (1997)

Study	Relative risk	95% CI
NUCA3001	0.389	0.206; 0.733
NUCA3002	0.674	0.393; 1.156
NUCB3001	0.492	0.183; 1.328
NUCB3002	0.452	0.226; 0.902

pooling model (see Section 6.2.3)

$$\begin{aligned} x_l = \log(\text{RR}_l) &\sim \text{Normal}(\theta_l, sd_l) \\ \theta_l &\sim \text{Normal}(\mu_\theta, \sigma_\theta) \\ \mu_\theta &\sim \text{Normal}(0, \text{sd} = 2) \\ \sigma_\theta &\sim \text{Exponential}(2). \end{aligned}$$

Here, we first rescale the observed RRs using the log transformation – this makes the assumption of a Normal sampling distribution more plausible. Then, we derive an estimate of the individual study standard deviation as

$$sd_l \approx \frac{\log(\text{RR}_l^{upp}) - \log(\text{RR}_l^{low})}{2z_{0.05}},$$

where RR_l^{low} and RR_l^{upp} are the lower and upper limit of the 95% interval, respectively, while $z_{0.05} \approx 1.96$ is the 97.5 percentile in the standard Normal distribution (see also Section 1.2.5).

We construct the partial pooling at the level of the mean RR, so that $\rho = \exp(\mu)$ is the estimate for the pooled RR, across the four studies. We model μ_θ using a minimally informative Normal distribution, in which the prior sd of 2 implies that a prior 95% range of $[0.02; 50.4]$, on the exponentiated scale (as is easy to check using the properties of the Normal distribution).

Finally, we use a PC prior for σ_θ – this implies that 95% of the prior mass lies below 1.5 (see Section 2.2.3), which is in fact a rather "relaxed" assumption, when translated on the natural scale for the RR.

Treatment effect waning

Chancellor et al. (1997) assume that the treatment effect lasts for *exactly* 2 years, after which all individuals revert to the same level as the ZDV arm. This implies that the RR is applied for the transition probabilities and that the costs of treatment are inflated by the acquisition of 3TC only for the first two Markov cycles. Nonetheless, they also acknowledge obvious uncertainty in this assumption by stating that '*the extent of the duration of effect of 3TC/ZDV is not known, although surrogate marker data from trials NUCA 3001, NUCB 3001 and NUCA 3002 indicate that an effect persists for at least 1 year, and blinded follow-up data to week 76 suggest that effects may persist for closer to 2 years*'.

To account for this, here we construct a survival model for the treatment effect duration. We create pseudo-aggregated data in the form of Binomial counts to inform the proportion of people who would still be on active treatment effect after j (see Section 8.5.2).

For instance, we could imagine a situation such as that depicted in Table 9.2. Here, we pick $I = 8$ intervals, in correspondence of which we make informed guesses at the number of individuals who may reasonably still be under effective treatment (of course, in a "real" analysis, these guesses would be informed by clinical expertise and subject to thorough sensitivity analysis). In the table, the column labelled δ shows the width of the discrete time intervals (e.g. $\delta_1 = 0.5$ for the first interval, between times 0 and 0.5) and we encode the information provided in the original paper by assuming that very few events happen before 2 years and that by the end of year 3 the treatment effectiveness has waned off for everyone.

Table 9.2: Pseudo-data to encode the assumptions about the treatment effectiveness duration for the combination therapy

Interval	Width δ	Events r	At risk nr
0 – 0.5	0.5	0	100
0.5 – 1	0.5	0	100
1 – 1.5	0.5	3	100
1.5 – 2	0.5	7	97
2 – 2.5	0.5	60	90
2.5 – 3	0.5	30	30
3 – 4	1.0	0	0
4 – 5	1.0	0	0

The observed counts in each interval are modelled as $r_i \sim \text{Binomial}(\phi_i, nr_i)$, where nr_i is the number of people at risk. The parameter ϕ_i indicates the probability that treatment wanes off, i.e. that it fails for at least one individual, in the i–th interval, which is equivalent to $1 - S_i$, the underlying interval-specific survival in effective treatment. Exponentiating and re-arranging Equation 8.6, we can write S_i in terms of the cumulative hazard $H_i = h_i\delta_i$, where h_i is the hazard function in interval i, which in turn allows us to express

$$\phi_i = 1 - S_i = 1 - \exp(-h_i\delta_i).$$

If we assume that within each interval the underlying time-to-event is modelled with a Weibull(α, μ) sampling distribution, using the results in Table 8.4 and recalling Equation 8.3, we can write

$$\log(h_i) = \log(\alpha) - \alpha\log(\mu) + (\alpha - 1)\log(u_i),$$

where u_i is the end point of the i–th interval. We can complete the model by setting suitable prior distributions for the Weibull parameters – for instance, we consider here $\alpha, \mu \sim \text{Exponential}(2)$, independently, to provide reasonably vague priors.

Under this formulation, the pseudo-data (r_i, nr_i) allow us to update the priors for (α, μ) and with these we can construct for any time point j the survival curve

$$S(j) = \exp\left(-\left(\frac{j}{\mu}\right)^{\alpha}\right)$$

(cfr. again Table 8.4), which can be used to modulate the estimated RR from the evidence synthesis, by defining the time-varying RR

$$\rho^*_j = 1 - S(j)(1 - \rho). \qquad (9.7)$$

Here, if $S(j)$ is large (close to 1), then the actual, time-varying RR is close to ρ. However, with smaller values of $S(j)$, going down to 0 to indicate the point in time when the treatment effect completely wanes off, then the time-varying RR gets increasingly close to 1. Notice that while Equation 9.7 is linear both in ρ and $S(j)$, it is highly non-linear in j.

9.2.2 Rescaling transition probabilities

Once the posterior distribution for ρ^*_j becomes available, we can then combine it with the estimates from the Multinomial-Dirichlet component of the model to derive the time-varying transition matrix in the 3TC+ZDV arm – *in theory*, all we have to do is to multiply the baseline probabilities in $\mathbf{\Lambda}^{(1)}$ by the time-varying relative risk ρ^*_j.

In practice, however, things are more complicated than this simple multiplicative rescaling, for a number of reasons. Firstly, applying the RR to all the transition probabilities will break the sum-to-one constraint in each row of the resulting transition matrix for the 3TC+ZDV arm. This is *relatively* easy to overcome, for instance by considering a re-scaling of the resulting matrix such as the following.

$$\begin{aligned}
\mathbf{\Lambda}^{(2)}_j &= \mathbf{\Lambda}^{(1)}\rho^*_j + diag\left(1-\sum_{s'=1}^{S}\lambda_{ss'}\rho^*_j\right)\\
&= \begin{pmatrix} 1-(\lambda_{12}+\lambda_{13}+\lambda_{14})\rho^*_j & \lambda_{12}\rho^*_j & \lambda_{13}\rho^*_j & \lambda_{14}\rho^*_j \\ 0 & 1-(\lambda_{23}+\lambda_{24})\rho^*_j & \lambda_{23}\rho^*_j & \lambda_{24}\rho^*_j \\ 0 & 0 & 1-\lambda_{34}\rho^*_j & \lambda_{34}\rho^*_j \\ 0 & 0 & 0 & 1 \end{pmatrix}.
\end{aligned}$$

To ensure that the rows of $\mathbf{\Lambda}^{(2)}_j$ sum to 1, we add a diagonal matrix where the non-zero elements are equal to the quantity $\left(1-\sum_{s'=1}^{S}\lambda_{ss'}\rho^*_j\right)$. This is equivalent to adding this factor to the elements on the diagonal of the matrix $\mathbf{\Lambda}^{(2)}_j$ only, which implies that: $\lambda^{(2)}_{jss'} = \lambda_{ss'}\rho^*_j$, for $s' \neq s$; and

$$\begin{aligned}
\lambda^{(2)}_{jss} &= \lambda_{ss'}\rho^*_j + 1 - \sum_{s'=1}^{S}\lambda_{ss'}\rho^*_j \\
&= 1 - \sum_{s'\neq s}\lambda_{ss'}\rho^*_j \\
&= 1 - \sum_{s'\neq s}\lambda^{(2)}_{jss'},
\end{aligned} \tag{9.8}$$

as required.

However, in addition to this issue, there are other, potentially more subtle and complex quirks that we must be aware of when rescaling a vector of transition probabilities. One of the trickiest in a situation such as the one we are describing here is the fact that we want to "transport" an estimate for the RR obtained by a number of studies to our specific population, essentially under the following assumptions: *i*) that we only have a "control" arm available in our data; and *ii*) that our population is *exchangeable* (see Section 6.2.4) with the ones from which the pooled RR estimate is derived.

These two assumptions may be critical because, *mathematically*, two generic probabilities p_1 and p_2 are inextricably linked to a RR by the chain or relationships

$$\begin{aligned}
\text{RR} = \frac{p_2}{p_1} &\Rightarrow 1 \geq p_2 = \text{RR}p_1 \\
&\Rightarrow \text{RR} \leq \frac{1}{p_1} \Leftrightarrow p_1 \leq \frac{1}{\text{RR}}.
\end{aligned} \tag{9.9}$$

From a statistical point of view, however, when we "transport" the estimated distribution for RR onto our own study, we do not necessarily have a guarantee that Equation 9.9 holds for the baseline probabilities estimated from the data at hand (as in $\mathbf{\Lambda}^{(1)}$ above).

Thus, if in the example above an entry $\lambda_{ss'} > \frac{1}{\rho^*_j}$, then the resulting rescaled value for $\lambda^{(2)}_{jss'}$ will exceed 1. Applying Equation 9.8 will still guarantee that the row-wise sum of the entries is 1, but some will be above 1 and others, by necessity, will be below 0, which is simply nonsensical. This mathematical impossibility should be taken as an indication that the assumption of exchangeability between the evidence synthesis data and our study is violated.

Finally, to avoid numerical instability in the resulting estimates, it may be helpful to work the problem on an unbounded scale. Considering again two generic probabilities p_1 and p_2 and the definition of RR, we can express

$$\text{OR} = \frac{p_2}{1-p_2}\Big/\frac{p_1}{1-p_1} = \frac{p_2}{p_1}\frac{1-p_1}{1-p_2} = \text{RR}\left(\frac{1-p_1}{1-\text{RR}p_1}\right). \tag{9.10}$$

Therefore, recalling Equation 6.4 and using Equation 9.10, we can define

$$\begin{aligned}
\tilde{\boldsymbol\Lambda}^{(2)}_j &= \underbrace{\text{logit}^{-1}\left(\underbrace{\text{logit}\left(\boldsymbol\Lambda^{(1)}\right) + \log(\text{OR})}_{\text{rescales in } (-\infty;\infty)}\right)}_{\text{rescales back to } [0;1]} \\
&= \text{logit}^{-1}\left(\text{logit}\left(\boldsymbol\Lambda^{(1)}\right) + \log(\rho^*_j) + \underbrace{\log\left(1-\boldsymbol\Lambda^{(1)}\right) - \log\left(1-\rho^*_j\boldsymbol\Lambda^{(1)}\right)}_{\text{adjusts RR to derive OR}}\right) \\
&= \begin{pmatrix} \tilde\lambda^{(2)}_{j11} & \cdots & \tilde\lambda^{(2)}_{j1S} \\ \vdots & \ddots & \vdots \\ \tilde\lambda^{(2)}_{jS1} & \cdots & \tilde\lambda^{(2)}_{jSS} \end{pmatrix}
\end{aligned}$$

and then compute

$$\boldsymbol\Lambda^{(2)}_j = \tilde{\boldsymbol\Lambda}^{(2)}_j + diag\left(1 - \sum_{s'=1}^{S}\tilde\lambda^{(2)}_{jss'}\right) \tag{9.11}$$

to ensure that the transition probabilities sum to 1 in each row of the resulting transition matrix. Again, if the assumption of exchangeability is broken and $\boldsymbol\Lambda^{(1)}$ is not consistent with the estimated values for ρ^*_j, even Equation 9.11 may produce nonsensical estimates for the transition probabilities in $\boldsymbol\Lambda^{(2)}_j$ – but note that Equation 6.4 is not affected by this problem, which can occur because of the adjustment factor $\log\left(1-\boldsymbol\Lambda^{(1)}\right) - \log\left(1-\rho^*_j\boldsymbol\Lambda^{(1)}\right)$.

Note also that, in the HIV example above, it makes sense to further rescale the elements on the diagonal of $\boldsymbol\Lambda^{(2)}_j$ because the model assumes that only "forward" progressions are allowed – individuals can either remain in the current state, or progress to a more severe health state. But because the RR is specifically estimated to determine the effectiveness of 3TC+ZDV in preventing these transitions, it is reasonable to apply it to those probabilities and simply rescale the elements on the diagonal, which indicate the chance that an individual does not progress from the current state, to ensure that each row of the transition matrix sums to 1.

In other problems, this may be more complex and, in general, we need to be very careful about rescaling, when obtaining probabilities using procedures such as the one highlighted above.

Table 9.3: Cost estimates (in 1995 £). Source: Chancellor et al. (1997)

Mean cost per patient per year	CD4 ∈ [200; 500]	CD4 < 200	AIDS
Direct care	1701	1774	6948
Community care	1055	1278	2059

Example 9.3. *HIV (continued): Bayesian modelling (2).* The original analysis in Chancellor et al. (1997) reports estimates for a set of relevant costs of care, as shown in Table 9.3.

In the original model, these are considered as fixed, although a scenario sensitivity analysis uses a set of alternative values for the cost of direct care (specifically set at 2938, 4398 and 11 223 for the three states respectively).

We instead use this information to build a model encoding the uncertainty over the cost of direct care. We use trial-and-error and the `bmhe` function `gammaPar()` (see Example 7.4) to get values for the parameters of a Gamma distribution for which most of the mass is approximately between the two extremes.

For example, we could use something like the following code (see Note 22 in Example 7.4 for more detail on using shortcuts for functions in `R` "pipes").

```
# Trial and error to get the parameters of a suitable Gamma (approximately!)
bmhe::gammaPar(2300,350) |>
  (\(x) rgamma(100000,shape=x$shape,rate=x$rate))() |> bmhe::stats()
```

```
     mean        sd      2.5%    median     97.5%
2298.0812  348.3887 1662.6087 2280.4737 3029.3360
```

to obtain a *reasonably* close interval for a Gamma(43.184, 0.019) distribution to model the cost of direct care in "Compromised CD4" with 95% of the mass approximately in the interval [1701; 2938]. Similar calculations can be made for the other two states, to give Gamma(19.905, 0.007) for "Low CD4" and Gamma(66.942, 0.007) for "AIDS".

Figure 9.4 shows graphically these three Gamma distributions. The horizontal segment below the x–axis indicates the observed extremes for the data, while the shaded area under the curves is the 95% interval under these priors. As is possible to see, all are pretty much aligned.

The cost of community care is informed by the data presented in Table 9.3. Ideally, we would have hard evidence (and perhaps a combination of sources) to be able to account for some uncertainty around these estimates. In the absence of this, we could use expert knowledge to elicit some plausible range and then follow a similar mechanism as above to derive suitable parameters for a Gamma distribution. Alternatively (and somewhat less satisfactorily), often HTA practitioners tend to add noise to the mean estimates by setting the standard deviation to a fraction of the mean – see Example 7.4 for another example of this practice.

Here, we follow this strategy and set the standard deviations to 20% of the point estimates. Using again `bmhe::gammaPar()`, we find that Gamma(25, 0.0237), Gamma(25, 0.0196) and Gamma(25, 0.0121) are suitable models for the states "Compromised CD4", "Low CD4" and "AIDS", respectively.

Finally, as for the acquisition of the two drugs, the cost of a year of treatment with ZDV is estimated at c_{mono} = £2278, while 3TC adds an annual cost of £2086. Chancellor et al.

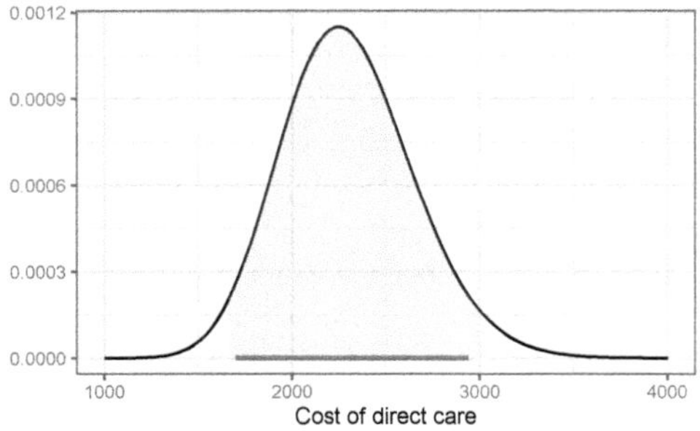

(a) CD4 $\in$ [200; 500].

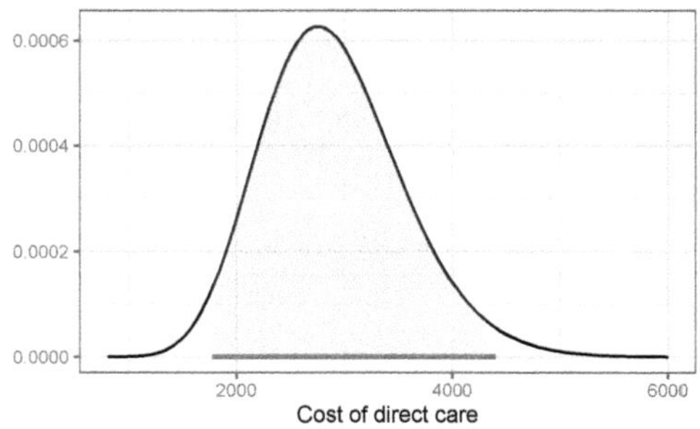

(b) CD4 < 200.

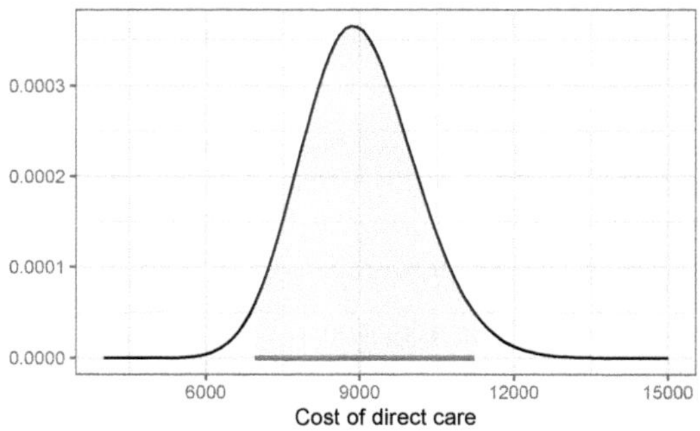

(c) AIDS.

Figure 9.4: Gamma priors for the cost of direct care.

(1997) assume three deterministic scenarios for the cost of the combination therapy, dictated by the treatment effectiveness duration.

In the base-case scenario, the treatment effect is assumed to last for exactly 2 years, during which the annual cost of 3TC+ZDV is given by c_{comb} = £(2278 + 2086)=£4364. After that, patients switch back immediately to monotherapy at an annual cost of c_{mono}, for the rest of the virtual follow-up (until $J = 20$ years). We take a similar approach, but consider an annual cost of c_{comb} for as long as the treatment effectiveness is estimated to be above 0, i.e. as a function of the survival curve $S(j)$ defined above.

At this point, we can finally code up all the modelling assumptions into a suitable JAGS code and then run it to obtain the estimates for the posterior distributions. We can do so using the following code.

```
model=function(){
# Multinomial-Dirichlet model for the observed transitions in the ZDV arm
  for (s in 1:S) {
    y[s,1:S] ~ dmulti(lambda[s,1:S],n[s])
    lambda[s,1:S] ~ ddirch(a[s,1:S])
  }

# Evidence synthesis for the RR in 3TC+ZDV vs ZDV
  for (l in 1:L) {
    x[l] ~ dnorm(theta[l],prec.x[l])
    theta[l] ~ dnorm(mu.theta,tau)
  }
```

```
  mu.theta ~ dnorm(0,0.25)
  sigma.theta ~ dexp(2);        tau <- pow(sigma.theta,-2)
  rho <- exp(mu.theta)

# Treatment effectiveness duration
  for (i in 1:I) {
    r[i] ~ dbin(phi[i],nr[i])
    phi[i] <- 1 - exp(-h[i]*delta[i])
    log(h[i]) <- log(alpha) -alpha*log(mu) + (alpha-1)*log(u[i])
  }
  alpha ~ dexp(2)
  mu ~ dexp(2)

# Estimates time-varying RR with treatment effect waning
  for (j in 1:(J+1)) {
    surv[j] <- exp(-pow(((j-1)/mu),alpha))
    rho.star[j] <- 1-surv[j]*(1-rho)
  }

# Model for the cost of direct care and for the cost of community care
  for (s in 1:(S-1)) {
    c.direct[s] ~ dgamma(shape.dir[s],rate.dir[s])
    c.comm[s] ~ dgamma(shape.comm[s],rate.comm[s])
  }
  c.direct[S] <- 0;             c.comm[S] <- 0

# Model for the annual cost of combination therapy
  c.comb[1] <- c.mono+c.3tc
  for (j in 2:(J+1)) {
    c.comb[j] <- ifelse(surv[(j-1)]>eps, c.mono+c.3tc, c.mono)
  }
}
```

This code is fairly straightforward and modular. We first include the Multinomial-Dirichlet model for the observed data in the ZDV arm. Then, we perform the evidence synthesis on the four studies to estimate the RR of progression for the combination therapy. Next, we use the aggregated pseudo-data to model the treatment effect duration and use the resulting survival curve (the node `surv`, defined for each Markov cycle, $j = 0, \ldots, J$ and thus for a total of $J + 1$ points) to compute the time-varying RR, `rho.star[j]`.

Finally, we model the various costs, taking care of setting the cost associated with the state "Death" to 0. Notice also that `JAGS` allows the use of a number of vector- and array-valued functions, much as `R` would do. In this case, we use the `ifelse()` function to define the cost of the combination therapy as a function of the treatment effectiveness, as mentioned above. Notice that we assume that the combination therapy fails whenever the estimated survival curve for the treatment effectiveness duration goes below a small threshold `eps`, set at 0.001 in the data list defined using the code below.

```
# Defines the data list and runs the model
library(R2jags)
datalist=list(
```

```
  y=y,S=S,n=n,x=x,prec.x=1/sd^2,L=length(x),J=20,
  a=matrix(c(3,3,3,3,0,3,3,3,0,0,3,3,0,0,0,3),nrow=S,byrow=T),
  shape.dir=c(43.184,19.905,66.942),rate.dir=c(0.019,0.007,0.007),
  shape.comm=c(25,25,25),rate.comm=c(0.027,0.0196,0.0121),
  u=c(.5,1,1.5,2,2.5,3,4,5),r=c(0,0,3,7,60,30,0,0),I=8,
  nr=c(100,100,100,97,90,30,0,0),delta=c(0.5,0.5,0.5,0.5,0.5,0.5,1,1),
  c.mono=2278,c.3tc=2086,eps=0.001
)

hiv=jags(
  data=datalist,parameters.to.save=c(
    "lambda","c.direct","rho.star","c.comb","c.comm","surv"
  ),model.file=model,n.chains=2,n.iter=10000,n.burnin=5000
)
```

In this case, the model is very quick to run and convergence does not pose any issues. The summary statistics for the posterior distribution of the RRs are shown in Figure 9.5a. The RR at time $j = 0$ (which is identical to the estimate from the evidence synthesis ρ – cfr. Equation 9.7) is estimated to be 0.513 with a 95% interval of $[0.307; 0.78]$, indicating a substantially beneficial effect of the combination therapy over ZDV only.

As time passes, this quickly decreases: at year $j = 3$, the RR is estimated as 0.917 (with a 95% interval of $[0.869; 0.966]$) and then it goes to 1, indicating that, by then, the treatment is no longer effective and thus produces no benefits.

This is consistent with the graph in Figure 9.5b, which is based on the posterior summaries for the survival curves induced by the Binomial model for the pseudo-counts r_i. Here, initially, the treatment effectiveness is almost identical to 1 (this holds for years $j = 0, 1, 2$), in line with the assumptions in Chancellor et al. (1997). After that, the treatment effectiveness starts to decrease sharply and by year $j = 4$ it is effectively below the threshold eps (indicated by the horizontal dashed line).

We can also post-process the simulations from the posterior distributions to construct Figure 9.6, which depicts the probabilities for the possible transitions, in the 3TC+ZDV arm.

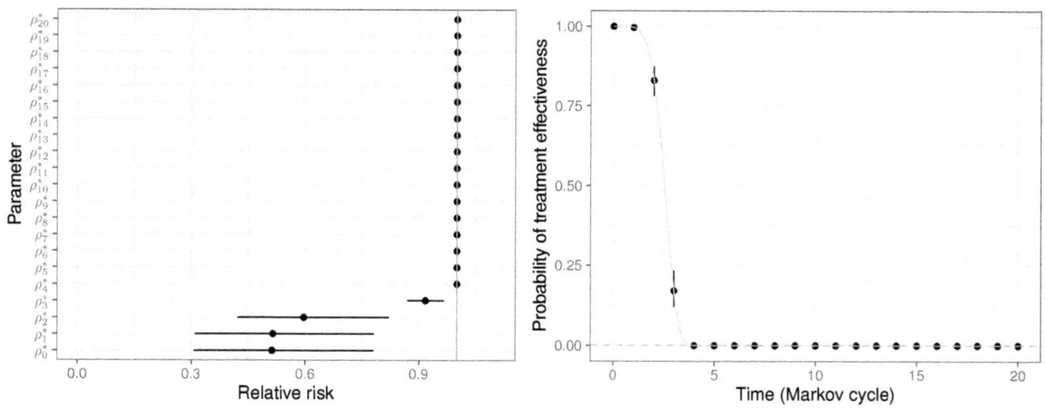

(a) ρ_j^*. (b) $S(j) = \Pr(\text{treatment effective at time } j)$.

Figure 9.5: Posterior distribution summaries for selected nodes.

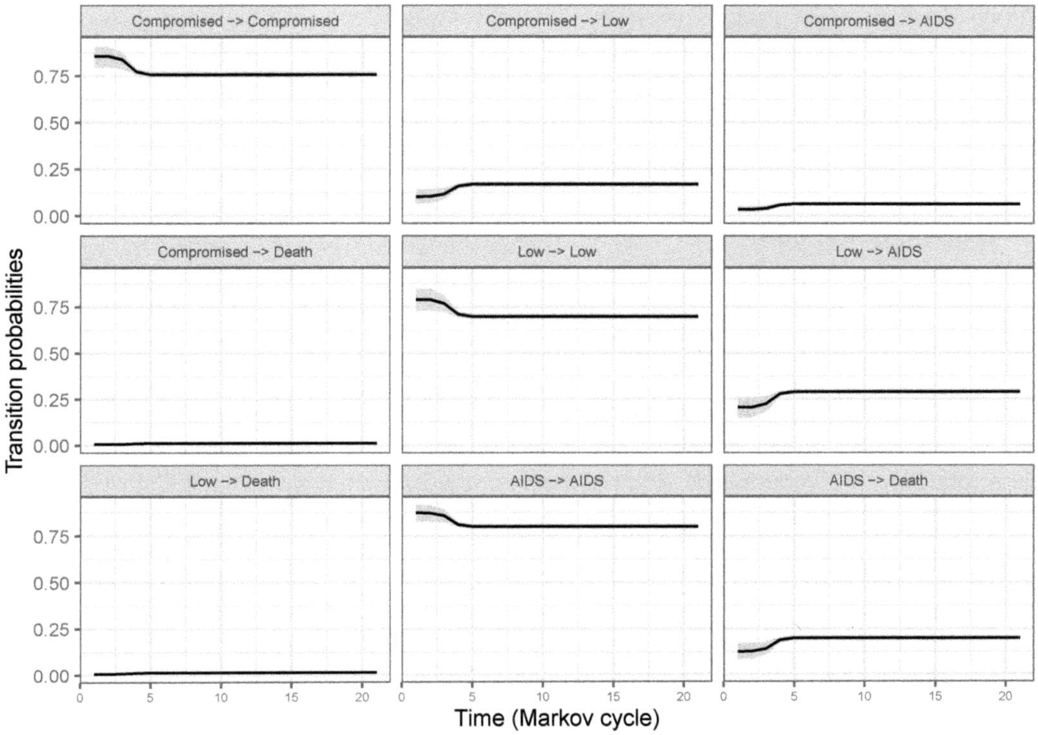

Figure 9.6: Estimates for the posterior distribution of the transition probabilities in the combination therapy arm. These are obtained by applying the time-varying RR to the estimates for the transition probabilities in the ZDV arm. Initially, the treatment is estimated to be effective and thus there is a reduction in the probability of the progressions; over time, the treatment effect wanes out and the probabilities switch back to the same levels as in the mono-therapy arm.

We present here the mean (dark curve) and the 95% interval (the grey ribbon), across the $J = 20$ years of virtual follow-up for the Markov model.

As long as the treatment is effective, the combination arm shows benefits in decreasing the progressions (from $s = 1$ to $s' = 2, 3, 4$; from $s = 2$ to $s' = 3, 4$ and from $s = 3$ to $s' = 4$). Once the treatment effect wanes down to 0 (around year 5), then the transition probabilities stops varying over time and revert to the same value as the ZDV arm.

9.2.3 Running the Markov model

Once we have obtained the estimates for the relevant posterior distributions, we need to post-process the results and apply the matrix algebra in order to run the Markov model. The real complexity in this case is that we need to apply the matrix algebra of Equation 9.2 or Equation 9.3 for each MCMC simulations for the model parameters (i.e. the number `n.sims`, in this case set at 2000).

In order to do so, it is often useful to consider `R` "arrays", which are multi-dimensional extensions to simpler matrices. For example, we may need to create an array `lambda`, with dimension $n_{sims} \times (J+1) \times S \times S$, in which, for each MCMC simulation $i = 1, \ldots, n_{sims}$ and for each Markov cycle $j = 0, \ldots, J$, we store a $S \times S$ transition matrix.

> **Indexing vectors and times**
>
> Notice the slight inconsistency between the pure mathematical notation and the computer one used in the rest of the chapter. As mentioned above, we consider here Markov cycles $j = 0, \ldots, J$.
>
> However, `R` does not allow to define a vector using the index 0 and thus in the code below we use `j=1,...,J+1` instead, where the index `j=1` indicates time $j = 0$, the index `j=2` indicates time $j = 1$ and so on.

We demonstrate how to "wrangle" the results from the `JAGS` model in Example 9.4.

Example 9.4. *HIV (continued): Markov model and economic evaluation.* We start the post-processing by defining the number of Markov cycles ($J = 20$, in this case, in line with the original analysis of Chancellor et al., 1997) and then a vector `start`, in which we set up the initial conditions in terms of states occupancy. Often, we assume that all the "virtual cohort" starts in one state, in this case "Compromised CD4", but we could distribute the individuals across the states, already at time $j = 0$. In this case, we consider a virtual cohort of 1000 individuals (but, again, we could choose any number we like).

Next, we initialise the $n_{sims} \times (J+1) \times S$ arrays `m1` and `m2`, in which we will store the occupancy matrices. These have three dimensions – the first one indicates the MCMC simulations for the model parameters, the second one the number of the Markov cycles (as mentioned above, we consider from $j = 0$ to $j = J = 20$, i.e. a total of $J+1$ time points) and the third one indicates the S states characterising the Markov model. In this case, we set up the arrays to 0, but this is also not essential and, for instance, we could create and fill them with `NA`s.

In `R` we can use the function `array()` to create a multidimensional array – note in the code below that we also use the optional argument `dimnames` to pass a list of names for each of the three dimensions. This is not essential, but it does help to navigate the objects we are creating and thus we recommend doing so.

Finally, for each MCMC simulation, we initialise the first row of the arrays `m1` and `m2` to the starting position – this means that at time $j = 0$ every individual is in the state "Compromised CD4".

```
# Time horizon for the Markov model
J=20

# Virtual cohort: everyone starts in State A
start=c(1000,0,0,0)

# Initialises the array for the number of individuals in each state
m1=m2=array(
  0,c(hiv$BUGSoutput$n.sims,(J+1),S),
  dimnames=list(1:hiv$BUGSoutput$n.sims,paste0("j=",0:J),states)
)
for (s in 1:S){
    m1[,1,s]=start[s]
```

```
    m2[,1,s]=start[s]
}
# Visualises the 'm1' array for the first MCMC simulation (first few rows)
m1[1,,] |> head()
```

```
    Compromised CD4 Low CD4 AIDS Death
j=0            1000       0    0     0
j=1               0       0    0     0
j=2               0       0    0     0
j=3               0       0    0     0
j=4               0       0    0     0
j=5               0       0    0     0
```

At this point, we can use the MCMC simulations for $\boldsymbol{\Lambda}_s$ and ρ^*_j to construct the actual transition matrices for the two treatment arms, which we indicate as $\boldsymbol{\Lambda}^{(1)}$ and $\boldsymbol{\Lambda}^{(2)}_j$, for the ZDV and the 3TC+ZDV arm, respectively. In line with the assumptions specified in Example 9.2, the former does not vary with the Markov cycle, while the latter does (and hence is indexed by j).

We first extract the simulations for the node `lambda` from the `JAGS` object `hiv` into the variable `lambda1`, which represents the transition matrix for the ZDV arm, $\boldsymbol{\Lambda}^{(1)}$. Then, we define a new array `lambda2`. This is temporarily filled with 0s and we specify its size to be the same as for `lambda1`, but with an additional fourth dimension, to account for the fact that this will vary with the Markov cycle j.

Once this is done, we can loop over the MCMC simulations `i` and the Markov cycles `j` to apply the estimated time-varying RR `rho.star[i,j]` to the ZDV transitions – for numerical stability and in line with the discussion in Section 9.2.2, we do this using Equation 9.11, which also ensures that each row must sum to 1:

```
# Formats the simulations for the transition probabilities in matrix format
lambda1=hiv$BUGSoutput$sims.list$lambda
lambda2=array(0,dim=c(dim(lambda1),(J+1)))

# Makes time-varying transition matrix for combination therapy
for (i in 1:hiv$BUGSoutput$n.sims) {
  for (j in 1:(J+1)) {
# Applies the time-specific RR to the transition probabilities for the ZDV arm
# NB: for numerical stability works on logit(lambda) + log(RR) + adjustment and
#     then applies the inverse logit transformation to go back to [0-1] scale
    lambda2[i,,,j]=bmhe::ilogit(
      bmhe::logit(lambda1[i,,]) + log(hiv$BUGSoutput$sims.list$rho.star[i,j]) +
        log(1-lambda1[i,,]) -
        log(1-lambda1[i,,]*(1-hiv$BUGSoutput$sims.list$rho.star[i,j]))
    )
# Rescales the diagonal of the transition matrix, so that each row sums to 1
    diag(lambda2[i,,,j])=diag(lambda2[i,,,j]) + (1-rowSums(lambda2[i,,,j]))
# Ensures that Death is an absorbing state
    lambda2[i,S,S,j]=1
  }
}
```

— this code makes use of the bmhe functions `logit()` and `ilogit()` that compute the logit and inverse logit transformations, respectively.

Sense-checking the transition probabilities

Once the array `lambda2` is computed, we can check that all the entries behave using code like the following.

```
which(lambda2<0,arr.ind=TRUE)
```

```
     dim1 dim2 dim3 dim4
```

Here, we are checking for negative transition probabilities – note that adding the option `add.ind=TRUE` will explicitly print the indices for all the array dimensions in which the condition we specify is encountered.

Luckily, in our problem there are no such cases – hence the output for `dim1 dim2 dim3 dim4` (indicating respectively the MCMC simulations, row, column and time point in the transition matrices), is empty. This broadly suggests that the data used to obtained the pooled RR estimate are reasonably consistent with those observed to obtain the estimates for $\mathbf{\Lambda}^{(1)}$.

Nonetheless, this type of check is actually very helpful and we recommend embedding it in the workflow, because in case there were unacceptable estimates, we may need to "fix" the resulting transition probabilities.

At this point, we can apply the R version of Equation 9.3 and fill the arrays `m1` and `m2` with the number of individuals that at each time point visit each of the states, for each MCMC simulation of the model parameters. We can do this compactly (and efficiently) using the R matrix multiplication operator `%*%`.

```
for (i in 1:hiv$BUGSoutput$n.sims) {
  for (j in 2:(J+1)) {
    m1[i,j,]=m1[i,j-1,] %*% lambda1[i,,]
    m2[i,j,]=m2[i,j-1,] %*% lambda2[i,,,j-1]
  }
}
# Visualises the two array for the first MCMC simulation (first few rows)
cbind(m1[1,,],m2[1,,]) |> head() |> round(2)
```

```
    Compromised CD4 Low CD4   AIDS  Death Compromised CD4 Low CD4   AIDS Death
j=0         1000.00    0.00   0.00   0.00         1000.00    0.00   0.00  0.00
j=1          720.38  198.82  71.38   9.43          892.41   77.30  26.81  3.48
j=2          518.94  258.25 186.22  36.59          795.50  133.40  61.44  9.65
j=3          373.83  252.59 282.23  91.34          684.10  184.46 109.48 21.95
j=4          269.30  220.47 341.54 168.70          529.67  237.48 182.26 50.60
j=5          194.00  181.10 365.40 259.51          401.60  253.46 249.97 94.98
```

As is possible to see from the output of the above R code, now the two arrays have been filled with numeric values for all the time points. Here, we bind the columns for `m1` to those of `m2`. The right-most four columns of the output above show the number of people transiting in each of the four states in the combination therapy, in correspondence of the first MCMC simulation of the model parameters – as is possible to see, more people tend to remain in the less severe state and fewer die.

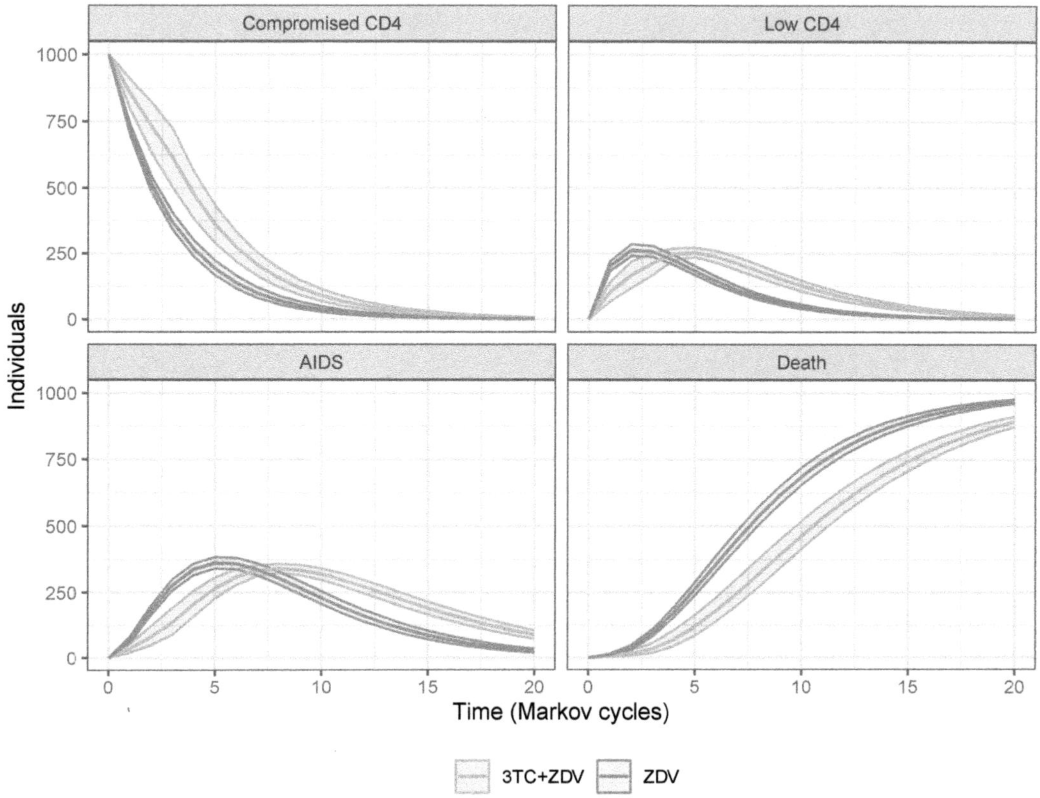

Figure 9.7: Number of individuals in each of the four states, for the two treatment arms.

The Markov model simulations can be visualised over the $J+1$ time points used, in what is often termed as the "Markov trace". We show the results for the HIV model in Figure 9.7. Over time, the combination therapy consistently maintains a higher number of individuals in the less severe state ("Compromised CD4") and, crucially, reduces the number of people who die.

Initially, the benefits extend to the other two states too, although at about time $j = 6$, more people remain in the combination than in the mono-therapy arm – this is because at that stage, most people have transitioned out of the "Compromised CD4" state and in the 3TC+ZDV arm fewer people die (and hence more remain in the either "Low CD4" or "AIDS").

In Chancellor et al. (1997), the cost-effectiveness analysis is based on life-years gained, meaning that each health state is implicitly assigned a utility value of 1. Again, a more "modern" analysis would focus on utility values associated with each of the states and then QALYs, but here we replicate the original framework, for simplicity.

We can easily obtain the occupancy probability arrays (as in Equation 9.2) by simply rescaling the objects `m1` and `m2` by the number of individuals in the virtual cohort, set at 1000. These are helpful to continue the post-processing of the results, as we show in the following code – note that we use the `lapply()` function (see Note 6 in Example 2.6), which compactly applies a function over a vector or a list, to ensure that the commands are repeated for each MCMC simulation $i = 1, \ldots, n_{sims}$.

```
# Defines the occupancy probability arrays
pi1=m1/1000
pi2=m2/1000
# Creates objects with "length of stay" in each state
los1=lapply(1:hiv$BUGSoutput$n.sims,function(i) {
  pi1[i,,] |> apply(2,sum)
}) |> bind_rows()

los2=lapply(1:hiv$BUGSoutput$n.sims,function(i) {
  pi2[i,,] |> apply(2,sum)
}) |> bind_rows()
```

We can use these objects to summarise the results and compute the expected length of stay in years for each treatment arm and for each of the S states of the Markov model, e.g. using the following simple R code.

```
los1 |> bmhe::stats()
```

```
                      mean         sd      2.5%    median     97.5%
Compromised CD4   3.554879 0.13219958  3.309164  3.550126  3.831981
Low CD4           1.703731 0.07416047  1.565027  1.702799  1.858641
AIDS              3.640974 0.14405413  3.377061  3.639726  3.936975
Death            12.100416 0.20535556 11.707869 12.100169 12.512958
```

```
los2 |> bmhe::stats()
```

```
                    mean         sd     2.5%   median     97.5%
Compromised CD4 5.158696 0.33665869 4.470759 5.170626  5.809213
Low CD4         2.350635 0.08875243 2.175183 2.351304  2.522376
AIDS            4.215254 0.12652896 3.977279 4.213221  4.470550
Death           9.275415 0.35772752 8.643653 9.260342 10.006364
```

We can see from these summary statistics that the combination therapy tends to have longer expected time in the less severe state and again, consistently with the findings above, shorter expected years in the state "Death".

We can also produce an estimate for the overall number of years alive (or Life Years Gained, LYG) in the two treatment arm and, by difference, a measure of treatment effectiveness, Δ_e.

```
los1 |> select(-Death) |>
  mutate(LYG1=rowSums(across(everything()))) |> select(LYG1) |>
  bind_cols(
    los2 |> bind_rows() |> select(-Death) |>
      mutate(LYG2=rowSums(across(everything()))) |> select(LYG2)
  ) |> mutate(Delta.e=LYG2-LYG1) |> bmhe::stats()
```

```
              mean        sd      2.5%    median     97.5%
LYG1      8.899584 0.2053556  8.487042  8.899831  9.292131
LYG2     11.724585 0.3577275 10.993636 11.739658 12.356347
Delta.e   2.825001 0.3024662  2.163359  2.838842  3.377800
```

In comparison to Chancellor et al. (1997), our model returns a larger differential in terms of years of life gained – this is because we allow for the treatment effect to wane off beyond the hard cutoff of two years set in the original analysis.

Similar analyses can be performed by combining the occupancy array `pi1` and `pi2` with the estimated posterior distributions for the various costs. We do this using the following `R` code, which returns the output in the form of a "tibble" that can be further aggregated to obtain relevant summaries.

```
# Define discount rate
d=0.06

# ZDV arm
c1=lapply(1:hiv$BUGSoutput$n.sims,function(i) {
  # Probability of occupancy with dimension: (J+1) rows x S columns
  pi1[i,,] |> as.data.frame() |> cbind(
    # Vector of times and drug cost
    j=0:J,c_drug=rep(2278,(J+1)),
    # Matrix with cost of community care with dimension: (J+1) x S
    matrix(
      rep(hiv$BUGSoutput$sims.list$c.comm[i,],(J+1)),
      (J+1),S,byrow=T,dimnames=list(0:J,paste0("c_comm_",states))
    ),
    # Matrix of cost of direct care with dimension: (J+1) x S
    matrix(
      rep(hiv$BUGSoutput$sims.list$c.direct[i,],(J+1)),
      (J+1),S,byrow=T,dimnames=list(0:J,paste0("c_direct_",states))
    )
  ) |> as_tibble()
}) |> bind_rows() |>
  # Applies discounting to all costs
  mutate(across(starts_with("c_"),~ .x/(1+d)^j)) |>
  # Computes the cost for each state
  mutate(
    `Compromised CD4`=`Compromised CD4`*
      (`c_drug`+`c_comm_Compromised CD4`+`c_direct_Compromised CD4`),
    `Low CD4`=`Low CD4`*(`c_drug`+`c_comm_Low CD4`+`c_direct_Low CD4`),
    `AIDS`=`AIDS`*(`c_drug`+`c_comm_AIDS`+`c_direct_AIDS`),
    sim=rep(1:hiv$BUGSoutput$n.sims,each=(J+1))
  ) |>
  # Selects only the relevant columns
  select(sim,j,`Compromised CD4`,`Low CD4`,`AIDS`)
```

First, we define the value of the discount rate, d (see Equation 5.2) – Chancellor et al. (1997) use a value of 6% for costs, although perhaps a more "modern" analysis would apply a smaller rate (see the discussion in Section 5.1).

Then, we start creating an object `c1`, in which we want to store the costs incurred in each state for each time point and derived by using different MCMC simulations for the model parameters. Firstly, we use again the `lapply()` function to repeat the commands for each MCMC simulation $i = 1, \ldots, n_{sims}$ and then we build a data frame, including the relevant variables. We start by including the $i-$th element of the occupancy probability array `pi1`, which we augment with a vector j, to keep track of the Markov cycle. Then, we add the various costs: the column c_drug is a vector in which the value 2278 is repeated for J+1 times: this is because the cost of ZDV is fixed for each Markov cycle. Next, we add the cost of community care: the JAGS object outputs a matrix with n_{sims} rows and S columns for this variable, which is assumed to not vary over the Markov cycles. Thus, we select the first row of values from the JAGS object hiv and create a matrix with J+1 rows and S columns using the code

```
matrix(
  rep(hiv$BUGSoutput$sims.list$c.comm[i,],(J+1)),
  (J+1),S,byrow=T,dimnames=list(0:J,paste0("c_comm_",states))
)
```

the first few rows of which look like the following.

```
  c_comm_Compromised CD4 c_comm_Low CD4 c_comm_AIDS c_comm_Death
0               1432.601       1290.595    1780.041            0
1               1432.601       1290.595    1780.041            0
2               1432.601       1290.595    1780.041            0
3               1432.601       1290.595    1780.041            0
4               1432.601       1290.595    1780.041            0
5               1432.601       1290.595    1780.041            0
```

Notice, again, the use of the option dimnames to associate meaningful names to the dimensions of the matrix – once more, this is not essential, but it is a helpful sanity check and will facilitate further wrangling of the data, later. The same reasoning applies for the cost of direct care, which are also estimated as a matrix of $n_{sims} \times S$ simulations in the JAGS model. Finally, for all MCMC simulations, we store the resulting data frame as a tibble, for ease of post-processing. At this stage, c1 is still a list with n_{sims} elements, each of which looks like the following

```
# A tibble: 21 x 14
  `Compromised CD4` `Low CD4`  AIDS Death     j c_drug `c_comm_Compromised CD4`
              <dbl>     <dbl> <dbl> <dbl> <dbl>  <dbl>                    <dbl>
1              1         0     0     0        0   2278                    1514.
2              0.72      0.2   0.07  0.01     1   2278                    1514.
3              0.52      0.26  0.19  0.04     2   2278                    1514.
4              0.37      0.25  0.28  0.09     3   2278                    1514.
5              0.27      0.22  0.34  0.17     4   2278                    1514.
6              0.19      0.18  0.37  0.26     5   2278                    1514.
# i 15 more rows
# i 7 more variables: `c_comm_Low CD4` <dbl>, c_comm_AIDS <dbl>, c_comm_Death <dbl>,
#   `c_direct_Compromised CD4` <dbl>, `c_direct_Low CD4` <dbl>, c_direct_AIDS <dbl>,
#   c_direct_Death <dbl>
```

(this output is for i=1 and, as such, it only has $J + 1 = 21$ rows, one for each time point).

Outside the lapply() function, we add the dplyr function bind_rows(), which is used to combine all the 2000 elements of the list into a single tibble. The resulting object has $n_{sims} \times (J + 1) = 2000 \times 21 = 42\,000$ rows.

Next, we apply discounting to all the cost variables. Here, we have made sure to follow a specific naming convention, where all the cost variables are labelled as c_XXX. Thus, we can use the command

```
mutate(across(starts_with("c_"),~ .x/(1+d)^j))
```

to compactly apply the discounting formula `x/(1+d)^j` (cfr. Equation 5.2) to each variable whose name starts with the string `"c_"`.

Finally, we first compute the overall cost associated with each state as the product of the probability of occupancy and the sum of the relevant item costs and then select only the relevant columns, which produces the object of interest, `c1`, the first few rows of which look like the following.

```
# A tibble: 42,000 x 5
    sim     j `Compromised CD4` `Low CD4`  AIDS
  <int> <int>             <dbl>     <dbl> <dbl>
1     1     0             6080.        0     0
2     1     1             4132.     1078.  968.
3     1     2             2808.     1321. 2383.
4     1     3             1908.     1219. 3407.
5     1     4             1297.     1004. 3890.
6     1     5              881.      778. 3926.
# i 41,994 more rows
```

As for the combination therapy arm, to create another object `c2`, we can basically copy and paste the code used above, with the two differences that: *i*) we use the occupancy probability array `pi2` (instead of `pi1`); and *ii*) we define the drug costs as `c_drug=cbind(hiv$BUGSoutput$sims.list$c.comb[i,])` because, in this case, the cost of acquisition of the drug does vary with the Markov cycles and thus, for each MCMC simulation, we obtain a vector of `J+1` values, which we add as a column to the data frame using the `R` built-in function `cbind()`.

Once these tibbles are available, we can wrangle them further to produce any relevant summary or to build a graph using `ggplot2`. For instance, we can use the following `R` code to derive summary statistics for the total cost by states across all years.

```
c1 |> group_by(sim) |> summarise(across(`Compromised CD4`:`AIDS`,~ sum(.x))) |>
  select(-sim) |> bmhe::stats()
```

```
                     mean        sd      2.5%    median    97.5%
Compromised CD4 17048.108 1352.2825 14578.474 16962.720 20000.67
Low CD4          8368.117  947.9769  6705.437  8325.948 10359.62
AIDS            32918.036 3078.9051 26985.268 32853.414 39044.47
```

```
c2 |> group_by(sim) |> summarise(across(`Compromised CD4`:`AIDS`,~ sum(.x))) |>
  select(-sim) |> bmhe::stats()
```

```
                    mean       sd      2.5%   median    97.5%
Compromised CD4 30610.17 2455.609 25876.633 30570.40 35486.50
Low CD4         11559.09 1170.714  9477.499 11522.48 14089.16
AIDS            34482.96 3183.027 28511.195 34431.35 40977.95
```

Similarly, we can summarise the total costs across both states and years as well as the incremental value for the combination therapy, Δ_c, using the following `R` code.

```
c1 |> mutate(tot.cost=rowSums(across(`Compromised CD4`:`AIDS`))) |>
  select(sim,tot.cost,j) |> group_by(sim) |> summarise(ZDV=sum(tot.cost)) |>
  select(ZDV) |> bind_cols(
```

```
  c2 |> mutate(tot.cost=rowSums(across(`Compromised CD4`:`AIDS`))) |>
select(sim,tot.cost,j) |> group_by(sim) |>
  summarise("3TC+ZDV"=sum(tot.cost)) |> select("3TC+ZDV")
) |> mutate(delta.c=`3TC+ZDV`-ZDV) |> bmhe::stats()
```

```
             mean        sd     2.5%   median    97.5%
ZDV      58334.26 3467.8189 51514.22 58255.94 65294.51
3TC+ZDV  76652.22 3782.0465 69220.32 76590.00 84123.95
delta.c  18317.96  869.8709 16615.61 18306.57 20002.90
```

Figure 9.8 shows the progression of the total cost per patient over the course of the virtual follow-up.

As is possible to see in Figure 9.8a, while at the beginning the combination therapy is more expensive, the two curves tend to get closer and closer. The combination therapy is still more expensive, but much less so and, interestingly, the interval estimates are on top of each other. Figure 9.8b shows the progression of the overall cumulative costs, which highlights the fact that the combination therapy does accrue larger costs by the end of the virtual follow-up. Finally, Figure 9.8c shows how annual costs are split, on average, across the states, indicating again that the combination therapy has higher costs mostly for the less severe states, especially for the first few years of the Markov model simulation.

In comparison to Chancellor et al. (1997), the costs are substantially higher, because we assume a larger cost for direct medical care (to account for the uncertainty in the hospital data, including the values observed in the alternative source). In addition, the full cost of the combination therapy generally occurs for longer periods (more or less up to $j = 4$), while the base-case analysis in the original model assumes that after two years the combination therapy reverts to mono-therapy with no uncertainty whatsoever.

9.3 Three-state Markov model

Another case in which Markov models are particularly popular in HTA is to evaluate a specific disease history, typically related to cancer and often referred to as "Three-state Markov model".

In this specific setup, the relevant population is made by individuals who are in the state of "Pre progression", i.e. they have already been diagnosed with cancer. In future times, their condition may deteriorate further in two ways: either they move into a state of "Progression" (e.g. through metastases or a general worsening of the cancer), or to the absorbing state of "Death". From "Progression", the clinical representation of the disease does not allow individuals to revert to a less severe state and the only available move is towards "Death". Figure 9.9 shows this natural history of the disease, graphically.

While it may look like a rough simplification, this structure is often suitable to describe the life-course of cancer patients, especially for aggressive tumours, where, effectively, there is no cure and thus it is not possible to reverse to less severe states of the illness.

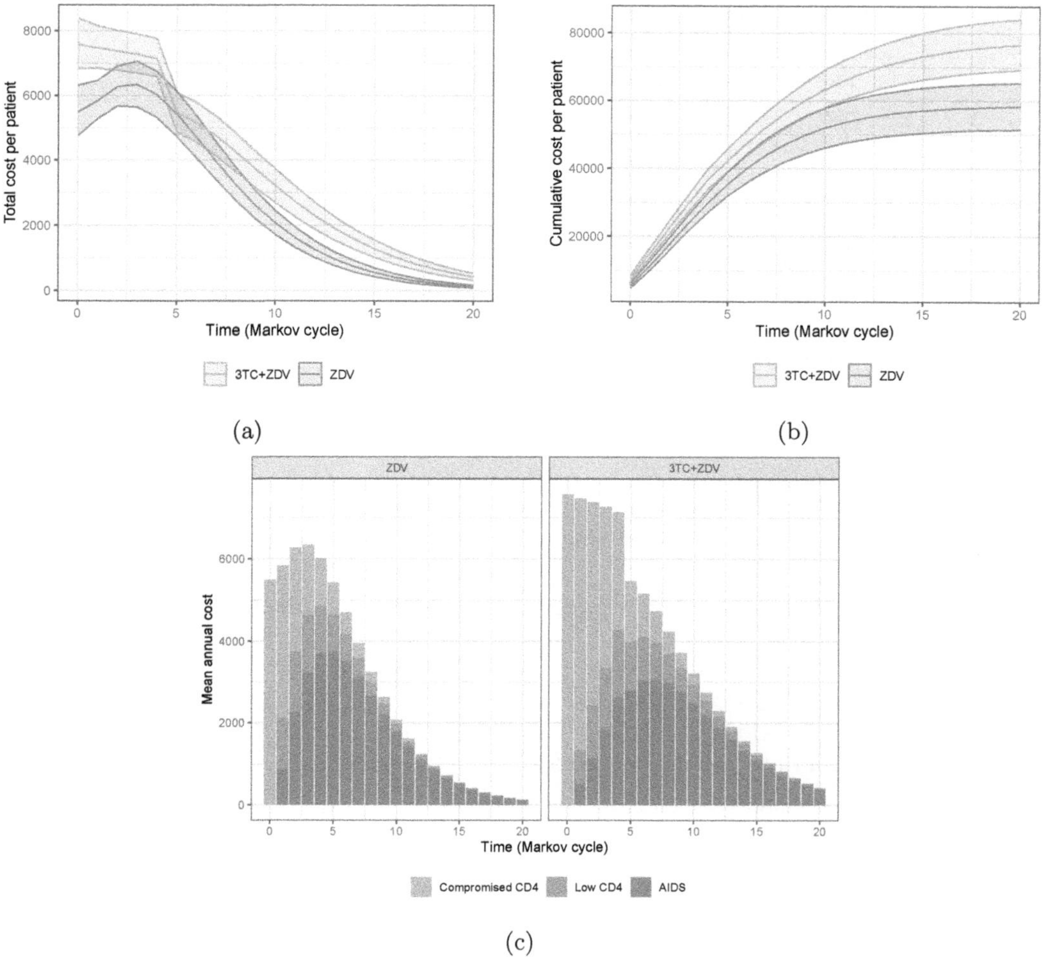

Figure 9.8: Analysis of the total costs over the course of the virtual follow-up. Panel (a) shows the estimated total cost per patient over the time of the Markov simulation, while panel (b) depicts the overall cumulative costs over time, for the two treatment arms. Panel (c) shows a barplot with the contribution of each state to the yearly costs in the two treatment arms.

When dealing with these situations, we often link the output of a survival analysis (as presented throughout Chapter 8) to the Markov model machinery. We showcase two ways of doing this, depending on the nature of the available data.

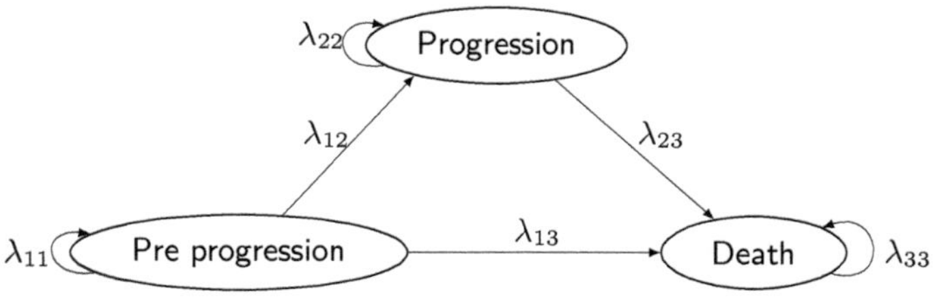

Figure 9.9: A graphical representation of the "Three-state cancer Markov model".

Table 9.4: A snippet of the data included in the TA 174. Source: Williams et al. (2017b)

Patient	Treatment	Progression?	Death?	Progression time	Death time
1	RFC	1	0	31.99	32
2	RFC	1	0	30.55	30.6
...	...	...	...	...	...
9	FC	1	0	35.73	36
10	RFC	1	1	0.17	0.46
...	...	...	...	...	...

9.3.1 Three-state Markov models with individual-level data

As mentioned in Section 8.3.2, *ideally*, we have access to individual-level data (e.g. from a randomised trial), describing the "event history" for each patient. Table 9.4 shows an example of this sort of data – in fact this is the same dataset considered in Example 8.1.

Digitising well is hard work (and comes with assumptions)...

As mentioned in Note 24 in Example 8.1, the data are obtained through digitisation and substantial post-processing to recreate all the individual trajectories in terms of all the relevant transitions – from pre-progression to progression; from pre-progression to death; and from progression to death.

The death times generated for patients who had a corresponding progression time matched closely the event times from the scanned pre-progression curve. This works if we assume a "*semi-Markov*"/clock-reset approach for the transition from progression to death. With this terminology, we indicate the assumption that continuous transitions rates can also depend on the time spent in the current state. This relaxes the more stringent Markov(1) assumption (see Equation 2.12), under which the transitions are "memory-less" and all that matters to determine the next state is the current one and not the full history (see also the discussion in Thom et al., 2025b, sec. 9.3.3).

In the case of the NICE TA174 synthetic data generated by Williams et al. (2017a), the semi-Markov assumption is fundamental because it lets the risk of moving to the next health state depend not only on the current state (e.g. progressed) but also on how long a patient has been in that state. In other words, the clock resets at progression and time since progression, not the total time since baseline, governs the hazard of death.

This flexibility is crucial when reconstructing synthetic individual-level data from digitised survival curves. If we assumed a strict Markov(1) process, the transition from progression to death could only depend on being in the progressed state, ignoring for how long each individual had sojourned there. This, in turn, would make it impossible to align reconstructed death times with the observed post-progression survival pattern, because the real data show that the risk of death changes with time since progression.

By using a semi-Markov model, we can model the post-progression hazard separately directly from the digitised post-progression survival curve, without having to match every progression event exactly to an individual's pre-progression time. The clock-reset assumption lets us treat the progression to death process independently, which greatly simplifies reconstruction while remaining realistic.

Ultimately, under a pure Markov(1) assumption, it may be near-impossible to generate individual-level data with event times for each patient, because of the lack of the complete history. Relaxing this to a semi-Markov approach does offer more possibilities, especially if we can complement the limited information from the survival curves with additional evidence.

This type of data would allow us to estimate directly all the relevant transition probabilities, because they contain information about the complete history of each individual and so we can use them to construct the "risk set" for each possible transition and then estimate the time-to-event.

Specifically, once the survival curves are estimated for each of the relevant subsets, we can provide estimates of the transition probabilities from a state s to another state s' at time j, using the survival curve computed for two consecutive times j and $j+\delta_j$ (where δ_j constitutes the length of the Markov cycle) as

$$\lambda_{jss'} \approx 1 - \frac{S(j+\delta_j)}{S(j)}. \tag{9.12}$$

This is because the ratio $\frac{S(j+\delta_j)}{S(j)}$ indicates the proportion of individuals who still have not experienced the event of interest (either progression or death) at time $j+\delta_j$, out of those individuals who were still at risk at the beginning of the interval $[j; j+\delta_j]$. Thus, the complement to 1 represents the proportion of individuals who between times j and $j+\delta_j$ have indeed experienced the event of interest.

If the Markov cycle is too wide, then the approximation based on the survival curve is very coarse and possibly quite biased in comparison to the underlying, continuous transition probability $\lambda_{jss'}$ for any given time j. But if the width of the interval is reasonably small, then Equation 9.12 is an acceptable discrete approximation of the continuous value – of course, what is "reasonably small" depends on the context.

If we have the full history of all the individuals, we can subset the data to derive the relevant risk sets (see in details the computations in Example 9.5):

- Subset 1: individuals at risk of making the transition from "Pre-progression" to "Progression"
- Subset 2: individuals at risk of dying from "Pro-progression" (without first transiting in "Progression")
- Subset 3: individuals at risk of dying from "Progression".

We can use these data to perform the survival analysis and apply Equation 9.12 to **directly** estimate λ_{j12}, from Subset 1; λ_{j13}, from Subset 2; and λ_{j23}, from Subset 3.

Moreover, using the fact that the transitions are mutually exclusive and exhaustive, we can estimate **indirectly**

$$\begin{aligned} \lambda_{11j} &= 1 - \lambda_{12j} - \lambda_{13j} \\ \lambda_{22j} &= 1 - \lambda_{23j}. \end{aligned}$$

and thus, since "Death" is an absorbing state, we can complete the transition matrix

$$\boldsymbol{\Lambda}_j = \begin{pmatrix} \lambda_{j11} & \lambda_{j12} & \lambda_{j13} \\ 0 & \lambda_{j22} & \lambda_{j23} \\ 0 & 0 & 1 \end{pmatrix}.$$

Once the transition matrix is obtained for each relevant time period (Markov cycle), we can simply run the Markov model of Figure 9.9 to derive all the relevant outputs.

Example 9.5. *NICE TA174 (adapted and expanded from Williams et al., 2017b): three-state modelling.* We consider again the data for NICE TA174; in particular, we can target the two underlying events (progression and death). The analysis based on the time until a progression is observed determines the so-called "progression-free survival" (PFS), while the analysis targeting death as the event of interest determines the so-called "overall survival" (OS) – see the discussion in Section 8.3.2.

It is possible to use the `survHE` function `make_data_multi_state()` to wrangle the original dataset and create the relevant indicator to then define the "risk sets".

```
# Uses survHE to restructure the dataset
risk_set=survHE::make_data_multi_state(data)
# Shows the first few rows of the resulting dataset. Here, treat=1 is RFC
risk_set |> as.data.frame() |> head() |> print(digits=2)
```

```
  id from to trans Tstart Tstop    time status treat prog death prog_t death_t
1  1    1  2     1      0    32 31.9908      1     1    1     0     32      32
2  1    1  3     2      0    32 31.9908      0     1    1     0     32      32
3  1    2  3     3     32    32  0.0092      0     1    1     0     32      32
4  2    1  2     1      0    31 30.5524      1     1    1     0     31      31
5  2    1  3     2      0    31 30.5524      0     1    1     0     31      31
6  2    2  3     3     31    31  0.0476      0     1    1     0     31      31
```

The object `risk_set` contains the information in Table 9.4, but restructured to account for the possible transitions. These are described in the columns labelled `from` and `to` (or, more compactly, in the column labelled `trans`); for instance, the first row of the dataset describes the time necessary for the patient indexed by the `patid` 1 to move from "Pre-progression" to "Progression, which happens in 32 time units (e.g. months).

The variables `Tstart` and `Tstop` indicate the times at which the individual enters and exits the relevant risk set – in other words, the individual associated with `patid=1` is at risk of making the transition from "Pre-progression" to "Progression" immediately at enrolment (as is reasonable) and until the event actually happens.

The dataset also contains progression and death indicators, respectively in the variables `prog` and `death`, taking values 0 or 1 if that specific event is censored or fully observed. Finally, the progression and death times are also recorded separately in the variables `prog_t` and `death_t`.

We can filter the dataset to select specific cases and sub-risk sets, as shown in the following `R` code. For instance, filtering for `trans==1` selects all the individuals who are at risk of making the transition from "Pre-progression" to "Progression". In fact, there are different outcomes observed among them; for instance, the combination `trans==1,prog==0,death==0` returns the subset of patients who while in "Pre-progression" have been fully censored, i.e. those for whom we do not know the actual time to progression or to death. In this case, the reported data indicate the time of censoring.

```
# Selects patients in Pre-progression who are fully censored
risk_set |> dplyr::filter(trans==1,prog==0,death==0) |> slice(1:3) |>
  as.data.frame() |> head() |> print(digits=2)
```

```
   id from to trans Tstart Tstop  time status treat prog death prog_t death_t
1 249    1  2     1      0 0.058 0.058      0     1    0     0  0.058   0.058
2 250    1  2     1      0 3.797 3.797      0     1    0     0  3.797   3.797
3 251    1  2     1      0 5.466 5.466      0     1    0     0  5.466   5.466
```

Another subgroup is made by those who have died before progression by filtering `trans==1,prog==0,death==1`. Notice that, in this case, the indicator `prog` is set to 0 to indicate that these patients are censored, with respect to the event of interest (progression).

```
# Selects patients in Pre-progression who die before progression
risk_set |> dplyr::filter(trans==1,prog==0,death==1) |> slice(1:3) |>
  as.data.frame() |> head() |> print(digits=2)
```

```
   id from to trans Tstart Tstop time status treat prog death prog_t death_t
1 527    1  2     1      0   1.5  1.5      0     1    0     1    1.5     1.5
2 528    1  2     1      0   2.1  2.1      0     1    0     1    2.1     2.1
3 529    1  2     1      0   2.6  2.6      0     1    0     1    2.6     2.6
```

Similar reasoning and code allow us to select different subgroups for the other transitions. For instance, the code

```
# Selects patients in Pre-progression who move to Progression and haven't died
risk_set |> dplyr::filter(trans==2,prog==1,death==0) |> slice(1:3) |>
  as.data.frame() |> head() |> print(digits=2)
```

```
  id from to trans Tstart Tstop time status treat prog death prog_t death_t
1  1    1  3     2      0    32   32      0     1    1     0     32      32
2  2    1  3     2      0    31   31      0     1    1     0     31      31
3  3    1  3     2      0    28   28      0     1    1     0     28      28
```

retrieves the patients at risk of dying from "Pre-progression", who have progressed but have not been observed to die. For these individuals, `Tstop` identifies the time at which they have reached the state "Progression" and the indicator for `death` is set to 0, as they are censored to the main event for the underlying transition ("Pre-progression" to "Death"). This is confirmed by the fact that the indicator `status` is set to 0 for these patients.

We can use the three relevant risk sets identified by the full subsetting based on `trans==1` ("Pre-progression" to "Progression"), or `trans==2` ("Pre-progression" to "Death"), or `trans==3` ("Progression" to "Death") and fit suitable survival models, for example as in the following `R` code and using `survHE` (see Section 8.4).

```
# Sets up informative priors on the Gompertz parameters to stabilise inference
priors=list(gom=list(a_alpha=1.5,b_alpha=1.5))

# Runs survival models on the specific subsets to obtain estimate
# of the various transition probabilities
m_12=fit.models(
  Surv(time,status)~as.factor(treat),data=risk_set |> dplyr::filter(trans==1),
  distr="gom",method="hmc",priors=priors
)
m_13=fit.models(
  Surv(time,status)~as.factor(treat),data=risk_set |> dplyr::filter(trans==2),
  distr="gom",method="hmc",priors=priors
)
m_23=fit.models(
```

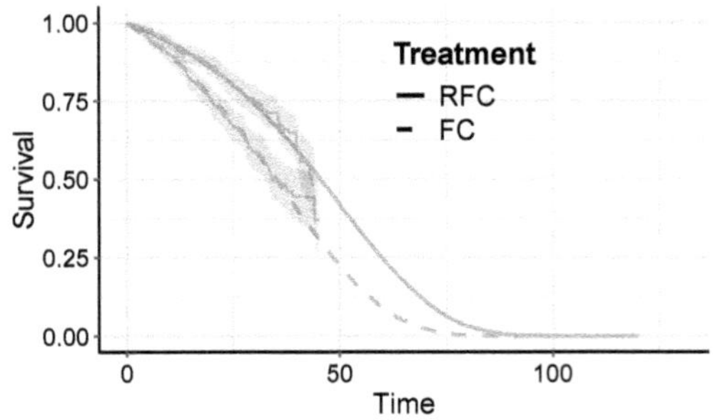

(a) Pre-progression to progression.

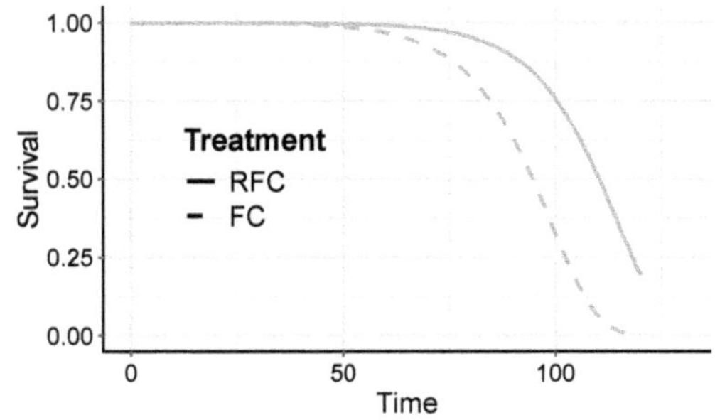

(b) Pre-progression to death.

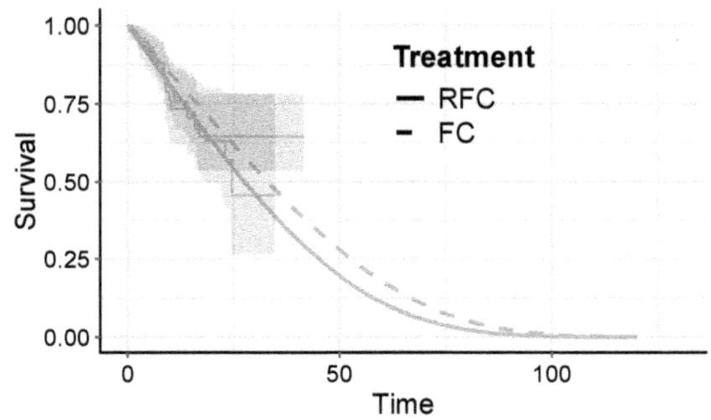

(c) Progression to death.

Figure 9.10: The survival curves estimated using a Gompertz model for the three subsets of the NICE TA174 data.

```
  Surv(time,status)~as.factor(treat),data=risk_set |> dplyr::filter(trans==3),
  distr="gom",method="hmc",priors=priors
)
```

Here, we choose a Gompertz model for all the transitions and specify informative priors to guard against the sparse information present in some of the risk sets (specifically for the transition from "Pre-progression" to "Death", which is characterised by large censoring – see Figure 9.10b).

While the model fit to the observed data is reasonably good for all three, the extrapolation to 120 months is not great for the "Pre-progression" to "Death" transition, where the curves barely reach median time. As mentioned above, this is due to the large amount of censoring (as evidenced from the KM curves in Figure 9.10).

We can use the `survHE` function `three_state_mm()`, which takes as inputs three model fit objects (such as `m_12`, `m_13` and `m_23`) obtained in the format of `survHE::fit.models()` and post-process the estimates to create a tibble with the progression of individuals over the three states. For instance, the command

```
mm=three_state_mm(m_12,m_13,m_23,t=seq(0,120),nsim=1000)
```

produces an object `mm`, which contains the resulting simulations in the tibble `mm$m`.

```
# A tibble: 242,000 x 11
   profile  time `Pre-progressed` Progressed Death sim_idx lambda_11 lambda_12
   <chr>   <dbl>            <dbl>      <dbl> <dbl>   <int>     <dbl>     <dbl>
```

```
 1 FC          0          1000       0    0         1      1       0
 2 FC          1           990.      9.94 0.150     1      0.990   0.00994
 3 FC          2           980.     19.9  0.457     1      0.990   0.0102
 4 FC          3           969.     30.0  0.927     1      0.989   0.0106
 5 FC          4           958.     40.1  1.57      1      0.989   0.0109
 6 FC          5           947.     50.2  2.38      1      0.989   0.0112
 7 FC          6           936.     60.3  3.39      1      0.988   0.0116
 8 FC          7           925.     70.5  4.58      1      0.988   0.0119
 9 FC          8           913.     80.7  5.98      1      0.987   0.0123
10 FC          9           902.     90.9  7.58      1      0.987   0.0127
# i 241,990 more rows
# i 3 more variables: lambda_13 <dbl>, lambda_22 <dbl>, lambda_23 <dbl>
```

Here, we have used `nsim=1000` simulations – in other words, for each simulated values from the posterior distribution of the transition probabilities $\boldsymbol{\lambda}$, we run the algebra to construct a version of the Markov model, in terms of how many people transit from each of the states at each given time points in the time horizon (from 0 to 120 months). To run the 1000 simulations, the model takes about 5 minutes – in comparison to the case shown in Example 9.4, this is much longer because, in the current model, the time horizon (120 months) is 10 times as long.

Figure 9.11 shows the Markov trace computed using the mean estimates for the state occupancy at different cycles. As is possible to see, the active treatment (RCF) seems to keep more patients for longer in the "Pre-progression" state, thus reducing the overall number of people who end up in the "Death" states, towards the end of the time horizon.

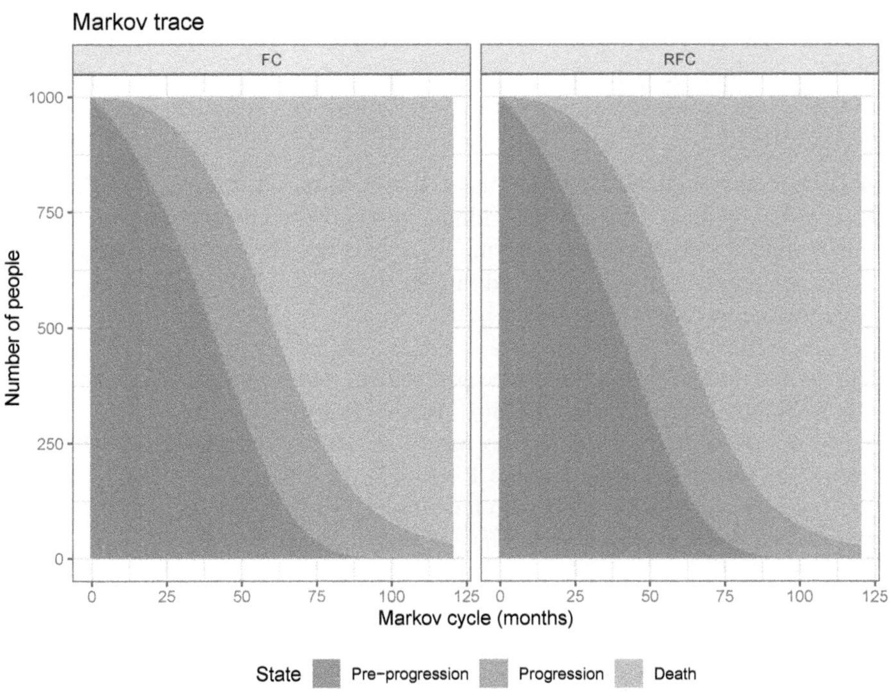

Figure 9.11: The Markov trace for the analysis of the NICE TA174.

We can also post-process the simulation results further to obtain a measure of "gain" in terms of the average time spent alive (and thus some measure of Life Years Gained) from the two treatments, for instance using the following R code.

```
(mm$m |> group_by(profile,sim_idx) |>
   summarise(los=sum(`Pre-progressed`)/1000 + sum(Progressed)/1000)) |>
  group_by(profile) |>
  summarise(
    mean=mean(los)/12,sd=sd(los)/12,
    `2.5%`=quantile(los,.025)/12,`97.5%`=quantile(los,.975)/12
  )
```

```
# A tibble: 2 x 5
  profile  mean    sd `2.5%` `97.5%`
  <chr>   <dbl> <dbl>  <dbl>   <dbl>
1 FC       5.06 0.705   3.96    6.56
2 RFC      5.36 0.669   4.33    6.90
```

As is possible to see, the RFC arm shows some gains over the FC arm, which confirms the visual inspection of Figure 9.11. Using the `nsim=1000` simulations, we can obtain a measure of uncertainty around this central estimate too.

9.3.2 Partition survival modelling

In cases where the full even history for each individual is not available, we need to resort to alternative methods in order to analyse a three-state cancer model. In these cases, one of the most popular workaround is to use "partitioned survival analysis" modelling (PSM, Woods et al., 2017).

The idea is that although we may not have access to a full dataset describing the times at which transitions occur for each individual, we typically can estimate (perhaps through digitisation from published studies) the survival curves for the main outcomes, OS and PFS. For instance, consider the curves depicted in Figure 9.12: at each time point j on the x–axis, we can read off the curves:

1. the proportion of individuals who are still in pre-progression as the area under the PFS curve (indicated as $\text{PFS}(j)$, in the figure);
2. the proportion of individuals who have died as the complement to 1 of the area under the OS curve (indicated as $1 - \text{OS}(j)$, in the figure); and
3. the proportion of individuals who have moved to progression as the area between the two curves (indicated as $\text{OS}(j) - \text{PFS}(j)$, in the figure).

Interestingly, this works in the specific circumstances of the three-state cancer Markov model, in which transitions only occur "forward" (i.e. it is not possible to revert to a less serious health state). This is often indicated as cumulative and non-reversible timeline. By definition, $\text{PFS}(t)$ and $\text{OS}(t)$ are monotonically decreasing, while backwards transitions

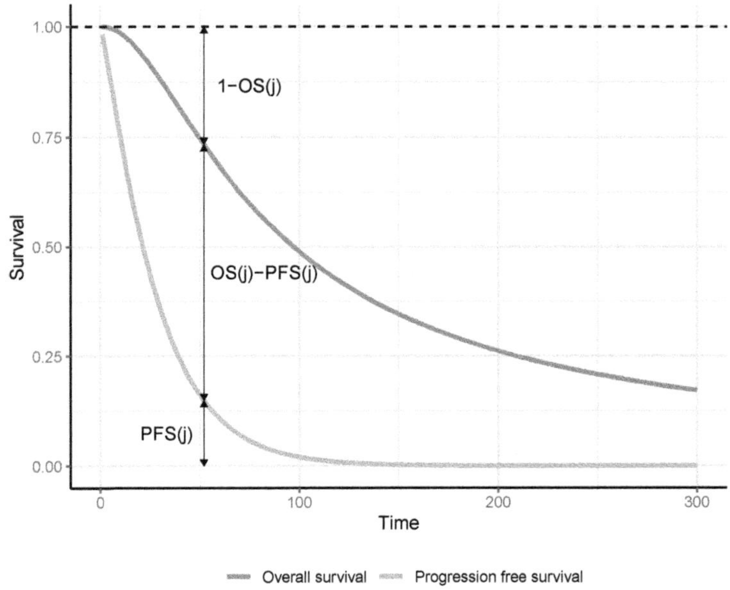

Figure 9.12: A graphical representation of the concept of partition survival analysis. Using PFS and OS, we can determine the proportion of individuals who are in each of the three states, at any given time.

would imply an increase in the curves over two consecutive times, which is not supported by the data. Thus, if the underlying disease/natural history suggests that individuals can move back and forth, we need to use different data (e.g. observed transition matrices)

In addition, by necessity, we must assume independence between the two curves, given that we do not observe the full individual history. This is almost invariably a critical point, because in fact, the same individuals generally contribute to both – the same person may have experienced a transition to progression and then die. However, only from the survival curves, there is no way to account for this underlying correlation.

One main limitation for PSM is that we cannot estimate the full transition probabilities, from the observed data. We cannot get the transition probabilities – only the occupancy probabilities, as indicated in Figure 9.13. The possible transitions and the relevant probabilities $\lambda_{ss'}$ are all greyed out, because we cannot directly identify them from the available data – what we can estimate are the proportion of individuals who, at each time period, transit in the three states, $\pi_s^{(j)}$.

Jackson et al. (2025) argue that perhaps the most critical limitation of PSMs is that because of the implied independence between OS and PFS, the necessary extrapolation from the observed curves to cover the longer-term follow for the three-state Markov model is likely to result in important bias.

An archetypical case is when extrapolated PFS probabilities end up being estimated with larger values than the corresponding OS probabilities, implicitly implying that a negative proportion of the cohort is occupying the progressed state. For this reason, Jackson et al. (2025) caution modellers and suggest care is needed in using PSMs uncritically.

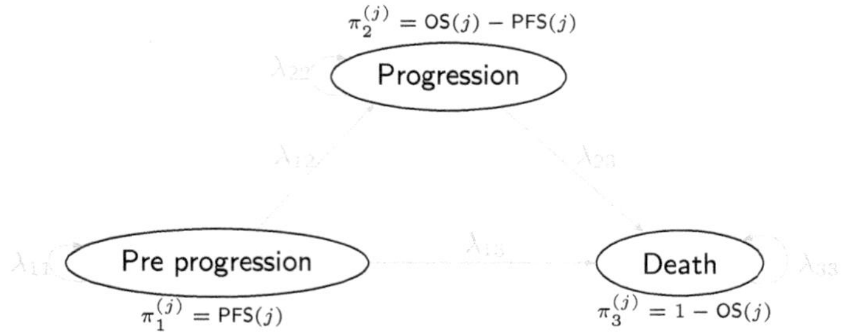

Figure 9.13: The partition survival representation of the three-state Markov model. Here, we cannot estimate the actual transition probabilities $\boldsymbol{\lambda}$ (which in fact are greyed out), but only the proportion of individuals that at each time point transit from the three states, $\boldsymbol{\pi}$.

9.4 Conclusions

This chapter has presented a detailed description of how multi-state (Markov) models are used in HTA applications. We have concentrated on two typical examples – the first one using a combination of data directly on the relevant transitions across a set of finite and mutually exclusive states, used to describe the "natural history of a disease" of interest. This structure naturally lends to a Bayesian modelling, which is particularly helpful to combine different sources of information into a principled framework to assess fully the underlying uncertainty in the model inputs and the associated one onto the economic outputs.

We have also linked up the use of MMs with survival modelling, in what is often termed a "three-state cancer Markov model". This is a special case of Markov model, in which transitions are informed by suitable survival models – we have showed the case where individual-level data are available to reconstruct the full event history and the one where we need to resort to simplifying assumptions (that often are harder to meet, in practice), which allow to get a Markov model-like structure, using partition survival modelling.

In the next part of the book, we will concentrate on more advanced problems and modelling frameworks, starting from methods to deal with missing data and then the increasingly important and popular topic of population adjustment and the analysis of the value of information.

Part III

Further modelling

10

Missing data and "structural values" in HTA

10.1 Introduction

This chapter expands mainly on concepts discussed in Chapter 5, when showcasing the use of Bayesian modelling for individual-level data in HTA.

In particular, we consider two important extensions that are often critical in health technology assessment alongside clinical trials: missing data and the presence of "structural" values. With this we encompass situations in which the observed data are characterised by "strange" values, which make the statistical analysis less straightforward. Examples include excess of zero costs, or perfect health utility (associated with a value of exactly 1).

Gabrio et al. (2025) present an extensive review of both frequentist and Bayesian modelling to handle missing data in HTA. More generally, Daniels and Hogan (2008) and Daniels and Xu (2020) are excellent references describing various Bayesian modelling strategies to deal with missing data (in the more general context of statistical modelling, rather than specifically in HTA).

In a nutshell, the problem with missing data is that we set out to observe n data points, but end up with a (much) lower number of fully observed individuals, n_{obs}. Of course, the fundamental issue is *how much lower* is the amount of data available – if the proportion of missingness is negligible, there is no point in agonising over it and we can just carry on with our modelling.

Conversely, if it is not (and often it is not!), then the next question to ask is whether it has a non-differential impact: are individuals in one treatment arm (or with a given exposure or individual characteristics) more likely to be missing? Is there a specific reason or explanation as to why data are not observed?

Of course, the very fact that information is not present when we originally planned to have it means that we cannot base all of our judgement and analysis on the empirical data – this is similar to the issues encountered in extrapolation (see Section 8.3); more importantly, this will have implications in terms of assessing how well a model does in terms of fitting, because, of course, information criteria based on the likelihood (see the discussion throughout Section 5.3) do not fully apply here – recall that the likelihood is conditional on the *observed* data and thus cannot tell us anything about data that are not observed.

The material and ideas presented and discussed in this chapter are far from exhausting and, in fact, they are purposely focused on providing a "bigger picture" idea of the main complexities and the possible advantages in using a full Bayesian approach to deal with them. Excellent and more comprehensive literature on the overall problem of handling missing data include van Buuren (2018), Little and Rubin (2019) and Carpenter et al. (2023).

DOI: 10.1201/9781003771050-10

10.2 Missing data mechanisms

Similarly to the discussion in Section 5.2.2, the main idea is to model jointly two relevant processes: the "*Model of Analysis*" (MoA) is the usual data-generating process in which we assume a set of relationships between observable data and unobservable parameters, while the "*Model of Missingness*" (MoM) describes the mechanism by which some of the observable data are, in fact, missing.

More technically, we can consider a set of data $\mathcal{D}_i = (y_i, \boldsymbol{x}_i, \boldsymbol{m}_i)$, where: y_i is the main outcome variable; $\boldsymbol{x}_i$ represents a (vector of) covariate(s); and $\boldsymbol{m}_i$ is a (vector of) missingness indicator variable(s). In general, we could face a situation in which missingness impacts both or either y and $\boldsymbol{x}$ and thus $\boldsymbol{m}_i$ would include as many elements as there are variables subject to missingness. Of course, the more structured missingness our dataset presents, the more complicated our overall analysis. For the sake of simplicity and to fix ideas, we consider here the simpler case in which missingness only affects the outcome variable – this means that there is only one missingness indicator $m_i = 1$ if y_i is not fully observed and $m_i = 0$ if it is.

Under the simplified scenario in which missingness only affects the outcome, another way to describe the data is to subset $\boldsymbol{y} = (\boldsymbol{y}^{\text{obs}}, \boldsymbol{y}^{\text{mis}})$, where $\boldsymbol{y}^{\text{obs}} = (y_1^{\text{obs}}, \ldots, y_{n_{\text{obs}}}^{\text{obs}})$ are the fully observed data (i.e. those indexes i for whom $m_i = 0$), while $\boldsymbol{y}^{\text{mis}} = (y_1^{\text{mis}}, \ldots, y_{n_{\text{mis}}}^{\text{mis}})$ are those subject to missingness and thus for whom $m_i = 1$. Naturally, $n = n_{\text{obs}} + n_{\text{mis}}$ is the overall sample size. The notation can be extended in the case of more structured missingness, e.g. also involving the covariates.

The goal is to model

$$p(y, m \mid \boldsymbol{\theta}[, \boldsymbol{x}]) = p\left(y \mid m, \boldsymbol{\theta}^{\text{MoA}}[, \boldsymbol{x}]\right) p\left(m \mid \boldsymbol{\theta}^{\text{MoM}}[, \boldsymbol{x}]\right) \tag{10.1}$$

$$= p\left(m \mid y, \boldsymbol{\theta}^{\text{MoM}}[, \boldsymbol{x}]\right) p\left(y \mid \boldsymbol{\theta}^{\text{MoA}}[, \boldsymbol{x}]\right), \tag{10.2}$$

where the whole set of model parameters can be partitioned as $\boldsymbol{\theta} = \left(\boldsymbol{\theta}^{\text{MoM}}, \boldsymbol{\theta}^{\text{MoA}}\right)$; we often assume that, for simplicity, the subsets $\boldsymbol{\theta}^{\text{MoM}}$ and $\boldsymbol{\theta}^{\text{MoA}}$ are distinct, but this may not be plausible (in which case, we may need to consider some form of correlation across them). In addition, the notation $[, \boldsymbol{x}]$ indicates that covariates may or may not be included in a particular distribution.

The factorisation in Equation 10.1 is often termed a "*pattern-mixture model*" (PMM, Little, 1993), while that in Equation 10.2 is referred to as a "*selection model*" (SM, Diggle and Kenward, 1994). PMMs define a marginal model for all possible missingness "patterns" and thus require the specification of the MoA conditionally on each – this may be more intuitive from a "causal" point of view, but may require a great amount of information. Conversely, SMs consider a marginal MoA (essentially, the one that we would use even in the absence of missingness) and then specifies a conditional model for the missingness mechanism. While both factorisations are viable, SMs are sometimes preferred because of the simpler way in which we can handle the MoA.

Broadly speaking, there are three potential mechanisms that we can use to explain how missingness is generated (Rubin, 1976). This is akin to the concept of "data-generating process" introduced in Section 1.1 and used throughout this book: it is about constructing

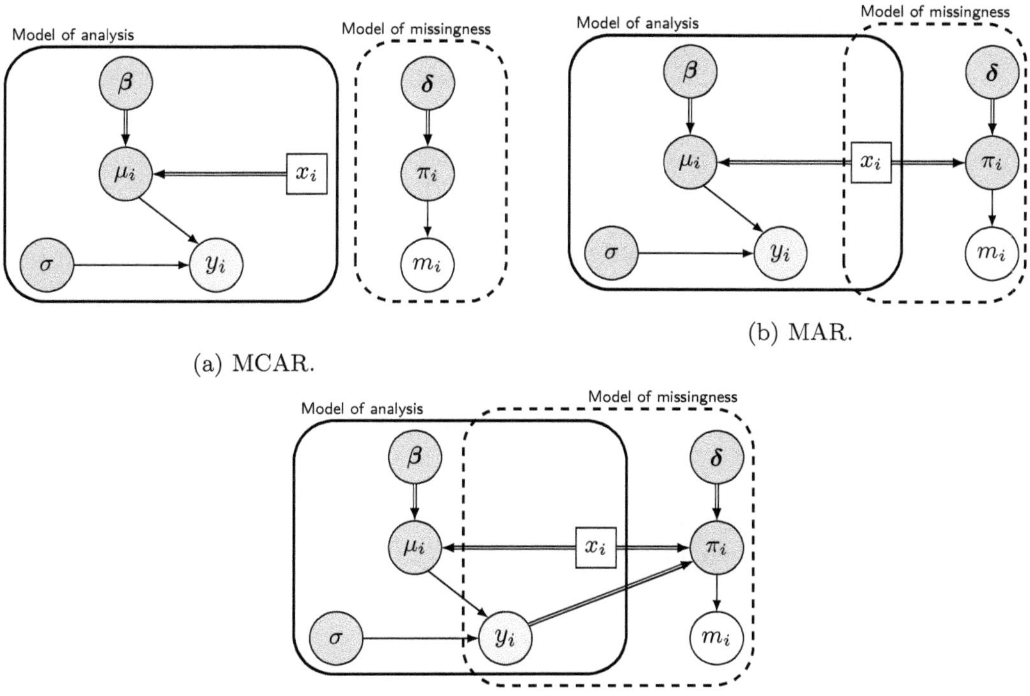

(a) MCAR.

(b) MAR.

(c) MNAR.

Figure 10.1: Graphical representation of the common missingness mechanisms. Each panel shows the Model of Analysis, used to describe the overall data-generating process for the observable outcome, y and the Model of Missingness, which shows our assumptions on how missingness arises.

a model that expresses our view in terms of relationships among suitable variables and how they influence the data we actually get to see (if only partially).

Figure 10.1 describes the three mechanisms using a SM representation. In each panel, the model parameters are shaded in dark colours and represented as circles; bold typesetting indicates that specific parameters may represent vectors. In addition, in line with Figure 3.1, double-edged arrows indicate logical relationships.

Unmodelled data (e.g. some covariate x_i), which we assume have been fully observed, are shown in a squared node with white background, while modelled data (e.g. the partially observed outcome y_i and the missingness indicator m_i) are also shown as circles – note that m_i is by necessity fully observed (because we *know* whether y_i is missing or not) and thus we represent it using a white background. Conversely, because we assume that y_i is subject to missingness, we depict it using a light coloured background.

In all panels, the solid boxes show the MoA, in this case defined, just to fix ideas, as a simple linear regression indexed by $\boldsymbol{\theta}^{\text{MoA}} = (\boldsymbol{\beta}, \sigma)$

$$
\begin{aligned}
y_i &\sim \text{Normal}(\mu_i, \sigma) \\
\mu_i &= \beta_0 + \beta_1 x_i
\end{aligned}
$$

– note that μ_i is just a deterministic function of $\boldsymbol{\beta} = (\beta_0, \beta_1)$ and x_i and thus we do not formally include it in $\boldsymbol{\theta}^{\text{MoA}}$ above.

Similarly, the dashed boxes present the MoM, which describes the alleged sampling process for a missingness indicator m_i. Without lack of generality, we can model $m_i \sim \text{Bernoulli}(\pi_i)$, where π_i is the "probability of missingness", typically centred at some value determined by $\boldsymbol{\delta}$, e.g. on the logit scale.

Figure 10.1a shows the "*Missing Completely At Random*" (MCAR) mechanism. This amounts to making the rather strong assumption that the two modules are completely separated, which implies that the way in which missingness is generated bears no impact on the model of analysis. Just to fix the ideas, we may use a simple model such as

$$\text{logit}(\pi_i) = \delta,$$

where the scalar δ represents the average probability of missingness on the logit scale, common to all individuals.

Irrespective of the actual MoM, the key point here is the assumptions that π_i does not depend on the data (y_i, x_i), or more prosaically that the MoA is independent on the MoM. Consequently, if this assumption is sensible (which it most often is not!), we can basically disregard the MoM and just carry on with our MoA as if missingness were not an issue: the estimates for the main parameters, i.e. $(\boldsymbol{\beta}, \sigma)$ in this case, will generally be unbiased – although they most likely will have lost precision, due to the lack of full information – see Example 10.1.

On a deeper level, the MCAR assumption also implies that we believe that the missing values occur just by total random chance and thus the value that we might have observed would have been generated by the exact same DGP that has produced the observed data.

Note 28: Complete case analysis and MCAR

Interestingly, when we analyse a dataset subject to missingness using standard statistical software, including R, the underlying (and often "silent") assumption is exactly MCAR, as the following simple example shows.

```
# 1. Generates 100 data points for a covariate x ~ Normal(mean=2,sd=5)
x=rnorm(100,2,5)

# 2. Generates 100 data points for the outcome y, with :
#  a. intercept (beta0) = 0.5
#  b. "effect" of x (beta1) = 1.5
#  c. error variance = 1, ie add 'rnorm(100)', which simulates 100
#       values from a Normal(0,1)
y=.5+1.5*x+rnorm(100)

# 3. Removes 20 values at random and replaces them with 'NA' (missing)
y[sample(1:100,20)]=NA

# 4. Runs a linear regression model (y on x) and print results
summary(lm(y~x))

Call:
lm(formula = y ~ x)

Residuals:
     Min       1Q   Median       3Q      Max
```

```
-1.99584 -0.72194  0.02039  0.75906  2.29681

Coefficients:
            Estimate Std. Error t value Pr(>|t|)
(Intercept)  0.35741    0.10963    3.26  0.00165 **
x            1.46922    0.02241   65.58  < 2e-16 ***
---
Signif. codes:  0 '***' 0.001 '**' 0.01 '*' 0.05 '.' 0.1 ' ' 1

Residual standard error: 0.9493 on 78 degrees of freedom
  (20 observations deleted due to missingness)
Multiple R-squared:  0.9822,    Adjusted R-squared:  0.982
F-statistic:  4300 on 1 and 78 DF,  p-value: < 2.2e-16
```

Here, we simulate 100 data points (y_i, x_i) and artificially remove 20% of the observations on the outcome y, while retaining the original values for x. The analysis performed by R using linear regression automatically considers only the "valid" cases (i.e. those completely observed on *all* the variables under consideration) – but note that other software such as Stata or SAS would proceed in exactly the same way. This method of analysis is often referred to as *Complete Case Analysis* (CCA), which is only valid if the underlying missingness generating mechanism is ignorable.

In fact, R explicitly tells us that it has deleted 20 observations (wasting the data on x, which were available even for these individuals) due to missingness – a message that sometimes goes unnoticed by the analysts. In this case, the sample size is still large enough and the model estimates for the intercept β_0 and the slope β_1 are not "significantly" different from their "true" value (0.5 and 1.5, respectively).

In Figure 10.1b we relax the rather unrealistic assumption of MCAR to consider the "*Missing At Random*" (MAR) mechanism: in this case, we assume that the probability of missingness does depend on the MoA, but only through the fully observed covariate x_i, for instance through a logistic regression model

$$\text{logit}(\pi_i) = \delta_0 + \delta_1 x_i.$$

In other words, we believe that the pair (m_i, x_i) includes all the information we need to determine the way in which missingness is generated. Pragmatically, this also means that, once we know the value of x_i, the MoM becomes essentially irrelevant because, if we "control" for the important covariates, we do not need any further information to avoid bias in the estimates of the relevant parameters, e.g. $(\boldsymbol{\beta}, \sigma)$, in this case. This can be also shown in Figure 10.1b as x_i "blocks" the pathway that connects y_i to π_i.

As an example, consider some blood pressure readings in a patient. Empirical evidence suggests that this variable may be missing more often for older patients or women (e.g. because of scheduling issues or different clinic attendance patterns). In this scenario, indicating: the partially observed data as y_i; the "true" value that would be observed if missingness had not occurred as y_i^*; and the observed characteristics as $\boldsymbol{x}_i = (\text{Sex}_i, \text{Age}_i)$, we then imply

$$\Pr(y_i \mid y_i^*, \boldsymbol{x}_i) = \Pr(y_i \mid \boldsymbol{x}_i),$$

or, in other words, that we believe that missingness in y_i is systematically related to observed patient characteristics $\boldsymbol{x}_i$, but not the unobserved measurement itself (the true blood pressure, y_i^*).

Finally, in Figure 10.1c we show what is most often the most likely description of the overall data-generating process, one in which the reason why an outcome is missing actually does depend on its unobserved value and termed "*Missing Not At Random*" (MNAR). In this case, the partially observed y_i also impacts on π_i, for instance through a more structured logistic regression

$$\text{logit}(\pi_i) = \delta_0 + \delta_1 x_i + \delta_2 y_i. \tag{10.3}$$

In the blood pressure example, we may consider that patients with higher levels may be more prone to missing measurements because they are sick and, for that reason, cannot attend a scheduled clinic. In the case of MNAR, ignoring the MoM is not possible and if we do so the resulting estimates obtained for the model parameters will be biased – see again Example 10.1.

The data *are*...?

Sometimes, there is a tendency to abuse the language and use phrasing such as "we assume that the data *are* MAR". This is not quite correct, because the data are just the data.

Much as they *are* not "Normal", or "Gamma" (which are just models we are willing to adapt to describe our understanding of the underlying sampling variability inherent in the data-generating process), they cannot *be* MAR or MCAR or MNAR. These are just labels that we may be comfortable using to describe how we feel that the missingness has been generated.

For this reason, perhaps a better phrasing would be "we assume that the underlying missingness mechanism is MAR". This is perhaps a mouthful and we *may* get away with the shortcut "the data are MAR" – but we should be fully aware of what that actually means...

Example 10.1. *Missing data simulation study.* We run a (ridiculously!) simple simulation study to demonstrate how different assumptions in the missingness mechanism can impact on the results of a model of analysis.

We start by considering a MNAR situation where the true MoM is

$$m_i \sim \text{Bernoulli}(\pi_i) \quad \text{with} \quad \text{logit}(\pi_i) = \delta_0 + \delta_1 x_i + \delta_2 y_i,$$

for set values $\boldsymbol{\delta} = (\delta_0, \delta_1, \delta_2) = (-0.5, 0.35, 0.83)$. The actual numbers are not that important, but note that we imply a relatively large value for the impact of the outcome y on the probability of missingness π – recall the interpretation of the coefficients of a logistic regression after Equation 6.2 and Note 17 in Example 6.3.

As for the "true" relationship between y and x, we imply a model

$$y_i = \beta_0 + \beta_1 x_i + \varepsilon_i$$

in which we set the coefficients $\boldsymbol{\beta} = (\beta_0, \beta_1) = (0.5, 1.5)$ and $\varepsilon_i \sim \text{Normal}(0, 1)$. This is the same MoA of Note 28 above, but we consider a larger sample size of $n = 2000$ individuals to reduce the impact of sampling variability in the estimates.

We use the simple R code below to encode these assumptions and run the simulations.

```
# Initialisation
mnar=list();  pmis=numeric();  S=1000;  set.seed(140873)
for (s in 1:S) {
  # Simulates full data with a large sample size (n=2000)
  x=rnorm(2000,2,5)
  y=0.5+1.5*x+rnorm(2000)
  # MoM: MNAR (depends also on unobserved y)
  pi=bmhe::ilogit(-0.5+0.35*x+0.83*y)
  m=rbinom(2000,1,pi)
  # Creates missing data
  y[m==1]=NA
  # CCA analysis (ignores the MoM): saves estimates for the coefficients
  mnar[[s]]=(lm(y~x) |> summary())$coefficients[,"Estimate"]
  # Proportion of missing data in each simulation
  pmis[s]=sum(m==1)/2000
}
```

Here, we first construct a large, fully observed dataset (y, x) – note that we set the random seed, to ensure replicability. Then, we code the true MoM, in which we set the probability of missingness to depend on both the covariate x and the outcome y, which we then set to NA according to this probability (or, equivalently, whenever m is equal to 1).

Finally, we analyse the data using a CCA, i.e. by simply letting the R function `lm()` remove the missing values, thus effectively ignoring the underlying MoM; note that although the CCA will discard the individual data affected by missingness, we use here the "correct" model – in reality, we may use a model that does not account for all the relevant factors (i.e. it is subject to residual confounding).

The estimated coefficients in each simulation are stored in the list `mnar` and this process is replicated for $S = 1000$ times. We also keep track of the proportion of missing data in the variable `pmis`: in this setup, the average proportion of missing data is around 65%. We can format the output into a tibble using the `dplyr` function `bind_rows()` so that we can apply the function `bmhe::stats()`, with which we compute some summary statistics, using the following command.

```
# Summarises the simulations
mnar |> bind_rows() |> bmhe::stats()
```

```
                mean         sd      2.5%    median     97.5%
(Intercept) 0.263245 0.05673721 0.1516397 0.2621029 0.3770304
x           1.457869 0.01344687 1.4301324 1.4579484 1.4833449
```

As is possible to see, in the long run, the estimates for both the intercept β_0 and the slope β_1 are not aligned with the "true" values (0.5 and 1.5, respectively): ignoring the informative missingness mechanism induces bias in our analysis.

Of course, if y had little influence on π, the bias implied in the CCA may not be meaningful and essentially we would revert to a MAR situation, assuming x *did* have a substantive impact on π and we had controlled for it in our MoA. In fact, re-running the simulation study above setting `pi=bmhe::ilogit(0.17+0.35*x+0*y)` gives the following results.

```
MAR analysis

                 mean          sd      2.5%    median     97.5%
(Intercept) 0.5011553 0.04039917 0.4257231 0.5008061 0.5806213
x           1.4998349 0.00938082 1.4817550 1.4997070 1.5182100
```

This time, the simulation suggests unbiased estimates of both β_0 and β_1. Notice that we change the value of δ_0 in the linear predictor for the MoM from -0.5 (used in the MNAR scenario) to 0.17, in order to keep consistency in the implied overall proportion of missing data, i.e. resulting in $m_i = 1$. We can use trial-and-error to tweak this parameter in order to achieve similar average values of `pmis`.

Similar results, with slightly increased precision, would hold if we re-defined `pi=bmhe::ilogit(0.5+0*x+0*y)`. This would set the impact of x to 0 and the intercept δ_0 to 0.5 (again, we can use trial-and-error to identify a suitable value to keep a similar proportion of missingness), thus implying a MCAR mechanism.

```
MCAR analysis

                 mean           sd      2.5%    median    97.5%
(Intercept) 0.4991814 0.040756329 0.4176532 0.5011247 0.577936
x           1.5002119 0.007355783 1.4855884 1.5001326 1.514239
```

Interestingly, if we modified the simulation to fix `pi=rep(0,2000)` to produce *no* missing values and replicated the analysis, the results would obviously present more precision in the estimates – note the progressive reduction in the standard deviation of the estimates, particularly in comparison to the MNAR and MAR cases shown above (about 3 times as large and more than double, respectively, for the slope).

```
No-missing analysis

                 mean           sd      2.5%    median     97.5%
(Intercept) 0.4995238 0.024870810 0.4481647 0.4993299 0.5458013
x           1.5000762 0.004445692 1.4917870 1.4999367 1.5085892
```

While the results presented in Example 10.1 intuitively confirms that we cannot simply analyse the MoA in the case in which we must assume MNAR, an important complication is that, because y_i is not fully observed, this model is not empirically identifiable. In particular, the parameter δ_2 cannot be estimated using the available data *only*. We return to this point in Section 10.3.2.

In addition, natural extensions to the models presented above adapt for when there are multiple fully observed covariates collected in a vector $\boldsymbol{x}_i$. Conversely, when missingness affect the covariates too, the model becomes a bit more convoluted, because we need to expand the presentation above to consider separate (but possibly correlated) MoMs, one for each variable that is affected by missingness. While, in theory, this is a reasonably straightforward extension, in practice, we need to have a large amount of *fully* observed data from which we can learn about the missing values, as well as be willing to make potentially untestable assumptions on the MoMs.

10.3 Missing data analysis methods

The discussion in Example 10.1 indicates that we should try and avoid using a CCA as our MoA, for two reasons: firstly (and most importantly), because this would only return estimates that are not biased in the case where the underlying missingness mechanisms are MCAR or MAR. In practice, this assumption may just not hold, as we may have strong knowledge of factors affecting missingness, which may well be beyond our control. More generally, we should not discard uncritically the possibility that, in fact, a MNAR mechanism may be more appropriate.

Secondly, even in the event that we may be willing to assume a MAR mechanism, we would obviously lose precision in our estimation, due to the lower observed sample size generated by the missingness. Coupled with the inevitable sampling variation affecting the data collection, this will likely contribute to producing unsatisfactory inference.

Although there are various methods suggested in the literature to handle the presence of missing data (including those based on "weighting" – see Section 11.3), we focus here on the most popular alternative, Multiple Imputation" (MI), in Section 10.3.1 and its fully Bayesian counterpart, in Section 10.3.2.

10.3.1 Multiple imputation

Suppose we observe a continuous variable y on $n_{\text{obs}} < n$ individuals; also, we completely observe an additional variable x on the n individuals in the sample. Figure 10.2a shows the dataset, where fully observed individuals are represented as dots, while those for whom the outcome y is not known (but the covariate x is) are presented as ? along the x–axis.

If we can assume MAR, full knowledge of x is sufficient to "explain away" the MoM and thus we do not need to formally model it in our analysis. In Rubin (1977) and then in Rubin (1987), the main idea is that we can use the fully observed data to describe the underlying relationship between them. Of course, the simplest way in which we can do this is through a linear regression

$$y_i = \beta_0 + \beta_1 x_i + \varepsilon_i \qquad \varepsilon_i \sim \text{Normal}(0, \sigma^2),$$

to derive model-based estimates for the parameters $\hat{\boldsymbol{\theta}} = (\hat{\beta}_0, \hat{\beta}_1, \hat{\sigma})$. The resulting linear fit is shown in Figure 10.2b.

With these, we can also obtain a *prediction* for all the individuals for whom the outcome is missing as

$$\hat{y}_i \sim \text{Normal}(\hat{\beta}_0 + \hat{\beta}_1 x_i, \hat{\sigma}^2).$$

The estimates for $\hat{\boldsymbol{\theta}}$ are obtained using the available data and thus are affected by the limited sample size (made even smaller by the presence of missingness), as well as the natural sampling variability. Consequently, a single prediction, or "imputation" in Rubin's original terminology, is just not good enough to account for both the sampling variability in the partially observed data and the underlying uncertainty in the model parameters.

However, if we replicate this process for a (relatively small) number R of times, then we effectively can obtain R "complete" datasets, as shown in Figure 10.2c, where different symbols indicate the predicted value for y for each of the $R = 5$ imputations. We can then use each of these datasets to estimate the target quantities, e.g. the mean and standard

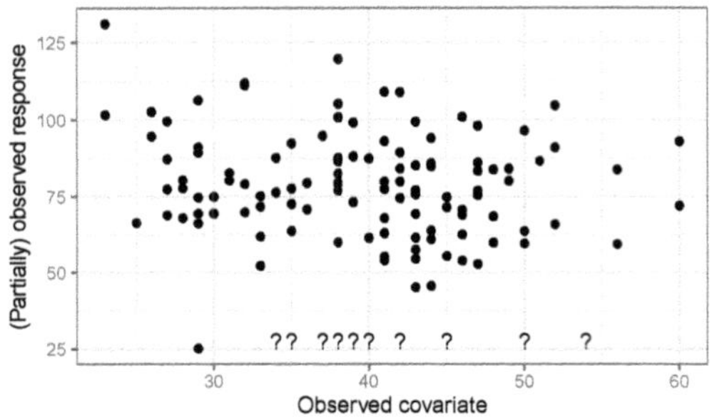

(a) (Partially) observed data for x and y.

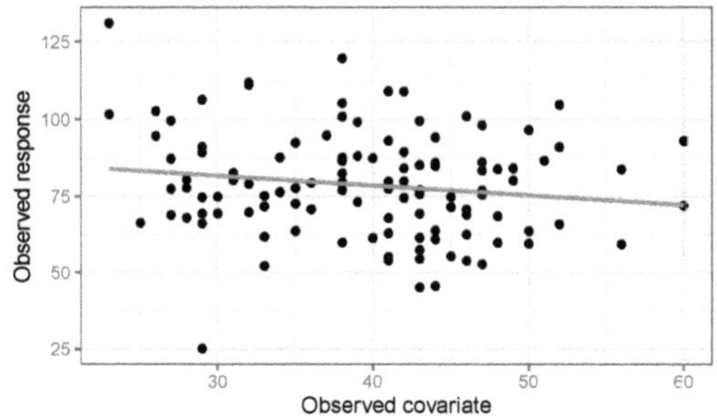

(b) Linear regression for the fully observed data.

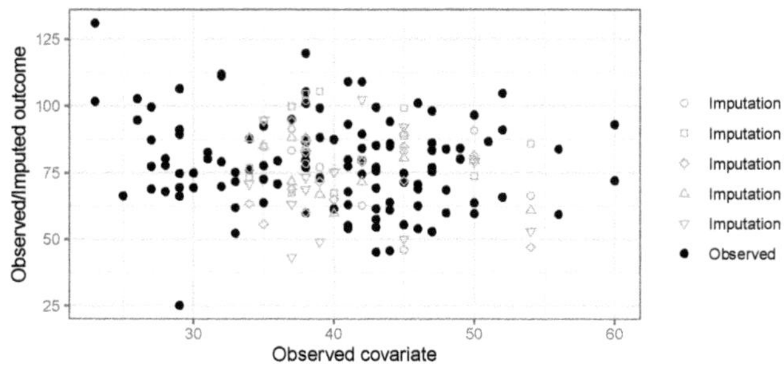

(c) Multiple imputation.

Figure 10.2: Graphical representation of the general principles underpinning multiple imputation. In panel (a) fully observed data are depicted as dots, while those for whom only the covariate on the x–axis is known are reported with a ? symbol. Under the assumption of MAR, in panel (b) the observed data are used to obtain predictions for the individuals for whom the covariate has been observed, but not the outcome. This is repeated a number R (= 5, in this case) of times to propagate uncertainty in the imputation, as shown in panel (c).

deviation of the outcome, which we indicate as $(\bar{y}_r, s_r)$, for each imputation $r = 1, \ldots, R$, fitting a suitable model.

Once the estimates $\bar{y}_r$ and s_r are obtained, then we can combine the R separate analysis results into a single final result, using “Rubin’s rule”

$$\hat{\mu}_{\text{MI}} = \frac{1}{R}\sum_{r=1}^{R}\bar{y}_r$$

with variance

$$\hat{\sigma}^2_{\text{MI}} = \underbrace{\left(1+\frac{1}{R}\right)}_{\substack{\text{finite sampling}\\ \text{correction}}} \underbrace{\left[\frac{1}{R-1}\sum_{r=1}^{R}\left(\bar{y}_r - \hat{\mu}_{\text{MI}}\right)^2\right]}_{\text{between imputation}} + \underbrace{\left[\frac{1}{R}\sum_{r=1}^{R} s^2_r\right]}_{\text{within imputation}}. \tag{10.4}$$

This formulation accounts for the correlation across the imputations, thus producing unbiased estimates of the target quantities. More specifically, the within-imputation variance describes the average uncertainty that would arise even if there were no missing data, i.e. the sampling variability inherent in the process of analysing a complete dataset. On the other hand, the between-imputation variance reflects the extra uncertainty introduced by the limited information in our data, due to the missing values.

If the imputations are very different, then this factor is also large; more importantly, if we could construct infinity replications, then the within-imputation variance would vanish – thus the finite sampling correction is included to inflate the within-imputation variance, to reflect the extra uncertainty from only using R imputations to estimate the between-imputation variance. If $R \to \infty$, then this factor disappears.

Think like a Bayesian, do like a frequentist

Rubin's ideas were very much grounded in a Bayesian perspective: the nature of multiple imputation is extremely similar to the simulation-based approach that characterises Bayesian modelling, of which Rubin himself has been a leading proponent, throughout his entire career.

Of course, back in the late 1970s and in the 1980s, researchers lacked both the computational power and the algorithms that have later allowed the "Bayesian revolution" of MCMC (see Section 2.3). Thus, his clever compromise was to "think like a Bayesian and do as a frequentist": instead of looking for a large number of simulations (which was hard to obtain, even for simple linear regression models), he settled for a limited number of complete datasets (typically 5 to 10 replicates) and then use meta-analytic techniques to pool the estimates together – again, a more Bayesian way to do this would perhaps be to apply a full hierarchical version of the model as in Section 6.2.3: each complete dataset statistics $(\bar{y}_r, s_r)$ could be used as "data" and a model constructed to pool them and obtain a single estimate.

In reality, since the computational advancements of MCMC, there is no need to keep the Bayesian/frequentist compromise, but the practice has stuck and "multiple imputation" has remained the gold standard in missing data analysis methods.

In principle, we do not need to restrict the MoA to a linear regression and could use different link functions $g(\cdot)$ for the linear predictor. It is also possible to relax MAR and produce versions of multiple imputation that, with some additional and typically untestable assumptions, can cater for MNAR. In any case, when relaxing the vanilla implementation of MI, the computational complexity of the "standard" hybrid imputation models increases substantially, thus suggesting that the marginal costs of implementing a full Bayesian version of the analysis is in fact decreasing. This is particularly relevant for the case of HTA, as we discuss more in detail in Section 10.4.

The basic caveat underpinning the extension of MI to more complex missingness mechanism scenarios is that we must preserve the property of *congeniality* (Meng, 1994) between the MoM and the MoA – in other words, if the model we use to impute the missing data is not fully consistent with the underlying data-generating process, then we would still imply bias in the final estimates. This has been addressed in different ways in the literature and, from a frequentist perspective, often using "robust" estimators[1].

[1]A large emphasis is often placed on estimators being "doubly-robust" in the context of frequentist modelling of missing data. With this terminology, we generally indicate methods that remain valid (i.e. provide unbiased estimates) if *either* the MoM or the MoA is (reasonably) correctly specified – of course, as indicated in Note 13 in Section 5.3, no model can be completely "correctly specified", but we can try to get as close as possible...

10.3.2 Bayesian modelling for missing data

From a Bayesian perspective, congeniality is less crucial, because there are no two separate steps (imputation and analysis); instead, using a single, unified structure to model the MoM and the MoA allows us to naturally handle the uncertainty from both the components. Thus, if the MoM is ignorable (e.g. under MAR), we can simply define the MoA and consider the missing data points as unobserved values to be estimated using the predictive distribution.

In other words, if MAR holds (meaning that we are prepared to assume its validity), then running a simple `JAGS` model such as the one sketched below would automatically take care of the missingness problem, by estimating a large number of samples from the predictive distribution of the outcome y. Passing data as `NA` instructs `JAGS` to do that calculation.

```
# Defines the data - the actual numbers do not matter here!
# NB: `NA` indicates the missing values in the vector y
x=c(1,2,3,4,5,6,7,8,9,10,...)
y=c(1,NA,2,NA,3,4,NA,NA,5,6,7,...)

model_mar= function() {
  for (i in 1:n) {
    # MoA
    y[i] ~ dnorm(mu[i], tau)
    mu[i] <- beta0 + beta1*x[i]
  }
  # Priors for beta0, beta1 and tau/sigma, e.g.
  beta0 ~ dnorm(0,0.1);    beta1 ~ dnorm(0,0.1)
  sigma ~ dexp(2)
  tau <- pow(sigma,-2)
}

# Runs the model in JAGS
m=jags(
  data=list(y=y,x=x,n=length(y)),
  # Note that we monitor y - the missing values will be "imputed" automatically
  parameters.to.save=c("beta0","beta1","sigma","y"),
  model.file=model_mar,n.chains=2,... # Other settings
)
```

When the MoM is non-ignorable, then it would need to be included formally in the full analysis – and more importantly, the impact of the partially observed data would need to be modelled. But in this case, being Bayesian does come alive as a very efficient way of doing things, as adding a (most likely subjective/informative) prior distribution, e.g. on the coefficient δ_2 in Equation 10.3 would help "make up" for the lack of full information in the covariate y.

```
# Defines the missingness indicator
m=ifelse(is.na(y),1,0)

model_mnar= function() {
  for (i in 1:n) {
  # MoA
    y[i] ~ dnorm(mu[i], tau)
    mu[i] <- beta0 + beta1*x[i]
```

```
  # MoM - *must* be explicitly modelled!
    m[i] ~ dbern(pi[i])
    logit(pi[i]) <- delta0 + delta1*x[i] + delta2*y[i]
  }
  # Priors for beta0, beta1, delta0, delta1 and sigma/tau: can be vague
  beta0 ~ dnorm(0,0.1);    beta1 ~ dnorm(0,0.1)
  delta0 ~ dnorm(0,0.1);   delta1 ~ dnorm(0,0.1)
  sigma ~ dexp(2)
  tau <- pow(sigma,-2)
  # Prior for delta2: *must* use substantive information, e.g.
  delta2 ~ dnorm(0.28,44)
}

# Runs the model in JAGS
m=jags(
  data=list(y=y,x=x,m=m,n=length(y)),
  # Note that we monitor y - the missing values will be "imputed" automatically
  parameters.to.save=c("beta0","beta1","delta0","delta1","delta2","sigma","y"),
  model.file=model_mnar,n.chains=2,... # Other settings
)
```

In the code above, we expand the model to account for a MNAR mechanism. In the absence of full data on y, the prior for δ_2 *must* include substantive information on the likely impact of the outcome on the missingness – here we use a Normal(mean $= 0.28$, sd $= 44^{-0.5} \approx 0.15$) to encode some relatively strong belief. As δ_2 is modelled on the logit scale, we can use simple MC analysis to derive that this implies an average OR for missingness of about 1.34 with a 95% interval of $[0.2; 1.78]$. This would imply that we are very confident about the fact that larger values of y would be associated with larger odds of missingness and that there would be very little chance of this relationship not being substantial (as the probability that $\exp(\delta_2) = \text{OR} < 1$ is tiny).

In addition, it is a good idea to include in the MoM as much information as possible: thus, if we had additional covariates we should add them to the linear predictor in Equation 10.3, as this would contribute to stabilise our inference and anchor it as much as possible to the available evidence. At the same time, we should always acknowledge that any inference would rely on the (generally) untestable assumptions we make about the effect of the missing data on the generation mechanism.

10.4 Missing data in HTA

The case of missing data in the HTA context is interesting because, in addition to all the "normal" complexity discussed above, there are other issues that must be taken into account, which contributes to both the computational as well as the conceptual aspects of the analysis.

Similarly to the discussion in Chapter 5, the first and perhaps biggest complication is the fact that we need to consider a bivariate outcome (e, c), made by two components that can show substantial correlation and non-linearity – and, notably, missingness can occur in either or both the two outcomes.

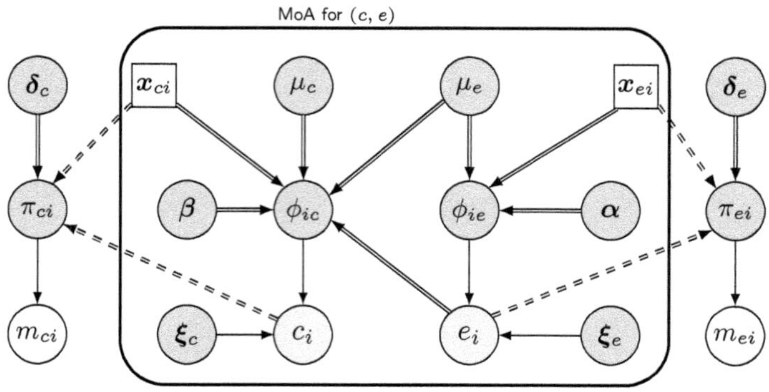

Figure 10.3: A (simplified) graphical description of the missingness mechanisms for a HTA problem. Here, *dashed* double-edged arrows indicate a logical relationship that may or may not be activated. For instance, the link between $\boldsymbol{x}_{ci}$ and π_{ci} can be present only if we are willing to assume a MAR process for the costs; similarly the link between e_i and π_{ei} would be present if we were willing to assume MNAR for the benefits, but not otherwise. The colour coding of the nodes is the same as described in Section 10.2 and Figure 10.1. The box shows the MoA for the (partially) observed data on costs and benefits, while there are now two MoMs, one for the costs and one for the benefits (in the left- and right-most part of the graph, respectively).

Figure 10.3 expands on the graphical representations presented above and provides a sketched version of the problem in the HTA context. Here, the MoA enclosed in the rounded rectangle embeds the marginal/conditional factorisation of the joint distribution $p(e, c \mid \boldsymbol{\theta}) = p(e \mid \boldsymbol{\theta}_e, x_e)p(c \mid \boldsymbol{\theta}_c, e, x_c)$ – see Section 5.2.2.

However, we also must include the potential MoM components; this time, we need to allow for two mechanisms, one to explain the missingness for the benefits and the other for the costs – in Figure 10.3, these are the two sub-modules at either side of the graph. We may consider a simplifying assumption whereby the two missingness mechanisms are independent, but more likely we may imply some level of correlation, perhaps by considering common covariates, or even more formally by linking the two probabilities of missingness.

Various assumptions on the two mechanisms can be encoded by considering the following basic specifications:

$$m_{ei} \sim \text{Bernoulli}(\pi_{ei}); \qquad \underbrace{\underbrace{\underbrace{\text{logit}(\pi_{ei}) = \delta_{e0}}_{\text{MCAR}} + \sum_{k=1}^{K} \delta_{ek} x_{eik}}_{\text{MAR}} + \delta_{eK+1} e_i}_{\text{MNAR}}$$

$$m_{ci} \sim \text{Bernoulli}(\pi_{ci}); \qquad \underbrace{\underbrace{\underbrace{\text{logit}(\pi_{ci}) = \delta_{c0}}_{\text{MCAR}} + \sum_{h=1}^{H} \delta_{ch} x_{cih}}_{\text{MAR}} + \delta_{eH+1} c_i}_{\text{MNAR}}.$$

The inclusion of more covariates in the linear predictors defines different assumptions: if only the intercept δ_{e0} or δ_{c0} is included, then we are assuming a MCAR mechanism, while adding fully observed covariates extends to MAR and, finally, adding the missing outcome e or c encodes MNAR. Of course any combination is in theory possible, i.e. we could assume MAR or effects and MCAR for costs, or MNAR for effects and MAR for costs. As discussed earlier, in a Bayesian context, we would need to embed some subjective information in the priors for δ_{eK+1} and δ_{cH+1}, to handle MNAR.

The multivariate and very structured nature of the modelling implies that in order to produce sensible results any form of MI must move away from simple and simplistic implementations, relying on Normality and independence. In turn, this suggests that the benefits of a full Bayesian approach may produce a very cost-effective alternative, particularly in light of the importance of the uncertainty analysis (which is even heightened in the face of limited information provided by the data).

Gabrio et al. (2025) present a thorough missing data analysis for the same TTT data discussed throughout Chapter 5 and we refer the reader that chapter as well as to the GitHub repository `https://github.com/giabaio/R-HTA-code` for more technical details and relevant `R` code.

10.4.1 Structural values

Another important quirk of HTA data is to do with the fact that the main outcomes may be subject to "structural values". We use this terminology to indicate the case in which a variable is observed with an excess of specific values. A typical example is when individuals present with an assessment of perfect health, as captured by suitable scales (e.g. the EQ-5D). Another perhaps less intuitive example is when we observe total costs accrued equal to 0 – this may happen for instance when patients are so sick that they immediately exit the follow-up without spending enough time under observation, or perhaps when they are substantially healthier than the rest of the population, thus failing to consume healthcare resources.

Either way, the fact that some individuals behave in a fundamentally different way than the rest of the target population may indicate the presence of distinct groups, leading to multimodality in the estimates for the average costs and benefits. Ignoring this mixture component typically will render the estimates biased and thus it is generally important to account for it in the modelling – particularly in presence of missing data.

Example 10.2. *MenSS (adapted from Gabrio et al., 2019).* The Men's Safer Sex (MenSS) pilot randomised trial (Bailey et al., 2016) evaluates the cost-effectiveness of a new digital intervention to reduce the incidence of Sexually Transmitted Infections (STI) in young men with respect to the standard of care, involving no other active intervention. QALYs are calculated from utilities based on the EQ-5D 3L questionnaire (see Note 10 in Section 4.2), while the total costs are calculated from different components (but include no baseline value). x' The study was originally planned with sample sizes of $n_1 = 75$ and $n_2 = 84$ in the control and active treatment, respectively and Table 10.1 shows some summary statistics of the available data, across the various points in the follow-up. Over the course of the study, there is substantial drop-out, with only as little as 23% completing the observation (and thus providing full data) in the treatment arm.

Figure 10.4 shows histograms for the distribution of QALYs and costs for the two treatment arms. As is possible to see, for both arms, the distribution of QALYs shows a marked "spike" at the value of 1, indicating a large proportion of participants in perfect health (the time horizon of the study is 1 year). This is not entirely surprising, given the nature of

Table 10.1: Summary statistics for the MenSS trial data. The study is initially planned with sample sizes of $n_1 = 75$ and $n_2 = 84$ in the control and active treatment, respectively. Source Gabrio et al. (2019).

Time	Type of outcome	observed (%)	observed (%)
Baseline	utilities	72 (96%)	72 (86%)
3 months	utilities and costs	34 (45%)	23 (27%)
6 months	utilities and costs	35 (47%)	23 (27%)
12 months	utilities and costs	43 (57%)	36 (43%)
Complete cases	utilities and costs	27 (44%)	19 (23%)

the study: the subjects are generally healthy and the underlying condition is typically not life-threatening.

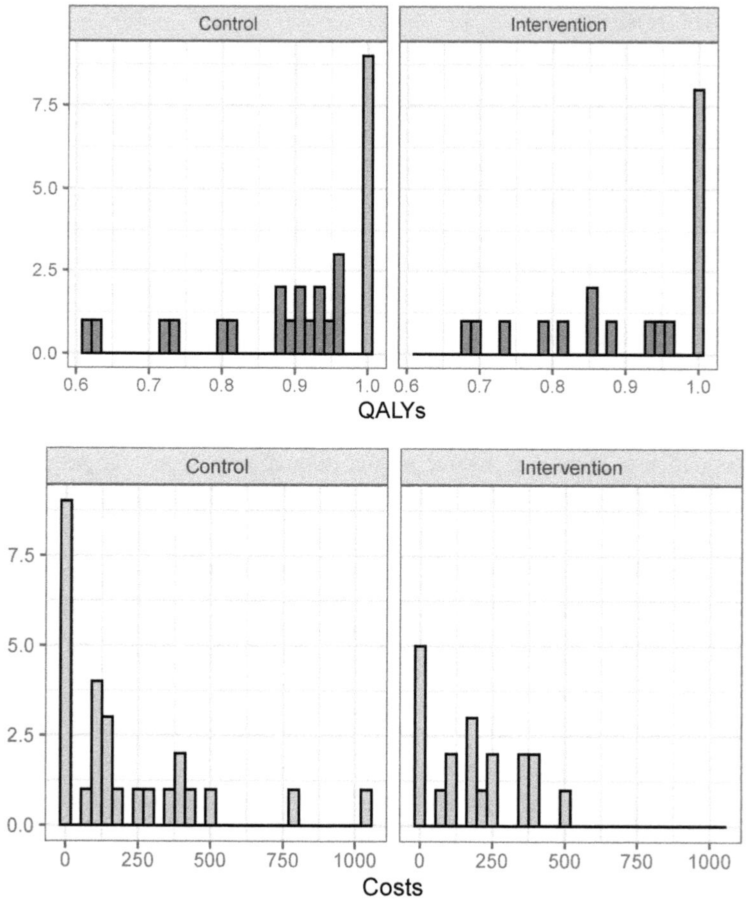

Figure 10.4: Empirical distribution for QALYs and total costs in the two treatment arms of the MenSS trial. The lighter coloured bars in the top panel show the "spike" at the value of exactly 1.

From the statistical point of view, however, this generates further problems, in addition to the presence of substantial missing data. Given the annual time horizon of the study, the theoretical distribution of the QALYs is capped at 1 and thus we could model the observed data using a Beta distribution; the spike of values at exactly 1, however, violates this assumption, since the Beta distribution is defined in the open interval $(0, 1)$.

Gabrio et al. (2019) compare three different models and present analyses for MAR and various MNAR assumptions. Here, we restrict our attention to the models assuming MAR for the effects and MNAR for the costs, for simplicity. This means that we assume that once the baseline utility values are observed, we can focus on the model of analysis and not worry about explicitly writing down further assumptions on the model of missingness. Of course, less restrictive (and more realistic!) assumptions would involve more complex modelling (see Gabrio et al., 2019; and Gabrio et al., 2025 for more detailed accounts).

The first model is a Normal-Normal MCF, similar to the one described in Example 5.3, in which the linear predictors are

$$\phi_{ei} = \alpha_0 + \alpha_1 \text{Trt}_i + \alpha_2(u_i - \bar{u}) \qquad \text{and} \qquad \phi_{ci} = \beta_0 + \beta_1 \text{Trt}_i + \beta_2(e_i - \mu_{et_i}),$$

where $t_i = 1, 2$ identifies the treatment arm to which the i−th individual belongs.

The second model is a Beta-Gamma MCF. This is theoretically more appropriate, because it correctly recognises the natural range of the two variables – the interval [0-1] for the QALYs and the open positive real line $(0, \infty)$ for the costs. Here, we have

$$\text{logit}(\phi_{ei}) = \alpha_0 + \alpha_1 \text{Trt}_i + \alpha_2(u_i - \bar{u}) \qquad \text{and} \qquad \log(\phi_{ci}) = \beta_0 + \beta_1 \text{Trt}_i + \beta_2(e_i - \mu_{et_i}).$$

While theoretically sound, this model has a fundamental, computational problem: the Beta distribution is constrained in the *open* interval $(0, 1)$, which clashes with the observed spike at 1 for the QALYs. The simplest way to limit this issue is to subtract a small constant $\varepsilon \to 0$ (say 0.01) to rescale all the QALYs, so that they actually can be modelled directly using a Beta. Note that this is possible because the observed range of the data is $[0.61; 1]$ and thus subtracting $\varepsilon = 0.01$ keeps all the values above 0.

This strategy is very easy to implement, but it feels a bit "hacky" and is potentially sensitive to the choice of the rescaling factor. In addition, much as the Normal-Normal MCF, it completely discards the fact that the observed spike may in fact indicate that the individuals have some fundamentally different features and thus the sampled data really are made by two potentially substantially different groups: the participants with QALY < 1, who experience some reduction in their QoL and those with perfect health.

We then develop a third model, based on a "hurdle" structure (Mullahy, 1986). The idea is to first model for each individual i an indicator $d_i = 1$ if $e_i = 1$ and 0 otherwise, using a logistic regression as a function of a set of relevant covariates $\boldsymbol{X}_i$. Following Gabrio et al. (2019), we use age, ethnicity, employment status and the treatment arm to estimate the probability that a participant is a "structural one", i.e. in perfect health, which is indicated as γ_i.

Then, we treat as fixed the observed participants with QALYs $= 1$, while we model those with QALYs < 1 using a Beta distribution, without the need to rescale the values. For each treatment arm, the average effectiveness is then constructed as a mixture

$$\mu_{et} = (1 - \bar{\gamma}_t)\mu_{et}^{<1} + \bar{\gamma}_t,$$

where $\bar{\gamma}_t$ is the average probability of structural ones and $\mu_{et}^{<1}$ is the average QALYs estimated for the data $e_{it}^{<1}$, i.e. for the individuals with QALYs < 1. This comes directly from the

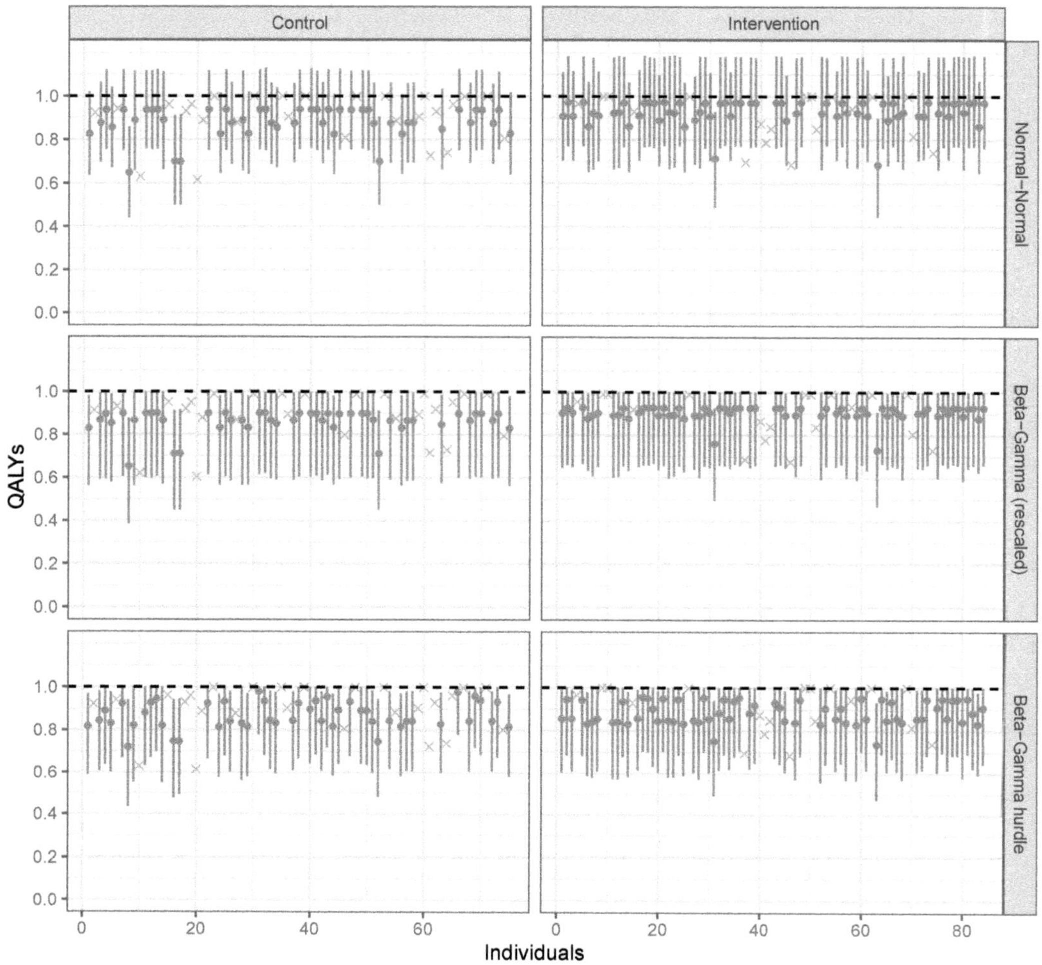

Figure 10.5: Bayesian posterior predictive estimates for the distribution of the missing data. In each panel, the lighter crosses indicate the observed data, while dots and segments show the posterior predictive mean and 95% interval. The Normal-Normal MCF model is naturally unconstrained, which fails to conform with the nature of the QALYs (which should lay below 1). This holds for Beta-Gamma rescaled model, but the rescaling means that the estimates are all shifted down. The Beta-Gamma hurdle model can cater for all the idiosyncrasies in the data

Beta model, which we can fit with no complications, as this subset is indeed constrained in $(0, 1)$.

Figure 10.5 shows the results of the model, in terms of the "Bayesian multiple imputation". Given the MAR assumption, the missing data are treated as unobserved values and are then sampled from the posterior predictive distribution.

In other words, the observed data and the assumptions in the model of analysis are used to first update the prior into the posterior distribution for the model parameters, which is in turn used to construct the posterior predictive distribution, averaging the sampling distribution $p(e^{\text{mis}} \mid \boldsymbol{\theta})$ with respect to the posterior $p(\boldsymbol{\theta} \mid e^{\text{obs}})$ – see Equation 1.7.

In Figure 10.5, for the three models, the dots represent the posterior predicted average for the unobserved QALYs, while the segment covers the 95% interval of the predictive distribution. The lighter crosses indicate the observed data, for which we do not obtain a prediction (or imputation).

The first notable finding is that, as expected, the Normal-Normal MCF fails to account for the natural range of the data, producing predictions that span well beyond the upper limit of 1. This tends to inflate the overall mean effectiveness – basically, the Normal distribution does not know that that it should be bounded at 1 and thus artificially pushes up towards higher values, when the observation is large enough.

The Beta-Gamma (rescaled) model behaves much more nicely and is correctly capped at 1. Generally speaking, the estimates are not massively different, in terms of the means, although obviously the uncertainty is affected. However, more importantly, the crosses fail to recognise the individuals in perfect health – in the rescaled data, there is no such thing, which may introduce some slight downward bias in the overall average effectiveness.

Finally, the Beta-Gamma hurdle model gets around the idiosyncrasy in the data. Individuals in perfect health are modelled to determine their chance of in fact having a value of 1 for the QALYs. Those directly observed at 1 are correctly identified as such, but in addition those estimated to belong in this category are also modelled and estimated with a value of QALYs at 1.

10.4.2 Further complications

For all the implied complexity, the discussion above only scratches the surface of the many issues that can arise with missing data in HTA. One further potential complication is the fact that in principle the observed data on (e, c) have in fact a longitudinal nature – in fact, the MenSS study is designed in this fashion.

While we often aggregate the longitudinal measurements into a cross-sectional summary, missingness may be "intermittent", e.g. individuals may be measured at baseline and at the first, but then not at the second follow-up, only to come back again at the third one. In a situation such as this, it is probably helpful to model these patterns and estimate the missing values at each time point in the follow-up – although, of course, this substantially complicates the modelling (see Gabrio et al., 2020; Mason et al., 2021).

From the computational point of view, the `R` package `missingHE` (Gabrio, 2024) simplifies the use of Bayesian modelling for missing data, based on `JAGS` code that is automatically created and run in the background, once the user specifies the main assumptions (on the missingness mechanism and the distributions for the partially observed data).

10.5 Conclusions

This chapter has given a very brief and sketched introduction to the philosophy underpinning statistical methods to deal with missing data, specifically for HTA. We have first reviewed the general mechanisms that we can use to describe the possible missingness generation and then moved to presenting typical modelling used to account for missingness in the analysis.

We have first discussed the gold standard of Multiple Imputation as a hybrid method – based on a Bayesian idea, but implemented within a frequentist approach. This was pretty much a historical accident, generated by the lack of suitable techniques that would allow a full Bayesian implementation.

Then, we have expanded to show how a Bayesian framework can be applied in general and specifically how it can prove particularly effective to deal with the several quirks of HTA data, including multivariate, non-Normal outcomes as well as structural values.

In the next chapter, we will discuss the ideas underpinning the principles of "population adjustment", an increasingly popular extension to NMA methods (presented in Chapter 7).

11

Population adjustment

11.1 Introduction

The methods described in Chapters 6 and 7 represent a progressive expansion from aggregated level summaries of a single pairwise comparison to the synthesis of an entire network of trials involving multiple treatments, simultaneously. Despite their differences in scope, these two frameworks share a common and consequential assumption, i.e. that the patient populations enrolled across the relevant studies are sufficiently exchangeable (see Section 6.2.4) and thus that pooling their results, whether directly or through a common comparator, yields estimates that are meaningful for the decision at hand.

However, when this is not tenable, naive pooling introduces bias into the indirect comparison, regardless of whether pairwise or network-based. This matters because, almost invariably, RCTs are designed with eligibility criteria that may differ substantially from one another and from the broader population of patients who will ultimately be treated, if the intervention is recommended. The network of evidence assembled through systematic literature review is therefore almost certain to comprise trials whose populations are heterogeneous in ways that matter for the estimated treatment effects.

In the case of fully available individual-level data, the wider biostatistics and causal inference literature has produced tools to deal with imbalance, e.g. using regression-based approaches such as propensity score (Rosenbaum and Rubin, 1983, 1984), as well as pure weighting-based tools, such as inverse probability weighting (Robins et al., 2000).

However, the structure of the data typically available for HTA submission exacerbates the problems even further: this is because while a sponsor may have direct access to the ILD from their own pivotal trial, the evidence on competing treatments exists, in the vast majority of cases, only in published aggregate form, typically consisting of average treatment effects and summary patient characteristics. This results in a structurally asymmetric evidence base: potentially rich, individual-level information on one arm of the comparison and only summary statistics on the other.

This asymmetry is precisely what creates both the motivation and the methodological challenge for the techniques we consider in this chapter, collectively referred to as *population adjustment methods*. The core objective of population adjustment is to produce estimates of relative treatment effect that are valid for a specific, well-defined target population, which is typically the population of patients for whom the healthcare decision is being made, rather than for the heterogeneous mix of trial populations from which the evidence happens to have been drawn, as described graphically in Figure 11.1.

Here, we consider an "anchored" comparison, where two active interventions (B and C) are separately compared to a common comparator (A). In the standard NMA framework of Chapter 7, we gain power by borrowing strength across the entire network of studies, under

DOI: 10.1201/9781003771050-11

the key assumption that relative treatment effects are "consistent" (Dias et al., 2013, 2018), i.e. the effect of a B versus C, whether estimated directly or inferred through the common comparator A, is the same across all study populations in the network.

Mathematically and with respect to Figure 11.1, this implies

$$d_{\text{BC(P)}} = d_{\text{AC(AC)}} - d_{\text{AB(AB)}}, \tag{11.1}$$

i.e. that the estimate for the effect of B vs C in the target population P can be obtained as the difference between the estimated effect of A vs C in the AC population and the estimated effect of A vs B in the AB population. In other words, under consistency, we can anchor the effect of the two treatments over the common comparator (placebo, in this case) and then by difference obtain the indirect treatment effect.

Of course, in reality, it is very possible that the two underlying populations AB and AC are fundamentally different, e.g. in terms of inclusion/exclusion criteria, or simply in terms of the distribution of the background characteristics (age, gender mix, co-morbidities, etc.), thus violating consistency. In addition, in Equation 11.1, the target population P is implicitly defined as a mixture of the original AB and AC populations, which again may not be a reasonable or helpful assumption in the HTA context.

To overcome these fundamental issues, the main idea of population adjustment is then to somehow rebalance the underlying characteristics of the populations in which the studies have been conducted, so that the resulting estimates of relative treatment effect are valid for a well-defined target population, rather than reflecting the potentially biased mix of trial populations from which the evidence was drawn.

11.2 Effect modifiers and collapsibility

One of the compounding issues in a general NMA framework such as that described in Figure 11.1 is that the unbalance in the background characteristics is generated by the

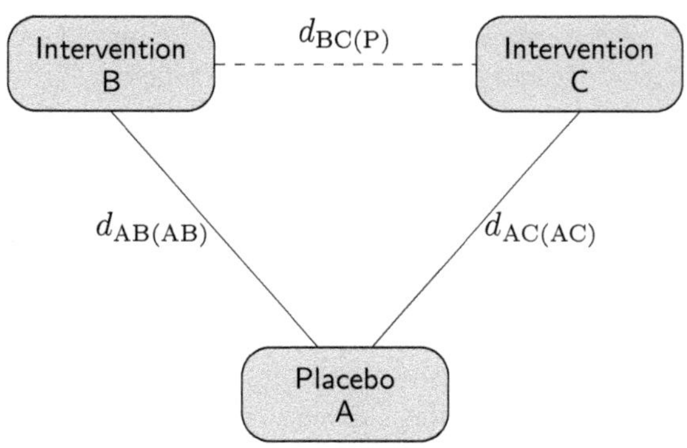

Figure 11.1: A graphical representation of the concept of population adjustment. The solid lines indicate observed studies, which we use to obtain estimates of the direct treatment effects. For instance $d_{\text{AB(AB)}}$ is the underlying effect of treatment B over placebo A, in the population investigated in the AB study. The dashed line indicates the absence of direct evidence; the target treatment effect is $d_{\text{BC(P)}}$, which indicates the benefits of treatment B over treatment C, in the target population P.

presence of *effect modifiers*, as well as prognostic factors – see among others Phillippo et al. (2025a) and Phillippo et al. (2025b) for more details.

Prognostic factors are covariates that affect absolute outcomes, regardless of treatment. Typically, these are balanced in a RCT, which means that they pose no concerns in terms of NMA and indirect comparisons.

Conversely, effect modifiers are defined as covariates that do affect the treatment and thus impact on the estimators for the relative effects, e.g. $\hat{d}_{\text{AC(AC)}}$ or $\hat{d}_{\text{AB(AB)}}$. This means that relative effects obtained from different populations may not be the same and thus, if there is imbalance in the effect modifiers, then

$$\hat{d}_{\text{AC(AC)}} - \hat{d}_{\text{AB(AB)}} \neq \hat{d}_{\text{AC(P)}} - \hat{d}_{\text{AB(P)}},$$

which in turns implies that we cannot "transport" the indirect treatment effect to the target population P.

Perhaps even more importantly, the scale in which the analysis is performed may also lead to problematic results in terms of comparisons across different population – we explore these issues in Example 11.1.

Example 11.1. *Effect modifiers and collapsibility.* Consider the hypothetical (and, as usual, ridiculously simplified!) situation described by Table 11.1.

In this study, smoking status is a prognostic factor because overall response rates differ between smokers and non-smokers, regardless of treatment:

$$\Pr(\text{Success} \mid \text{Non-smokers}) = \frac{185}{250} = 0.74 \quad \text{and} \quad \Pr(\text{Success} \mid \text{Smokers}) = \frac{51}{150} = 0.34$$

and thus smoking status predicts the outcome.

Moreover, treatment is evenly distributed across the two strata of the smoking status variable:

$$\Pr(\text{Treatment} \mid \text{Non-smokers}) = \frac{150}{250} = \Pr(\text{Treatment} \mid \text{Smokers}) = \frac{90}{150} = 0.6.$$

Consequently, smoking is not a confounder and, in addition, for the purposes of this silly example, we assume that there are no other unobserved or unobservable confounder either.

Now, if we consider as a measure of the treatment effect the risk difference

$$\text{RD} = \Pr(\text{Success} \mid \text{Treatment}) - \Pr(\text{Success} \mid \text{Placebo})$$

Table 11.1: A fictional example of a study in which a treatment is contrasted to Placebo and we have information about smoking status as a covariate. Adapted from Remiro Azócar (2025).

	Non-smokers		Smokers		Total	
	Success	Failure	Success	Failure	Success	Failure
Treatment	135	15	45	45	180	60
Placebo	50	50	6	54	56	104
Total	185	65	51	99	236	164

and compute it in the strata (NS and S for Non-smokers and Smokers, respectively), we get

$$\text{RD}_{\text{NS}} = \frac{135}{150} - \frac{50}{100} = 0.4, \quad \text{and} \quad \text{RD}_{\text{S}} = \frac{45}{90} - \frac{6}{60} = 0.4$$

and so the treatment does not have a differential effect across different levels of smoking, which is thus *not* an effect modifier.

Similarly, if we use the OR as a measure of treatment effect (and recalling Equation 6.8), we get that

$$\text{OR}_{\text{NS}} = \frac{135/150}{15/150} \Big/ \frac{50/100}{50/100} = 9 \quad \text{and} \quad \text{OR}_{\text{S}} = \frac{45/90}{45/90} \Big/ \frac{6/60}{54/60} = 9,$$

so that, again, the effect of the treatment does not vary across strata defined by smoking, which again is *not* an effect modifier.

Conversely, when considering the risk ratio

$$\text{RR} = \Pr(\text{Success} \mid \text{Treatment})/\Pr(\text{Success} \mid \text{Placebo})$$

we have in the two subgroups

$$\text{RR}_{\text{NS}} = \frac{135}{150} \Big/ \frac{50}{100} = 1.8 \neq \text{RR}_{\text{S}} = \frac{45}{90} \Big/ \frac{6}{60} = 5,$$

indicating that, *on this scale*, smoking is indeed an effect modifier.

The interpretation across different scales becomes in fact more complex, because even in situations seemingly identical we may get further differences. For instance, for both the RD and the OR, the data in Table 11.1 suggest treatment effect homogeneity (i.e. no confounding, as well as perfect balance and no effect modification).

In the case of the RD, the crude overall effect

$$\text{RD}_{\text{crude}} = \frac{180}{240} - \frac{56}{160} = 0.4$$

coincides with the weighted average of the stratum-specific ones

$$\begin{aligned}\text{RD}_{\text{weighted}} &= w_{\text{NS}}\text{RD}_{\text{NS}} + w_{\text{S}}\text{RD}_{\text{S}} \\ &= \frac{250}{400}0.4 + \frac{150}{400}0.4 = 0.4,\end{aligned}$$

where w_{NS} and w_{S} are the proportion of the total sample size in each of the strata. This property is referred to as *collapsibility* (Greenland et al., 1999) and thus we say that the RD is *collapsible*.

On the other hand, collapsibility does not hold for the OR, because the crude value is

$$\text{OR}_{\text{crude}} = \frac{180/240}{60/240} \Big/ \frac{56/160}{104/160} = 5.6,$$

which differs from the weighted average among the strata

$$\begin{aligned}\text{OR}_{\text{weighted}} &= \exp\left(w_{\text{NS}} \log(\text{OR}_{\text{NS}}) + w_{\text{S}} \log(\text{OR}_{\text{S}})\right) \\ &= \exp\left(\frac{250}{400} \log(9) + \frac{150}{400} \log(9)\right) = 9\end{aligned}$$

– this quantity averages the stratum-specific effects *on the scale of the linear predictor* (i.e. log OR rather than directly OR). The crude estimates identify the population *marginal* effects, while the weighted estimates are the population *conditional* effects.

In the absence of effect modification, for non-collapsible measures the direction of the treatment effect aligns, but the magnitude generally varies when considering the population average marginal vs conditional effects. More problematically, when there is effect modification, the rank ordering of the treatments may even flip.

Interestingly, an effect modifier may still be collapsible. For instance, even if smoking were an effect modifier for the RD, the crude and weighted estimates would still coincide. This is due to the mathematical form of the estimand, which in the case of the RD is linear. It is for this reason that measures such as the OR or the HR are non-collapsible (see also the discussion in Note 27, in Section 8.4.6).

Similarly, effect modification is not a key factor for an RR to be collapsible: in fact, the requirements are that a covariate is not a confounder and that the baseline risk is balanced across its strata. In the specific context of the data in Table 11.1, if we had that

$$\Pr(\text{Treatment} \mid \text{Non-smokers}) = \Pr(\text{Treatment} \mid \text{Smokers})$$

and

$$\Pr(\text{Success} \mid \text{Placebo, Non-smoker}) = \Pr(\text{Success} \mid \text{Placebo, Smoker}).$$

then even if smoking were an effect modifier for the RR, this would still be collapsible.

In the next sections, we consider specific methods that are prevalent in the HTA context that are used to perform population adjustment.

11.3 Methods for population adjustment

Historically, the two most widely used population adjustment methods in HTA practice are *Matching-Adjusted Indirect Comparison* (MAIC, Signorovitch et al., 2010, 2012) and *Simulated Treatment Comparison* (STC, Caro and Ishak, 2010; Ishak et al., 2015).

MAIC is a propensity score-like reweighting approach that adjusts the individual-level data from one trial (typically the sponsor's study) to match the aggregate summary statistics reported from the comparator trial. Specifically, it assigns weights to individuals in the ILD trial such that the weighted means of the observed covariates align with the published means from the aggregate data study. The weighted outcomes are then used to estimate the treatment effect in the reweighted (now "matched") population.

Conversely, STC is a regression-based method that models the relationship between covariates and outcomes in the ILD trial and then uses this fitted model to predict the expected outcomes, had the ILD trial enrolled a population with the covariate distribution of the comparator study.

Despite their widespread adoption (particularly for MAIC), both methods have well documented limitations. Similarly to other weighting procedures, MAIC can suffer from extreme or unstable weights, when covariate overlap between the trials is poor, leading to high variance and potentially unreliable estimates. This problem worsens as the number of adjustment covariates increases, relative to the effective sample size[1] (Phillippo et al., 2016, 2018). As for STC, due to its nature as a regression-based method, it avoids the weighting instability of MAIC. However, it is affected by other important limitations: its typical implementation directly targets conditional treatment effects on the scale of the outcome model, rather than marginal effects. As discussed above, this can lead to bias when the outcome model is non-linear or when non-collapsible effect measures such as ORs or HRs are used (Remiro Azócar et al., 2021).

In addition, both standard MAIC and STC crucially target the population of the comparator trial, which may not be the one relevant to the decision-maker, while also failing to naturally accommodate network structures involving more than two treatments without performing multiple pairwise adjustments and then pooling them in a secondary meta-analysis (thus introducing further, most likely untestable, assumptions).

To overcome these problems, research in the area of population adjustment has been particularly active in the past few years, producing important contributions. Among these, notable examples are *multilevel network meta-regression* (ML-NMR, Phillippo et al., 2020, 2025a), which extends population adjustment to arbitrary network structures and allows inference in any specified target population; and *outcome regression standardisation*, based on g-computation (Remiro Azócar et al., 2022) or marginalisation via multiple imputation (MIM, Remiro Azócar et al., 2024), which address the marginalisation problem in STC by constructing marginal effect estimates through imputation of missing covariate data in the aggregate trials.

Interestingly, these methods have a very strong Bayesian flavour, as well as marked computational complexity, which is however limited by the availability of suitable `R` packages to perform the underlying analyses – respectively `multinma` (Phillippo, 2024) and `outstandR` (Green et al., 2026). In the next sections we present the general modelling structure, highlighting relevant issues in terms of the target estimands and then review the basic assumptions and computational working of the two methods.

11.3.1 Multilevel Network Meta-Regression

The main idea underlying ML-NMR is to build a model capable to connect the two modules, one for the ILD and the other for the ALD evidence, so as to ensure that population-level parameters are derived consistently, avoiding aggregation bias and accounting for non-collapsibility, all well established problems in the wider evidence synthesis literature (Sutton et al., 2008; Saramago et al., 2012; Donegan et al., 2013).

The general individual-level data modelling structure proceeds as follows. We typically have data on individuals $i = 1, \ldots, n_{st}$ under each treatment arm $t = 1, \ldots, T$ in study $s = 1, \ldots, S$. Each study s is typically conducted in a specific population, which may differ from the others in terms of eligibility criteria, demographic characteristics and the distribution of prognostic factors and effect modifiers. The target population P may be one of these, or an entirely different one.

Almost invariably, in the notation of Figure 11.1, at least one study involves a comparison between interventions A vs B, where $t =$ A is some kind of placebo or standard of care and $t =$ B is the active intervention, to be contrasted with another active intervention C,

[1] In the context of MAIC, the effective sample size quantifies the loss of information due to reweighting – essentially, how many "independent" observations remain after adjustment/matching.

considered in other studies. The data are modelled as

$$y_{ist} \sim p\left(y_{ist} \mid \boldsymbol{\theta}_{ist}\right),$$

with parameters $\boldsymbol{\theta}_{ist} = (\mu_{ist}, \boldsymbol{\alpha}_{ist})$, where μ_{ist} is the individual mean outcome (which typically depends on some relevant covariates) and $\boldsymbol{\alpha}_{ist}$ are a set of possible ancillary parameters (e.g. standard deviations, scales, shape parameters, etc.); the ancillary parameters may or may not be made to depend on the covariates and in fact may or may not be present, depending on the functional form of the sampling distribution $p(\cdot)$. This is similar to the description given in Section 5.2.2 and Section 8.3.3.

We then construct a (generalised) linear predictor

$$g\left(\mu_{ist}\right) = \eta_{st}(\boldsymbol{x}_{ist}) = \beta_{0s} + \boldsymbol{x}_{ist}^{\top}(\boldsymbol{\beta}_1 + \boldsymbol{\beta}_{2t}) + \gamma_t \tag{11.2}$$

where: $g(\cdot)$ is the link function; β_{0s} is the study-specific intercept, representing baseline risk or outcome level in study s (stratified to preserve randomisation); $\boldsymbol{x}_{ist}$ are the observed covariates for individual i in study s on treatment t; $\boldsymbol{\beta}_1$ identifies the prognostic effects (covariates that affect absolute outcomes but not treatment effects); $\boldsymbol{\beta}_{2t}$ are treatment-covariate interaction terms capturing effect modification (with $\boldsymbol{\beta}_{2\text{A}} = \mathbf{0}$ for the reference treatment A); and γ_t is an individual-level treatment effect for an individual with $\boldsymbol{x}_{ist} = \mathbf{0}$, with $\gamma_{\text{A}} = 0$.

As for studies where only aggregated summaries are published, ML-NMR constructs the likelihood by integrating Equation 11.2 over the joint distribution of covariates within each study arm. For each aggregated outcome $y_{\bullet st}$ observed in study s and for arm t, the model is specified as:

$$\begin{aligned} y_{\bullet st} &\sim p(y_{\bullet st} \mid \boldsymbol{\theta}_{\bullet st}) \\ \mu_{\bullet st} &= \int_{\mathcal{X}} g^{-1}(\eta_{st}(\boldsymbol{x})) f_{st}(\boldsymbol{x})\, d\boldsymbol{x}, \end{aligned} \tag{11.3}$$

where $\boldsymbol{\theta}_{\bullet st} = (\mu_{\bullet st}[, \boldsymbol{\alpha}_{\bullet st}])$ – again, ancillary parameters may or may not exist, depending on the distributional form chosen for the aggregated level data. In Equation 11.3, $f_{st}(\boldsymbol{x})$ denotes the joint covariate distribution in that study arm and $\mathcal{X}$ is its possible range.

The model is completed by specifying suitable prior distributions for the parameters – in the most basic structure implemented in the `R` package `multinma`, $\beta_{0s} \sim \text{Normal}(0, \text{sd} = 100)$ and $\gamma_t, \boldsymbol{\beta}_1, \boldsymbol{\beta}_{2t} \overset{iid}{\sim} \text{Normal}(0, \text{sd} = 10)$. The models are constructed in `Stan` using a process akin to that shown for `survHEhmc` and `survextrap` in Sections 8.4 and 8.5.1, respectively.

There are several advantages to using a Bayesian framework, even in the face of the underlying computational complexity. Firstly, using a Bayesian approach allows us to propagate fully the uncertainty in the marginalisation integral, as part of the posterior sampling. In addition, as the model naturally assumes some forms of (conditional) exchangeability in the ILD and ALD components, the Bayesian framework makes it easier to, at least conceptually, handle the underlying correlation across the modules.

On the other hand, the need to evaluate the marginalisation integral (once at each MCMC iteration) does impose a computational burden on this modelling structure. To limit this, ML-NMR uses numerical approximation based on Quasi-Monte Carlo (QMC) integration. This is a form of approximation for multidimensional integrals, obtained by averaging a function over a carefully chosen deterministic sequence of points, rather than exploring the full space randomly.

Unlike standard pseudo-random numbers-based Monte Carlo (see Section 1.2.4), QMC exploits numerical sequences designed to fill the target space more uniformly, with fewer gaps

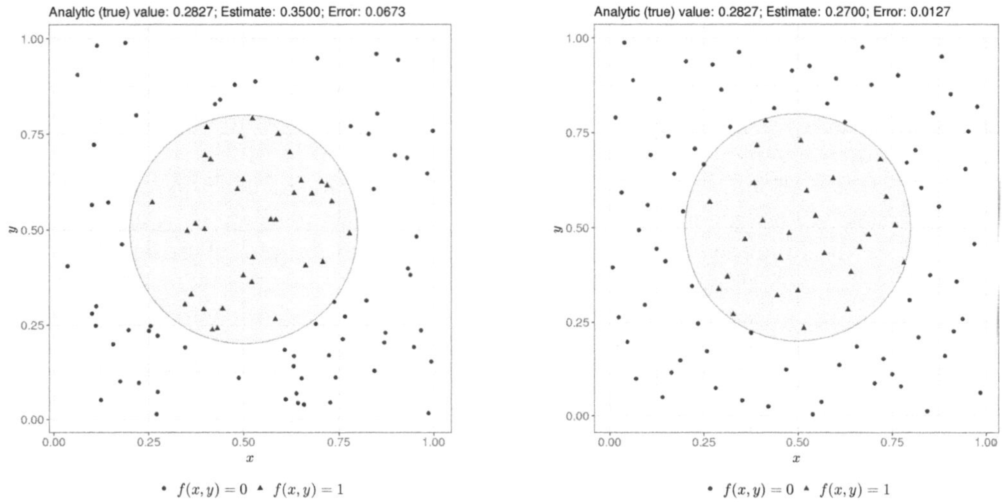

(a) Monte Carlo Integration. (b) Quasi-Monte Carlo Integration.

Figure 11.2: Comparison of Monte Carlo and Quasi-Monte Carlo integration methods for approximating the two-dimensional integral $\iint f(x, y)dxdy$ by evaluating the function at $n = 100$ sample points and computing the average: $\frac{1}{n}\sum_{i=1}^{n} f(x_i, y_i)$. The shaded region represents the integration domain, a circle of radius 0.3 centred at (0.5, 0.5), where $f(x, y) = 1$ inside the circle (points shaped as triangles) and $f(x, y) = 0$ outside (dots). The integral estimate equals the proportion of lighter points. Figure 11.2a: Monte Carlo uses pseudo-random sampling, which creates clusters of points in some regions and leaves gaps in others, leading to inefficient coverage of the integration domain. Figure 11.2b: Quasi-Monte Carlo uses a deterministic low-discrepancy sequence that forces the points to be spread more uniformly across the space. This more even coverage typically yields more accurate estimates with the same number of evaluations.

and "clumps". For smooth functions, this can achieve convergence rates close to $\mathcal{O}(n^{-1})$ rather than Monte Carlo's $\mathcal{O}(n^{-1/2})$, although the advantage diminishes in very high dimensions or for non-smooth integrands – a simplified example of this comparison is shown in Figure 11.2.

The specification in Equation 11.3 assumes that the aggregated level sampling distribution has a tractable, known form, which holds for standard outcome types (Normal, Binomial, Poisson, Multinomial) but not universally. For outcomes such as survival times where no natural aggregate distribution exists, ML-NMR can instead work directly with the likelihood contributions from each data level, avoiding the need for an explicit aggregated distribution, thus enabling broader applicability including time-to-event models (Phillippo et al., 2024).

The crucial advantage of ML-NMR for healthcare decision-making is its capacity to produce treatment effect estimates in *any* specified target population P, not merely in the populations of the observed studies – that is, provided we can reliably estimate the covariate distributions!

Using again the slightly more verbose notation presented in Figure 11.1, for a target population with joint covariate distribution $f_{(\mathrm{P})}(\boldsymbol{x})$, the *population-average conditional treatment effect* between treatments B and C is derived from Equation 11.2 as

$$\begin{aligned} d_{\mathrm{BC(P)}} &= \int_{\mathcal{X}} \left(\eta_{\mathrm{B(P)}}(\boldsymbol{x}) - \eta_{\mathrm{C(P)}}(\boldsymbol{x})\right) f_{\mathrm{(P)}}(\boldsymbol{x})\, d\boldsymbol{x} \\ &= \bar{\boldsymbol{x}}_{\mathrm{(P)}}^{\top}(\boldsymbol{\beta}_{2\mathrm{B}} - \boldsymbol{\beta}_{2\mathrm{C}}) + \gamma_{\mathrm{B}} - \gamma_{\mathrm{C}}, \end{aligned} \tag{11.4}$$

where $\mathcal{X}$ is the support of the covariates and the closed-form expression in terms of mean covariate values $\bar{\boldsymbol{x}}_{\mathrm{(P)}}$ in population P derives from the linearity of the treatment contrast *on the linear predictor scale*. This estimator is in the same spirit of Equation 5.9, as discussed in Section 5.2.2 and it represents the average individual-level treatment effect when the entire population P is shifted from treatment C to treatment B.

Notably, computing the population-average conditional treatment effect requires only the means of effect-modifying covariates in the target population: neither the full joint distribution nor information about baseline risk is needed for conditional effects.

However, as discussed in Note 16 in Section 6.2, economic models are based on *absolute* outcome predictions, rather than *relative* treatment effects. Thus, for a generic treatment t, the target estimand in population P is

$$\bar{\mu}_{t\mathrm{(P)}} = \int_{\mathcal{X}} g^{-1}\left(\eta_{t\mathrm{(P)}}(\boldsymbol{x})\right) f_{\mathrm{(P)}}(\boldsymbol{x}) d\boldsymbol{x}. \tag{11.5}$$

Because the quantity inside the integral in Equation 11.5 depends on the typically highly non-linear function $g(\cdot)$, in this case we do require the full joint covariate distribution $f_{\mathrm{(P)}}(\boldsymbol{x})$, which is rarely reported in a meaningful way, since published aggregate data studies typically provide only marginal summaries such as means, standard deviations or frequencies, for each covariate separately.

ML-NMR addresses this by reconstructing plausible joint distributions using copula methods (originally introduced by Sklar, 1959; but see also Joe, 2014 for a more recent detailed account), which combine the reported marginal summaries with assumed correlation structures and marginal distributional forms borrowed from the individual patient data studies (Phillippo et al., 2020).

Once absolute outcome predictions are available, *population-average marginal treatment effects* can also be estimated as

$$\delta_{\mathrm{BC(P)}} = g\left(\bar{\mu}_{\mathrm{B(P)}}\right) - g\left(\bar{\mu}_{\mathrm{C(P)}}\right). \tag{11.6}$$

These differ from the conditional effects in Equation 11.4 whenever the effect measure is non-collapsible (see Example 11.1) and quantify the change in the overall population event occurrence, when shifting from one treatment to another. Importantly, they can only be computed if the distribution $f_{\mathrm{(P)}}(\boldsymbol{x})$ is reliably estimated.

Evidence from simulation work indicates that ML-NMR estimates tend to be reasonably stable under mis-specification of the estimated covariate distribution, although models with substantial non-linearity or analyses targeting directly marginal rather than conditional estimands may exhibit greater sensitivity.

Example 11.2. *Conditional vs marginal estimates.* We return to the overly-simplistic case of Example 11.1. From Table 11.1, we can compute the distribution of the covariate $x =$ Smoking status in the target population as $f(\mathrm{NS}) = 250/400 = 0.625$ and $f(\mathrm{S}) = 150/400 = 0.375$. The stratum-specific means (which in this case can be defined as probabilities) are

$$\mu_{\mathrm{B}}(\mathrm{NS}) = \frac{135}{150} = 0.9 \quad \text{and} \quad \mu_{\mathrm{A}}(\mathrm{NS}) = \frac{50}{100} = 0.5$$

and

$$\mu_{\mathrm{B}}(\mathrm{S}) = \frac{45}{90} = 0.5 \quad \text{and} \quad \mu_{\mathrm{A}}(\mathrm{S}) = \frac{6}{60} = 0.1,$$

where A indicates the placebo and B indicates the treatment arms. Assuming $g(\cdot) = \text{logit}(\cdot)$ and using these estimates, we can compute the average of Equation 11.4 as the discrete sum

$$\begin{aligned} d_{\mathrm{BA}} &= \sum_x \left[\eta_{\mathrm{B}}(x) - \eta_{\mathrm{A}}(x)\right] f(x) \\ &= \left[\text{logit}\left(\mu_{\mathrm{B}}(\mathrm{NS})\right) - \text{logit}\left(\mu_{\mathrm{A}}(\mathrm{NS})\right)\right] f(\mathrm{NS}) + \left[\text{logit}\left(\mu_{\mathrm{B}}(\mathrm{S})\right) - \text{logit}\left(\mu_{\mathrm{A}}(\mathrm{S})\right)\right] f(\mathrm{S}) \\ &= (2.1972 - 0)\, 0.625 + (0 + 2.1972)\, 0.375 = 2.1972. \end{aligned}$$

Conversely, in line with Equation 11.5, the population-average marginal treatment effect is computed with respect to the example in Table 11.1 as

$$\bar{\mu}_{\mathrm{B}} = \sum_x \mu_{\mathrm{B}}(x) f(x) = 0.9 \times 0.625 + 0.5 \times 0.375 = 0.75$$

and

$$\bar{\mu}_{\mathrm{A}} = \sum_x \mu_{\mathrm{A}}(x) f(x) = 0.5 \times 0.625 + 0.1 \times 0.375 = 0.35$$

– note that these quantities coincide with the crude estimates from the "Total" part of Table 11.1. Using these, we can compute the discrete version of Equation 11.6 as

$$\begin{aligned} \delta_{\mathrm{BA}} = g(\bar{\mu}_{\mathrm{B}}) - g(\bar{\mu}_{\mathrm{A}}) &= \text{logit}(\bar{\mu}_{\mathrm{B}}) - \text{logit}(\bar{\mu}_{\mathrm{A}}) \\ &= 1.0986 - (-0.619) \\ &= 1.7177 \end{aligned}$$

Because of the non-collapsibility of the logit, we get that $d_{\mathrm{BA}} \neq \delta_{\mathrm{BA}}$.

When few aggregate data studies are available for a particular treatment, insufficient information may exist to estimate the relevant treatment-covariate interaction terms, $\boldsymbol{\beta}_{2t}$. This situation may require a "shared effect modifier" assumption, in which interactions are constrained to be constant across a treatment set (Phillippo et al., 2020). Such an assumption might be defensible when treatments share pharmacological class and mechanism of action, but is otherwise restrictive. Under this constraint, interaction effects can be borrowed from treatments with individual patient data or pooled across multiple aggregate data treatments.

In a minimal two-study comparison with aggregate data for only one treatment, this reduces ML-NMR to the same limitation as MAIC and STC: estimates are constrained to the aggregate study population. However, in networks of moderate size, the shared effect modifier assumption can often be tested by selectively relaxing constraints or avoided entirely given sufficient data (Phillippo et al., 2023). Furthermore, the fundamental assumption underlying all population adjustment, conditional constancy of relative effects, can be evaluated within the ML-NMR framework using standard network meta-analysis diagnostics for heterogeneity and inconsistency, as discussed in Chapter 7.

Worked examples using ML-NMR are shown in Phillippo et al. (2025a) and in the `multinma` website `https://dmphillippo.github.io/multinma/`.

11.3.2 Outcome regression standardisation using g-computation

Both MAIC and STC, as well as ML-NMR, fundamentally address the problem of transporting treatment effect estimates to a target population when covariate distributions differ across studies. However, as mentioned above, a distinct challenge arises in the context of outcome regression methods like STC: the standard implementation targets conditional treatment effects on the scale of the outcome model, rather than the marginal effects required for population-level decision-making in HTA (Remiro Azócar et al., 2021, 2022).

As discussed in Example 11.1, when the effect measure is non-collapsible, conditional and marginal effects diverge, even in the absence of treatment-covariate interactions. Standard STC methods that simply plug predicted outcomes into the regression model therefore produce biased estimates of the marginal treatment effect in the target population.

To overcome this issue, Remiro Azócar et al. (2022) propose using parametric g-computation (where 'g' stands for 'generalised', as originally defined in Robins, 1986), a method borrowed from the causal inference literature, which predicts the natural-scale outcome under different treatment strategies by using a regression model and then averages those predictions over the covariate distribution in the population of interest, to obtain estimates for the relevant marginal effects. In a Bayesian context (and assuming the absence of unobserved confounding – see Daniels and Hogan, 2008), this essentially amounts to the discussion of Section 5.2.3 and the general model can be visualised as in Figure 11.3.

In the specific context of the HTA population adjustment case, we first fit an outcome regression model to the available individual patient data from the AB study, for instance using the same general structure as in Equation 11.2. This is indicated as 'First-stage regression' in Figure 11.3. In a Bayesian context, we thus obtain L samples from the posterior distributions of the parameters $\boldsymbol{\theta}$, including the regression coefficients $\boldsymbol{\beta}$ (which capture treatment effects and covariate relationships) and any relevant ancillary parameters $\boldsymbol{\alpha}$, such as variances or dispersion parameters.

We then use the published aggregate summaries from the AC study to reconstruct the joint covariate distribution $f_{\text{AC}}(\boldsymbol{x})$. This typically involves fitting parametric distributions

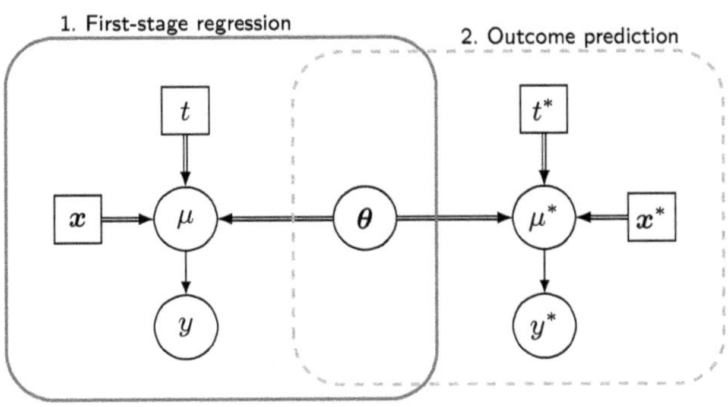

Figure 11.3: Synthetic data generation for parametric g-computation. Individual-level covariates $\boldsymbol{x}^*$ are sampled from parametric distributions fitted to the aggregate summaries from the AC study. For each treatment assignment $t^* \in \{A, B\}$, the regression model fitted to the AB individual patient data (with parameters $\boldsymbol{\theta}$, including the regression coefficients as well as any other ancillary parameter) is used to predict the natural-scale mean μ^*, which in turn is used to sample from the posterior predictive distribution for the outcome y^*. Adapted from Remiro Azócar et al. (2024).

(e.g. multivariate Normal for continuous covariates, or Multinomial distributions for categorical variables), with the correlation structure borrowed from the individual patient data, if needed. Alternatively, we can rely on copula-based methods, similarly to ML-NMR. Either way, we can use this distribution to simulate a full vector of covariates $\boldsymbol{x}^* \sim f_{\text{AC}}(\boldsymbol{x})$.

At this point, we can consider a sample of N^* *synthetic* individuals from the AC population with individual-level profiles $\boldsymbol{x}_i^*$ and use the output from the first-stage regression $\boldsymbol{\theta}$ to predict the outcome y^* that might be observed in the AC population, had those individuals be allocated to $t^* \in \{A, B\}$. In particular, we consider a sample where the covariates profile is balanced (in fact, identical in the specification of Remiro Azócar et al., 2024) across the intervention arms, so that the treatment effect can be identified without further issues.

The two steps of model fitting and outcome prediction can be embedded in a single Bayesian modelling operation. For each synthetic individual $i = 1, \ldots, N^*$, we can draw $l = 1, \ldots, L$ samples from the predictive distribution $y_{it^*}^{*(l)} \sim p\left(y_{it^*} \mid \boldsymbol{\theta}^{(l)}, \boldsymbol{x}_i^*\right)$. Averaging these predicted outcomes across the N^* synthetic individuals gives us marginal outcome predictions $\bar{y}_{t^*}^{(l)}$ from which we can compute a sample of L estimates of the marginal treatment effects such as the B vs A effect in the AC population, i.e.

$$\Delta^{(l)} = \bar{y}_{\text{B}}^{(l)} - \bar{y}_{\text{A}}^{(l)},$$

which can be used to provide summaries for the underlying distribution (e.g. mean and intervals).

The approach explicitly targets marginal estimands, ensuring compatibility in indirect comparisons when effect measures are non-collapsible and can extrapolate beyond observed covariate overlap, unlike propensity score methods such as MAIC.

On the other hand, parametric g-computation has some important limitations. First, the in its basic construction, it is restricted to pairwise indirect comparisons, similarly to the "vanilla" implementation of STC. While in principle the method could be extended to larger networks by performing multiple pairwise comparisons and synthesising the results, this requires additional assumptions and does not naturally leverage the full network structure in the way that ML-NMR does.

In addition, the validity of the marginal effect estimates depends critically on the correct specification of both the outcome regression model and the parametric distributions used to generate the synthetic covariate data. Mis-specification of either component can introduce bias and there is limited ability to check model fit in the aggregate data study, where individual-level observations are unavailable. This is particularly concerning when extrapolating to covariate regions poorly represented in the ILD.

Finally, the computational burden of running this approach can be substantial. The process requires generating a complete pseudo-ILD dataset and computing predictions for every synthetic individual at each iteration of the uncertainty quantification procedure. With typical choices of $L \approx 4000$ posterior draws and $N^* \approx 1000$ synthetic individuals, this results in millions of individual-level predictions.

The computational cost is further compounded when the outcome model is complex. For survival models with flexible baseline hazards (such as spline-based approaches), each prediction requires numerical integration to compute survival probabilities. For count or other generalised linear models with overdispersion, additional random draws are needed for dispersion parameters. When multiple treatments are being compared, the number of predictions scales linearly with the number of treatment arms.

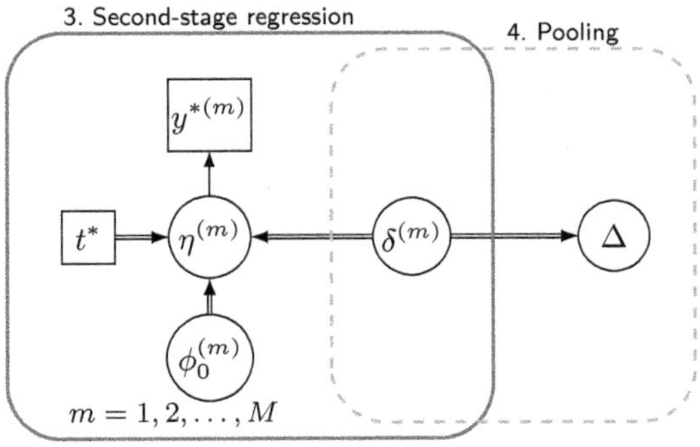

Figure 11.4: The analysis stage of multiple imputation marginalisation. For each of the M imputed datasets generated in the imputation stage (described in Figure 11.3), we perform a "second-stage regression" in which predicted outcomes $y^{*(m)}$ are regressed against the treatment assignments t^*. The marginal treatment effect $\delta^{(m)}$ is estimated for each imputed dataset and the M estimates are then summarised using Rubin's rule, to produce the pooled estimate Δ. Adapted from Remiro Azócar et al. (2024).

11.3.3 Multiple imputation marginalisation

Multiple imputation marginalisation (MIM) addresses both the computational limitations and some conceptual gaps of standard parametric g-computation by embedding the outcome regression standardisation process within the established framework of multiple imputation (Remiro Azócar et al., 2024).

The first part of MIM is essentially identical to the process described in Figure 11.3, in which we generate L samples from the predictive distribution for the outcome y^* that might be observed in N^* synthetic individuals from the AC population, if they were allocated to treatments in $t^* = \{A, B\}$ instead. However, to simplify the rest of the computation, MIM proceeds to "thin" the L simulations for $\boldsymbol{\theta}$ to only consider a number $M << L$ – typically, $M = 20$ to 50 "imputations", in missing data parlance (see Section 10.3.1).

These process basically amounts to create M "complete" versions of the full dataset that might be observed if a AB trial with N^* individuals were run in the AC population. In the analysis stage (depicted in Figure 11.4), each of these $m = 1, \ldots, M$ imputed datasets is analysed separately, by modelling the relationship between the predicted outcome $y^{*(m)}$ and the treatment assignment t^*, using a generalised linear regression such as

$$g\left(\eta_i^{(m)}\right) = \phi_0^{(m)} + \delta^{(m)} t_i^*, \tag{11.7}$$

where $\phi_0^{(m)}$ is the intercept and $\delta^{(m)}$ is the relevant marginal treatment effect – again, because we are constructing the N^* individuals as perfectly balanced in terms of background characteristics, we do not need to control for the effect of $\boldsymbol{x}^*$ in Equation 11.7.

Again, within a full Bayesian setting, we can obtain R samples from the posterior distribution of the relevant parameter $\delta^{(m)}$ – but this time the overall size $M \times R$ allows for a much more feasible computation. Using these we can pool the point estimates for $\delta^{(m)}$ and their resulting variances, e.g. using Rubin's rule, to produce the pooled estimate of the treatment effect, accounting for both within-imputation uncertainty (how much predictions vary within one synthetic dataset) and between-imputation uncertainty (how much the M datasets differ from each other due to the random sampling of covariates).

The R package outstandR (Green et al., 2026) implements both maximum likelihood and Bayesian versions of MIM, along with standard outcome regression standardisation using g-computation and other population adjustment methods – some examples are presented in the package website https://statisticshealtheconomics.github.io/outstandR/.

In particular, the Bayesian formulation for MIM offers several advantages: it naturally handles uncertainty in regression parameters without bootstrap resampling, readily accommodates missing data in the ILD study itself through standard multiple imputation techniques and allows incorporation of prior information about model parameters or covariate distributions. The full posterior distribution provides a natural input for probabilistic sensitivity analysis in downstream economic models (see Section 4.3).

11.4 Further challenges

While population adjustment is gaining increasing popularity in the HTA context and the established methods described above are becoming more and more relevant and used in applied analyses, there are still numerous research questions unresolved and possible extensions to the existing methods.

Among these, Gao et al. (2025) discuss the further complexity generated by the presence of heterogeneous treatment effects, while Campbell et al. (2026) extend the general framework of ML-NMR to consider subgroup-level summary statistics that may be available in published studies and potentially highly informative.

11.5 Conclusions

In this chapter we have discussed the general framework underpinning the important problem of population adjustment. This is particularly key in HTA, because naive indirect comparison may very easily produce biased (and irrelevant!) estimates for the relevant treatment effect parameters, which would of course have dire consequences in terms of the meaningfulness of the economic evaluation.

We have presented recent development in statistical methodology, which are gaining substantial traction and becoming very popular in the HTA context. These have all a very strong Bayesian nature and thus fit nicely with the overall Bayesian decision-making process.

In the next chapter, we will present the most important features (both in terms of methodology and applications) of the important analysis of the value of information, a suite of tools that can be used to measure the economic value of additional information.

12

Value of information

12.1 Introduction

We have seen throughout the many examples in the previous chapters that a fundamental component of the HTA process is the characterisation and full analysis of the impact of uncertainty in the model parameters on the decision-making. As mentioned in Note 12 in Section 4.3.3, this exercise cannot be made purely on probabilistic terms, because doing so (e.g. by using the CEACs) would fail to account for the potential *payoffs* associated with the decision.

In other words, there may be situations in which large uncertainty in the model parameters (and thus, potentially, on the probability that a given intervention is deemed to be the most cost-effective) is associated with very limited consequences. Similarly, it is possible that situations that, at face value, do not look highly uncertain may hide dire consequences – the (admittedly silly) example in Note 12 is a point in case.

These considerations suggest that, in fact, the process of "uncertainty analysis" as defined in Section 4.3 is a bit more complicated and involves more nuanced aspects. These can be better understood and more efficiently tackled under the framework of "Value of Information" (VoI) analysis (originally devised in Howard, 1966), an increasingly popular method in health economic evaluations.

More specifically, the process can be depicted graphically as in Figure 12.1, where the main point is the suggestion of the cyclical nature and evidence is hardly ever definitive. At the point of initiating a new HTA evaluation, researchers must look into the existing evidence basis, e.g. through a systematic review. All the available evidence must be combined (e.g. using the processes described in Chapters 6 and 7) to feed into the main cost-effectiveness analysis, based on current evidence. This determines the decision, which is not just binary in terms of adopt/reject, but also involves through the uncertainty analysis the explicit option of collecting more information and carrying out more research.

This is the stage in which the analysis of the "value of information" plays a fundamental role, as we will show in the rest of this chapter. In particular, this should drive the research priorities, in terms of what is the best design to collect new information and which quantities to target to reduce uncertainty. This leads to an increment in the evidence basis, which should be accounted for when the process can start over with a new systematic review. This characterisation suggests that the overall HTA process is inherently Bayesian – recall the mantra of Lindley (1972), as discussed in Section 1.2.2.

Heath et al. (2024) is the most recent and comprehensive textbook on the use of VoI in healthcare. The companion `voi` package (Jackson and Heath, 2024) can be used to perform the actual calculations – cfr. also the package website

DOI: 10.1201/9781003771050-12

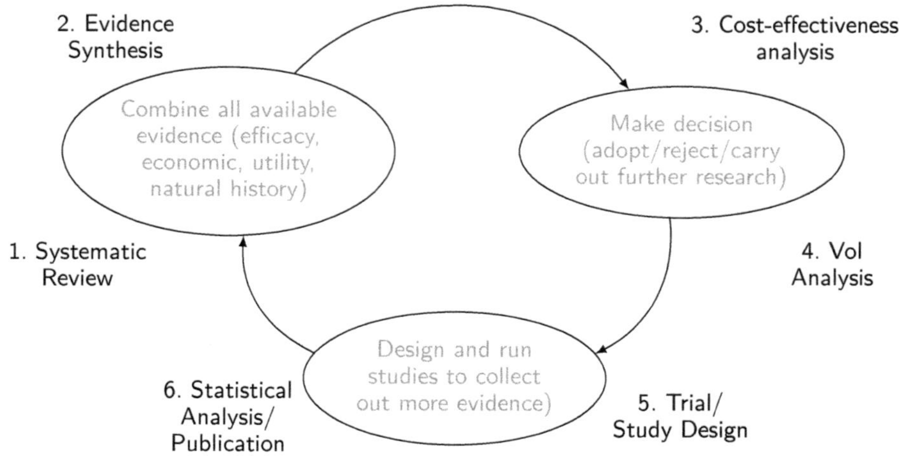

Figure 12.1: Evidence based decision-making and Value of Information. Source: Welton (2018)

`https://chjackson.github.io/voi/articles/book.html` for code to replicate the examples discussed in Heath et al. (2024).

12.2 Basic ideas

Generally speaking, at the point of considering the conduct of a new study before firmly committing to a new intervention, the main expectation is that the new evidence will contribute to reducing – or, in an ideal world, fully eliminating – uncertainty in at least a subset of the model parameters.

When updating the cost-effectiveness analysis, on the basis of the new evidence that becomes available, we may find that the optimal decision has changed – we may have thought that $t = 2$ was the most cost-effective treatment on the basis of the original evidence, but now $t = 1$ is deemed to be better value for money. In this case, we would generate a change in the monetary net benefit (MNB – cfr. Equation 4.3 and Section 4.2) through the acquisition of the new evidence.

Conversely, we may see no difference in the optimal decision-making before and after the collection of the new data – in that case, we would have produced no increase in the MNB. The *expected* VoI can be quantified by the average gain in MNB from the collection of new data.

In general, VoI measures are always expressed as something like

$$\begin{aligned}\text{VoI measure} = {} & \text{Value of an } \textit{idealised} \text{ decision-making process} - \\ & \text{Value of the } \textit{current} \text{ decision-making process.}\end{aligned} \tag{12.1}$$

VoI analysis in practice

The nature of VoI analysis intrinsically considers a hypothetical future scenario in which, somehow, we are able to *gain more information in order to reduce or eliminate uncertainty in some or all the model parameters.* In practice, this is most likely an idealised situation, which may be impossible to obtain. More importantly, we do this analysis *before* we get to see any new data – the point of VoI is exactly to quantify the potential benefits of running the extra analysis prior to actually investing the money to do it!

For this reason, in addition to performing uncertainty analysis, VoI is used as a tool for *research prioritisation* – the idea that we can identify what specific parameters we should investigate out of the many that characterise our model. Thus, when performing VoI, there are two important consequences.

Firstly, any VoI measure in itself is only meaningful in *expectation* – it is the various forms of *Expected* Value of Information that are helpful to us. This is because we do not have the actual new data yet, but we can try and quantify what we expect to gain from them, if we are actually able to collect them.

As a consequence, Equation 12.1 is meaningful (and drive how VoI measures are constructed) when we take relevant expectations on both sides. The second term on the right-hand side of Equation 12.1 is represented by

$$\max_t \mathrm{E}_{\boldsymbol{\theta}} \left[\mathrm{NB}_t(\boldsymbol{\theta})\right],$$

which determines the treatment that, given current evidence, is associated with the highest expected utility. The first term depends on the idealised process, as we clarify in Equations 12.2, 12.3 and 12.9. In all cases, however, it involves a suitable expectation of a relevant maximisation – essentially flipping around the order of the two operations, in comparison to the term related to the current decision-making process.

The second important point to make about VoI practical calculation is that it is essentially a predictive measure (see for instance the analysis in Example 3.1 in Section 3.2). In other words, we use the information arisen from the *current* analysis/modelling to obtain this expectation.

Even more specifically, this means that the basis for the computation of any measure of VoI is in the uncertainty analysis for the current model (see Section 4.3 and Table 4.1, in particular).

In terms of interpretation, the main complexity of Equation 12.1 is that there is no natural upper bound. VoI measures are positive (because, in the worst-case scenario, there is no gain in MNB), but it is not possible to define an absolute scale and thus it is hard to assess directly "*how low is a low VoI*".

This suggests that we must take other factors into account – for instance the actual cost of acquisition of the new evidence (e.g. the conduct of a confirmatory RCT). In addition, we should consider carefully what is the (subgroup in the) population that would be mostly affected both by the technology under evaluation and by the evidence collected. Finally, another important consideration is about the time horizon over which the new intervention/evidence are assumed to bear an impact. We return to these points particularly in Section 12.5.

Table 12.1: A tabular representation of the process of uncertainty analysis of a fictional decision-making model, including a VoI analysis to determine the EVPI

	Parameter simulations				Expected utility		VoI analysis	
Sims	θ_1	θ_2	...	θ_Q	$\text{NB}_1(\boldsymbol{\theta})$	$\text{NB}_2(\boldsymbol{\theta})$	$\text{NB}^*(\boldsymbol{\theta})$	$\text{OL}(\boldsymbol{\theta})$
1	0.58	0.38	...	0.42	*77480*	67795	77480	9685
2	0.51	0.02	...	0.08	87165	*106535*	106535	0
3	0.61	0.14	...	0.06	*58110*	38740	58110	19370
4	0.2	0.73	...	0.73	77480	*87165*	87165	0
...	...	...	...	...	...	...	...	...
$S = 1000$	0.03	0.2	...	0.56	48425	*87165*	87165	0
				Average:	72365.35	77403.49	91192.02	13788.53

In addition, from the pragmatic point of view, there are important computational and modelling issues, which have for a very long time impaired the establishment of VoI as a principled and applicable methodology to perform uncertainty analysis in HTA. These have been largely overcome in recent times, with a large body of literature devoted to devising methods for fast and reliable computation of various VoI measures, which we review particularly in Section 12.4 and Section 12.5.

12.3 Expected value of perfect information

There are, roughly speaking, three different measures for VoI. The simplest (and in many ways less useful) is the *Expected Value of Perfect Information* (EVPI).

We can think of this as a highly idealised scenario in which we are able to collect evidence that can completely remove all uncertainty in all the model parameters. Clearly, this is pretty much an impossibility, as it would amount to a study with infinite sample size to learn perfectly all the relevant parameters $\boldsymbol{\theta}$. Despite this, the EVPI is a useful measure to grasp the basic concept of VoI and it can be proved that it places an upper limit to the amount of money that we should be willing to invest to improve the decision-making process.

One effective way of thinking about this problem is to consider a PSA table, such as that described in Table 4.1, or, more specifically, the one shown in Table 12.1. Here, we assume that our economic model is characterised by Q parameters $\boldsymbol{\theta} = (\theta_1, \ldots, \theta_Q)$ and that we are able to produce a MCMC analysis in which we obtain $S = 1000$ simulations from the posterior distribution $p(\boldsymbol{\theta} \mid \boldsymbol{y})$, for some suitable data $\boldsymbol{y}$. For each simulated value of the parameters, we can construct the net benefit associated with two relevant options, a status quo $t = 1$ and the new intervention $t = 2$. Averaging over the S simulations allows us to compute the overall expected utilities, which are presented at the bottom of Table 12.1.

We can define

$$\begin{aligned} \text{EVPI} &= \text{E}_{\boldsymbol{\theta}}\left[\max_t \text{NB}_t(\boldsymbol{\theta})\right] - \max_t \text{E}_{\boldsymbol{\theta}}\left[\text{NB}_t(\boldsymbol{\theta})\right] \\ &= \text{E}_{\boldsymbol{\theta}}\left[\text{NB}^*(\boldsymbol{\theta})\right] - \mathcal{NB}^*, \end{aligned} \tag{12.2}$$

where, for each PSA simulation $s = 1, \ldots, S$ in Table 12.1, the quantity

$$\text{NB}^*(\boldsymbol\theta) = \max_t \text{NB}_t^{(s)}(\boldsymbol\theta)$$

is the row-wise maximum net benefit (i.e. the values typeset in italics in each row) and $\mathcal{NB}^*$ is defined in Equation 4.5. In this example, the EVPI amounts to $91\,192.02 - 77\,403.49 = 13\,788.53$.

In terms of Table 12.1, for each PSA simulation $s = 1, \ldots, S$, the *Opportunity Loss*

$$\text{OL}(\boldsymbol\theta) = \text{NB}^*(\boldsymbol\theta) - \text{NB}_{t^*}^{(s)}(\boldsymbol\theta)$$

is the row-wise difference between the maximum net benefit $\text{NB}^*(\boldsymbol\theta)$ and the net benefit for the overall most cost-effective intervention, $t^* = \arg\max \text{E}_{\boldsymbol\theta}\left[\text{NB}_t(\boldsymbol\theta)\right]$, which in this case is $t = 2$ – as is possible to see in the last row of Table 12.1, where the overall expected utilities are $\mathcal{NB}_2 = 77\,403.49 > \mathcal{NB}_1 = 72\,365.35$ (cfr. also Table 4.1).

Interestingly,

$$\begin{aligned}\text{E}_{\boldsymbol\theta}\left[\text{OL}(\boldsymbol\theta)\right] &= \text{E}_{\boldsymbol\theta}\left[\text{NB}^*(\boldsymbol\theta) - \text{NB}_{t^*}(\boldsymbol\theta)\right] = \text{E}_{\boldsymbol\theta}\left[\text{NB}^*(\boldsymbol\theta)\right] - \text{E}_{\boldsymbol\theta}\left[\text{NB}_{t^*}(\boldsymbol\theta)\right] \\ &= \text{E}_{\boldsymbol\theta}\left[\max_t \text{NB}_t(\boldsymbol\theta)\right] - \max_t \text{E}_{\boldsymbol\theta}\left[\text{NB}_t(\boldsymbol\theta)\right]\end{aligned}$$

and thus Equation 12.2 can be expressed equivalently as the average $\text{OL}(\boldsymbol\theta)$ – cfr. Table 12.1.

A typical EVPI analysis can be summarised against the grid of values for the willingness-to-pay, k, as in Figure 12.2.

Figure 12.2 shows a "kink" at around $k = 20100$, which indicates the "break-even point" (BEP), i.e. the value of the willingness to pay in correspondence of which the optimal decision changes. This explains why the EVPI is effectively a combination of two separate functions – one, increasing quite steeply and leading up to the BEP and the other, showing a much flatter shape, after the BEP. Generally speaking, expected VoI curves typically show behaviours such as this and may have multiple change-points, when the optimal decision changes over the range of willingness-to-pay thresholds selected.

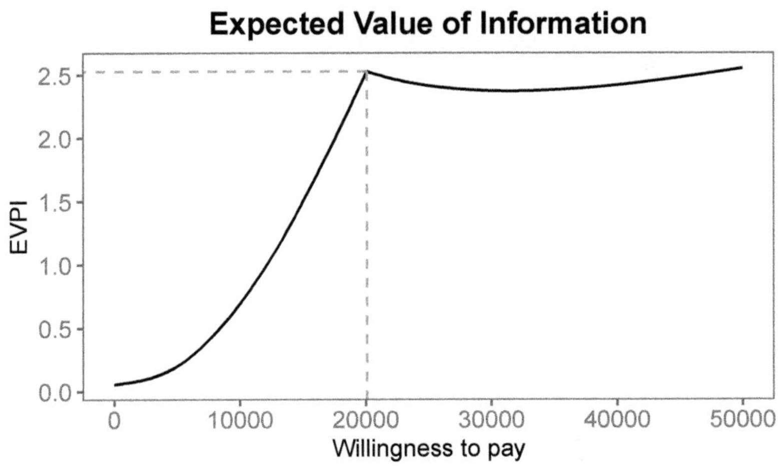

Figure 12.2: The analysis of the EVPI, as a function of different values for the willingness-to-pay threshold

In Figure 12.2, the y–axis represents the *monetary* value of expected information – in other words, the maximum amount that we should be prepared to pay to buy new data to completely eliminate the uncertainty on all the model parameters. In this particular case, this is at most £2.5 per individual, which is obviously very small, indicating that the impact of uncertainty in the decision-making process is probably negligible and thus we can use the current data to make a decision.

As mentioned above, however, in general it is a bit more complicated to interpret this value, because the absolute magnitude must be put in relation with the cost of acquisition of the new evidence. For instance, if EVPI = £1 000 000, we may argue that there is large value in reducing uncertainty and therefore we should consider deferring the decision until we get more data. But of course this depends on how much would the actual data-generating process cost – if, say, we could design a suitable trial at the cost of £3 000 000, then we would be in fact losing a substantial amount of money by doing it!

We return to this point more specifically in Section 12.5.1.

12.4 Expected value of partial perfect information

One of the ways in which we can relax the frankly unrealistic assumptions of the EVPI, i.e. that we can get all the information we need for all the model parameters, is to realise that, even if it were possible to completely eliminate the uncertainty, there may be some parameters that matter more to us. In other words, we can think of partitioning the vector of model parameters as $\boldsymbol\theta = (\boldsymbol\phi, \boldsymbol\psi)$, where $\boldsymbol\phi$ is the subset of the "parameters of interest" (often termed as "focal"), while $\boldsymbol\psi$ are the "remaining" or "nuisance" parameters.

The former may include quantities such as the prevalence of a disease, HRQL measures or length of stay in hospital, while the latter may be variables such as the cost of treatment with other established medications. The main idea here is that for some of the parameters, the uncertainty may just be beyond our control – for instance, if the cost of acquisition is not fixed, but determined by legal regulations, which we cannot modify.

In this particular scenario, the interest is in quantifying the value of gaining more information on $\boldsymbol\phi$, while leaving current level of uncertainty on $\boldsymbol\psi$ unchanged. The relevant VoI measure is referred to as *Expected Value of Partial Perfect Information* (EVPPI) and is defined as

$$\text{EVPPI} = \text{E}_{\boldsymbol\phi}\left[\max_t \text{E}_{\boldsymbol\psi|\boldsymbol\phi}[\text{NB}_t(\boldsymbol\theta)]\right] - \max_t \text{E}_{\boldsymbol\theta}[\text{NB}_t(\boldsymbol\theta)]. \qquad (12.3)$$

Intuitively, we think of this process along those lines: if we were truly able to learn *perfectly* the value of $\boldsymbol\phi$, while leaving $\boldsymbol\psi$ at the current uncertainty, the decision making process would be effected by looking at $\max_t \text{E}_{\boldsymbol\psi|\boldsymbol\phi}[\text{NB}_t(\boldsymbol\theta)]$, i.e. we would first compute the relevant expected utility associated with each treatment option and then we would maximise it to determine the most cost-effective option.

Of course, we cannot learn $\boldsymbol\phi$ with absolute certainty and thus the *idealised* decision process is in fact obtained by taking the average (with respect to the relevant parameters, $\boldsymbol\phi$) of this quantity. In line with Equation 12.1, we need to compare this with the current decision-making process, which is again defined as $\max_t \text{E}_{\boldsymbol\theta}[\text{NB}_t(\boldsymbol\theta)]$.

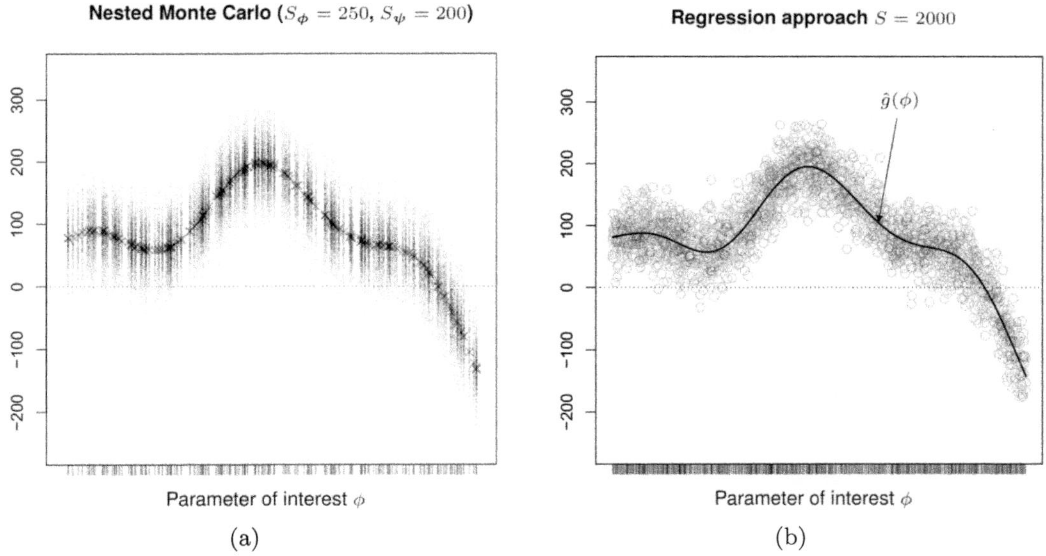

Figure 12.3: EVPPI as the relationship between the parameters of interest $\boldsymbol{\phi}$ and the conditional expectation of the *incremental* net benefit $\mathrm{E}_{\boldsymbol{\psi}|\boldsymbol{\phi}}[\mathrm{IB}_t(\boldsymbol{\theta})]$. Panel (a) shows the "brute force" approach based on nested Monte Carlo simulation, while panel (b) shows the regression-based approach. Source: Strong (2018)

In all but really trivial models, $\max_t \mathrm{E}_{\boldsymbol{\psi}|\boldsymbol{\phi}}[\mathrm{NB}_t(\boldsymbol{\theta})]$ is the element that contributes to the high computational complexity of this operation, because it involves a maximisation of an expectation, i.e. nested (typically complex and highly non-linear) integral operations.

For this reason, while the theoretical underpinning of the EVPPI is just as old as that of the much simpler EVPI, until very recently (particularly with the key contributions of Strong et al., 2014; and Heath et al., 2016) it has been virtually impossible to perform calculations for the EVPPI in realistically complex models.

12.4.1 Computing the EVPPI through brute force nested Monte Carlo

The simplest way of computing the EVPPI is through "brute force" and applying nested Monte Carlo integration. This assumes that we first simulate a large number of values, say S_ϕ from the marginal distribution of the parameters of interest, $\boldsymbol{\phi}$. Then, *conditionally* on each of these values, we simulate a further layer of nested simulation, say S_ψ values, from the conditional distribution $p(\boldsymbol{\psi} \mid \boldsymbol{\phi} = \boldsymbol{\phi}^{(s)})$, for each $s = 1, \ldots, S_\phi$.

For instance, assuming there are only two relevant interventions $t = 1, 2$ and thus $\mathrm{IB}(\boldsymbol{\theta}) = \mathrm{NB}_2(\boldsymbol{\theta}) - \mathrm{NB}_1(\boldsymbol{\theta})$, we can use these $S_\phi \times S_\psi$ simulations to characterise the distribution of the expected incremental benefit, as in Figure 12.3a.

Here, the ticks along the x–axis indicate the S_ϕ simulated values from the marginal distribution $p(\boldsymbol{\phi})$. For each of these values, the dots are the S_ψ simulations from the conditional distribution $p(\boldsymbol{\psi} \mid \boldsymbol{\phi} = \boldsymbol{\phi}^{(s)})$, which can be used to determine the expected incremental benefit, shown along the y–axis as the crosses. The decision-making process based on this representation would imply that whenever $\mathrm{E}[\mathrm{IB}(\boldsymbol{\theta})] > 0$ then the new treatment $t = 2$ would be deemed as more cost-effective, while in correspondence of values for $\boldsymbol{\phi}$ that are associated with $\mathrm{E}[\mathrm{IB}(\boldsymbol{\theta})] < 0$, then the status quo $t = 1$ would be preferred.

While this approach is reasonably easy to follow, it has the major drawback of being utterly inefficient, because in order to fully characterise both the marginal and the conditional distributions of interest, we will need a very large number of simulations for both layers – a typical recommendation is that S_{ϕ} and S_{ψ} should be in the order of 10 000 (Brennan et al., 2007), leading to a very large number of overall simulations.

Note 29: Non-additivity of the EVPPI

Another case in which the computation of the EVPPI is much simplified is when we consider a single parameter of interest, e.g. $\boldsymbol{\phi} = \theta_1$ and thus $\boldsymbol{\psi} = (\theta_2, \ldots, \theta_Q)$. In this case, we can probably use the nested MC approach discussed above; however, one additional complexity is that the EVPPI is a non-additive measure, i.e. in general

$$\text{EVPPI}(\phi_1, \phi_2) \neq \text{EVPPI}(\phi_1) + \text{EVPPI}(\phi_2).$$

Thus, the value of learning about multiple variables together can be higher, lower, or equal to the sum of their individual EVPPI values, due to potentially high dependencies in the decision-making process and interactions between uncertainties.

For this reason, while the univariate EVPPI analysis may be a helpful starting point, we should not rely on this if we are truly interested in groups of parameters.

12.4.2 Regression-based approximation to the EVPPI

Strong et al. (2014) introduced the idea of framing this problem within the context of non-linear regression. In this setup, we can consider the PSA simulations for the important parameters as a set of Q_{ϕ} "*observed* covariates" $\boldsymbol{X}$, while the resulting PSA simulations for the net benefit for each treatment considered as a vector of "*observed* outcomes" $\boldsymbol{y}$. Table 12.2 shows this situation using a fictional PSA simulation.

Notice that in this particular case, we slightly abuse the wording of our problem, since the "data" used to run the regression model are not really observed: rather, they are simulations

Table 12.2: PSA simulations from a fiction economic model. Here the full set of model parameters comprises of Q quantities, partitioned into Q_{ϕ} "important" and Q_{ψ} "remaining" parameters. The S simulations for the resulting net benefit function for treatment option t play the role of the "observed" outcome, $\boldsymbol{y}$, while the $S \times Q_{\phi}$ matrix of simulations for the important parameters is the "observed covariates", $\boldsymbol{X}$

	Outcome $\boldsymbol{y}$	Covariates $\boldsymbol{X}$				Nuisance parameters			
Sims	$\text{NB}_t(\boldsymbol{\theta})$	ϕ_1	ϕ_2	...	ϕ_{Q_ϕ}	ψ_1	ψ_2	...	ψ_{Q_ψ}
1	20814	0.97	0.39	...	0.01	0.02	0.24	...	0.57
2	41628	0.39	1.20	...	0.47	1.13	0.26	...	0.78
3	41628	0.19	0.70	...	0.18	-2.56	0.48	...	0.69
4	41628	0.53	0.44	...	0.02	0.08	0.57	...	0.01
...	...	...	...	...	...	...	...	...	...
S	48566	0.42	0.33	...	0.34	1.04	0.63	...	0.42

based on the current economic model, reflecting the current state of uncertainty about the model inputs.

In a nutshell, the idea is to model

$$\begin{aligned}\text{NB}_t(\boldsymbol{\theta}) &= \text{E}_{\boldsymbol{\psi}|\boldsymbol{\phi}}[\text{NB}_t(\boldsymbol{\theta})] + \varepsilon \\ &= g(\boldsymbol{\phi}) + \varepsilon, \end{aligned} \tag{12.4}$$

with $\varepsilon \sim \text{Normal}(0, \sigma_\varepsilon^2)$ and where $g(\boldsymbol{\phi})$ is an unknown, non-linear function that can be used to approximate as best as possible the unknown conditional expectation $\text{E}_{\boldsymbol{\psi}|\boldsymbol{\phi}}[\text{NB}_t(\boldsymbol{\theta})]$ – note that when taking the conditional expectation, the net benefit only depends on $\boldsymbol{\theta}$ through the subset $\boldsymbol{\phi}$ and hence so does the function $g(\cdot)$.

In comparison to the brute force approach, this can be *much* more efficient, because we only use a relatively small number of "data points", i.e. the S PSA simulations, which are usually in the order of a few thousands. Of course, we can extend the size of the MCMC simulations from the model parameters that we use to construct Table 12.2, but we would generally still require a much smaller sample size than in the nested MC case.

The main idea is shown graphically in Figure 12.3b: here, the circles represent the S PSA simulations from the distribution of $\boldsymbol{\phi}$ – notice that, in this case, we consider only $S = 2000$, as opposed to the $S_\phi \times S_\psi = 250 \times 200 = 50000$ nested MC simulations used in the brute force approach. We feed these "data points" to the regression model to estimate the function $\hat{g}_t\left(\boldsymbol{\phi}^{(s)}\right)$, which in turn can be used to approximate Equation 12.3 using the S PSA simulations as

$$\text{EVPPI} \approx \frac{1}{S}\sum_{s=1}^{S} \max_t \hat{g}_t\left(\boldsymbol{\phi}^{(s)}\right) - \max_t \frac{1}{S}\sum_{s=1}^{S} \hat{g}_t\left(\boldsymbol{\phi}^{(s)}\right).$$

Obviously, the main complexity of the regression-based approach is to effectively retrieve the underlying unknown, non-linear relationship that characterises the function $g(\cdot)$. Strong et al. (2014) and Heath et al. (2016) suggest either the use of Generalised Additive Models (GAMs, Hastie and Tibishirani, 1990; and Wood, 2017), or extensions based on Gaussian Process (GP) regression (Williams and Rasmussen, 2006), as very efficient options.

We quickly review both below, while Heath et al. (2024, specifically in sec. 3.4) present extended `R` code to use GAMs or GPs to compute the EVPPI in applied examples, using the `voi` package.

Generalised additive models

For each treatment option $t = 1, \ldots, T$, GAMs define

$$g_t(\boldsymbol{\phi}) = \sum_{q=1}^{Q_\phi} h_t\left(\phi_q^{(s)}\right), \tag{12.5}$$

where, again, Q_ϕ is the number of important parameters; $\phi_q^{(s)}$ is the $s-$th PSA simulation for the $q-$th important parameter; and the functions $h_t(\cdot)$ are piecewise polynomials, whose degree defines the smoothness of the $g_t(\cdot)$.

Much as splines (see Section 8.5.1), GAMs can be implemented as a frequentist or a Bayesian model. When using GAMs, the package `voi` is based on the implementation developed in the `R` package `earth` (Milborrow, 2011), which is in fact a frequentist analysis.

The "vanilla" implementation of GAMs uses one-dimensional splines for each parameter, which, as mentioned in Note 29 above, can be overly restrictive, particularly when parameters are highly correlated. To overcome this limitation, we can extend the formulation in Equation 12.5 to include interaction terms. This is generally very powerful, but tends to explode the computational complexity of the model, meaning that estimates should be based on a much larger PSA sample, thus reducing the advantages of the regression-based approach – see also Heath et al. (2024) and Baio et al. (2025a, pp. 113–124) for a much more technical and extensive description.

For this reason, when the number Q_{ϕ} of parameters included in $\boldsymbol{\phi}$ is sufficiently "large" say, above 5, GP regression can be used as an efficient alternative (Strong et al., 2014; Heath et al., 2016; Baio et al., 2025a).

Gaussian Process regression

The GP regression approach starts by considering for each treatment or intervention under consideration a multivariate regression model

$$\left(\text{NB}_t^{(1)}(\boldsymbol{\theta}), \text{NB}_t^{(2)}(\boldsymbol{\theta}), \ldots, \text{NB}_t^{(S)}(\boldsymbol{\theta})\right) \sim \text{Normal}(\boldsymbol{H}\boldsymbol{\beta}, \boldsymbol{\Sigma} + \sigma_\varepsilon^2 \boldsymbol{I}), \tag{12.6}$$

where

$$\boldsymbol{H} = \begin{pmatrix} 1 & \phi_1^{(1)} & \cdots & \phi_{Q_\phi}^{(1)} \\ 1 & \phi_1^{(2)} & \cdots & \phi_{Q_\phi}^{(2)} \\ \vdots & & \ddots & \\ 1 & \phi_1^{(S)} & \cdots & \phi_{Q_\phi}^{(S)} \end{pmatrix} \tag{12.7}$$

is a "design matrix" and $\boldsymbol{\phi}^{(s)}$ are the values of the s-th PSA simulations for the subset of important parameters, $\boldsymbol{\phi}$. The quantity σ_ε^2 is the residual variance from the regression construction, while $\boldsymbol{I}$ is a $(S \times S)$ identity matrix and $\boldsymbol{\beta} = (\beta_0, \ldots, \beta_{Q_\phi})$ is a vector of length $(Q_\phi + 1)$ of regression coefficients used to model the *linear* relationship between $\boldsymbol{\phi}$ and $\text{E}_{\boldsymbol{\psi}|\boldsymbol{\phi}}[\text{NB}_t(\boldsymbol{\theta})]$.

In a GP regression, the linear structure is rendered flexible by constructing the covariance matrix $\boldsymbol{\Sigma}$ in terms of a *covariance function* $\mathcal{C}(r,s)$, which can be used to describe the joint variability of any two "observed" points $\text{NB}_t^{(r)}(\boldsymbol{\theta})$ and $\text{NB}_t^{(s)}(\boldsymbol{\theta})$ – in our case, these are two PSA simulations for the net benefit.

The standard implementation of the GP regression model considers a squared exponential covariance function

$$\mathcal{C}_{\text{Exp}}(r,s) = \sigma^2 \exp\left[\sum_{q=1}^{Q_\phi}\left(\frac{\phi_q^{(r)} - \phi_q^{(s)}}{\delta_q}\right)^2\right]. \tag{12.8}$$

Here, σ^2 is the GP marginal variance, while the $q-$th element of the vector $\boldsymbol{\delta} = (\delta_1, \delta_2, \ldots, \delta_{Q_\phi})$ defines the "smoothness" of the relationship between two net benefit values with "similar" values for each of the $q-$th important parameter $\boldsymbol{\phi}_q$.

This model is more naturally Bayesian and we can specify a full set of prior distributions, including for the $(2Q_\phi + 3)$ hyperparameters $(\boldsymbol{\beta}, \boldsymbol{\delta}, \sigma, \sigma_\varepsilon)$. This, however, can still be very computationally intensive and thus, in practice, the estimates are obtained through numerical optimisation and, possibly, conjugate modelling (Strong et al., 2014).

Borrowing from the context of spatial and spatio-temporal modelling and Integrated Nested Laplace Approximation (INLA), Heath et al. (2016) suggest a revised version of the GP regression to speed up the computations – see for instance Blangiardo and Cameletti (2015); or Gómez-Rubio (2020), among others, as well as Section 3.1.2 for more details in INLA.

In a nutshell, the main idea is to re-formulate the regression model as

$$\left(\text{NB}_t^{(1)}(\boldsymbol{\theta}), \text{NB}_t^{(2)}(\boldsymbol{\theta}), \ldots, \text{NB}_t^{(S)}(\boldsymbol{\theta})\right) \sim \text{Normal}(\boldsymbol{H\beta} + f(\omega), \sigma_\varepsilon^2 \boldsymbol{I}),$$

in terms of the linear predictor $\boldsymbol{H\beta}$ and a "spatially structured" effect $f(\omega)$, which absorbs all the non-linearity and correlation among the parameters in $\boldsymbol{\phi}$. This spatial effect can be estimated efficiently using a combination of Stochastic Partially Differential Equations (SPDE – see Gómez-Rubio, 2020; Krainski et al., 2019; Lindgren et al., 2011 for more technical descriptions and insights) and INLA.

Intuitively, the main advantage of this process is that we can use a simple linear component and augment the model using, effectively, a specific random effect to obtain a non-linear, flexible estimate for the function $g_t(\cdot)$.

Spatial modelling and the EVPPI

Technically speaking, the spatial structure associated with ω implies that it should have a bi-dimensional nature – this is what happens in typical geostatistical analysis in which we model the correlation between points in the 2-d geographical space (e.g. two cities).

In the case of the EVPPI, the "space" is not so much a physical one, but rather is made by the $Q_{\boldsymbol{\phi}}$ important parameters. Heath et al. (2016) reconcile this by pre-processing the "covariates" (i.e. the simulations for the important parameters $\boldsymbol{\phi}$) using a data reduction technique referred to as *Principal Fitted Components* (Cook and Forzani, 2008), which effectively projects the $Q_{\boldsymbol{\phi}}$–dimensional space of the parameters into a smaller number of principal components – we can use the first two to recreate the spatial structure required to use efficiently the SPDE-INLA method.

If the correlation among the $Q_{\boldsymbol{\phi}}$ parameters is such that the first two components are not sufficient to fully explain all the non-linearity in $g_t(\cdot)$ (and thus to estimate the EVPPI sufficiently accurately), then we can add a number of bi-dimensional spatially structured effects, based on the first few principal fitted components (Heath et al., 2016).

Bayesian Additive Regression Trees

Bayesian Additive Regression Trees (BARTs) are a machine learning flexible and powerful tool used to make predictions and understand relationships in data, particularly suited to model problems such as those in Equation 12.4. We only provide here a very non-technical and sketched introduction to them and refer the interested reader to the original publication in Chipman et al. (2010), or the excellent review by Hill et al. (2020).

In a nutshell, BART predicts the function $g(\boldsymbol{\phi})$ by combining many simple binary decision trees, used to recursively partition the space of the "covariates" $\boldsymbol{\phi}$ into subsets, based on simple splitting rules, e.g. in the form $\phi_q < c$, for some randomly generated cutoff c. Each tree makes a small contribution to the overall prediction and thus estimating the function using only a single tree would result in a very rough approximation. However, using a large number of trees as an "ensemble" estimate allows to capture complex patterns without the need to specify them upfront.

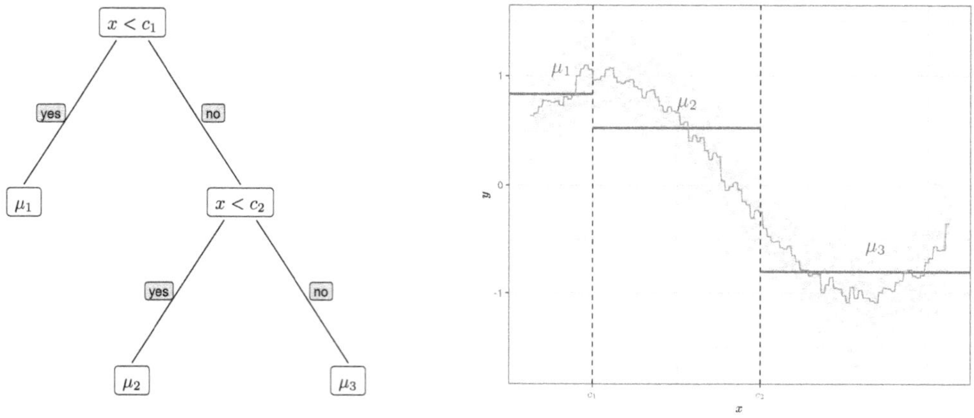

(a) (b)

Figure 12.4: A graphical overview of the BART process. Panel (a) shows how the tree splits the data, based on a randomly generated set of cutoffs (here, c_1 and c_2, for generality). Panel (b) shows the piecewise estimate (horizontal line, labelled as μ_1, μ_2 and μ_3), derived from a single tree and as the sample mean of the subsets of data in which $x < c_1$, $x \in (c_1, c_2)$ and $x > c_2$, respectively. The grey curve overlaid on the observed data (the grey points) is the "ensemble" estimate, obtained summing over all the trees (in this case, 200). Source: Martin et al. (2021)

Figure 12.4 shows this process graphically. Figure 12.4a depicts the decision tree for a fictional case in which we only consider a single covariate x and a decision rule based on cutoffs c_1 and c_2. For each tree that we decide to consider in the process, the parameters μ_1, μ_2, μ_3 are estimated by the data, e.g. using the observed sample mean for the outcome y in the subset where $x < c_1$, or where $x \in (c_1; c_2)$ or where $x > c_2$, respectively.

Figure 12.4b shows the estimated configuration for one particular run (i.e. a single tree). As is possible to see, this is a very rough approximation of the underlying relationship between x and y – in this case, we are basically fitting a piecewise function to the data. However, if we use a large enough number of trees, then the ensemble combination (which effectively is some kind of weighted average of all the trees) will be flexible enough to estimate the underlying sinusoidal relationship between x and y (shown by the grey points).

In order to avoid overfitting for any of the single trees used to approximate the function $g(\cdot)$, BART uses a naturally Bayesian approach and suitable "regularisation" priors, to ensure that each tree contributes to a limited part of the overall estimation, guaranteeing much flexibility in the resulting estimate. Posterior inference in BARTs can be done using suitable MCMC extensions, usually embedding Metropolis within Gibbs samplers (see Section 2.3).

In line with its machine learning nature, BART is specifically designed for regression models including a large number of predictors and thus it may work particularly well to compute the EVPPI when Q_ϕ is very large, thus overcoming some of the computational limitations of GAMs and GP regression, although this comes at the expenses of the smoothness with which the resulting estimated function is produced. The package voi implements BART as one of the strategies to compute the EVPPI.

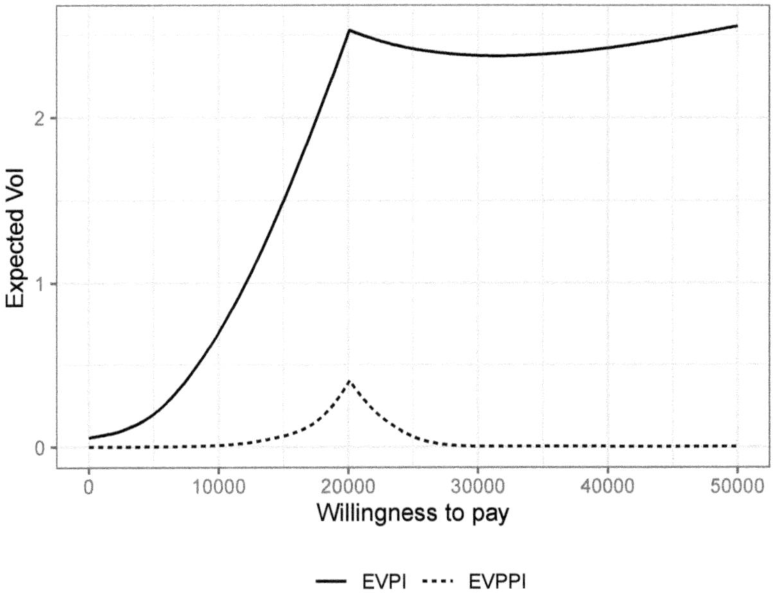

Figure 12.5: The analysis of the EVPPI, as a function of different values for the willingness-to-pay threshold.

12.4.3 Interpreting the EVPPI

Heath et al. (2024) and the `voi` package website `https://chjackson.github.io/voi`, as well as the help functions for the package `BCEA` contain several worked examples on how to compute the EVPPI (note that objects created by `BCEA` are in the correct format and can thus be passed as input to the `voi::evppi()` function). We focus here more on the interpretation of the results.

Figure 12.5 shows the analysis of the EVPPI for three of the model parameters[1]. We can compare the EVPPI (the dashed curve) with the EVPI, computed in Figure 12.2. In fact, the EVPI is the theoretical upper bound for the EVPPI.

In this case, the three parameters contribute relatively marginally to the overall uncertainty – recall that the overall EVPI was perhaps already rather limited (cfr. the discussion in Section 12.3) and thus, given the large number of parameters characterising the model, the combination of this three only determines a fraction of the overall EVPI.

We can also quantify the individual impact of each model parameter in terms of the "single-parameter" EVPPI. `BCEA` terms this the "Info Rank plot" (Baio et al., 2025a), shown in Figure 12.6.

This gives a general indication of the ranking of the various parameters, in terms of their contribution to the overall EVPI and can then be used as a guide to identify which ones are those that should be investigated further. Note however that, as suggested earlier, VoI measures are *not* additive and thus it is possible that a parameter is associated with a very

[1]Technically, this is the "Vaccine" model considered in the `BCEA` package and described in Baio et al. (2025a). The model includes 56 parameters.

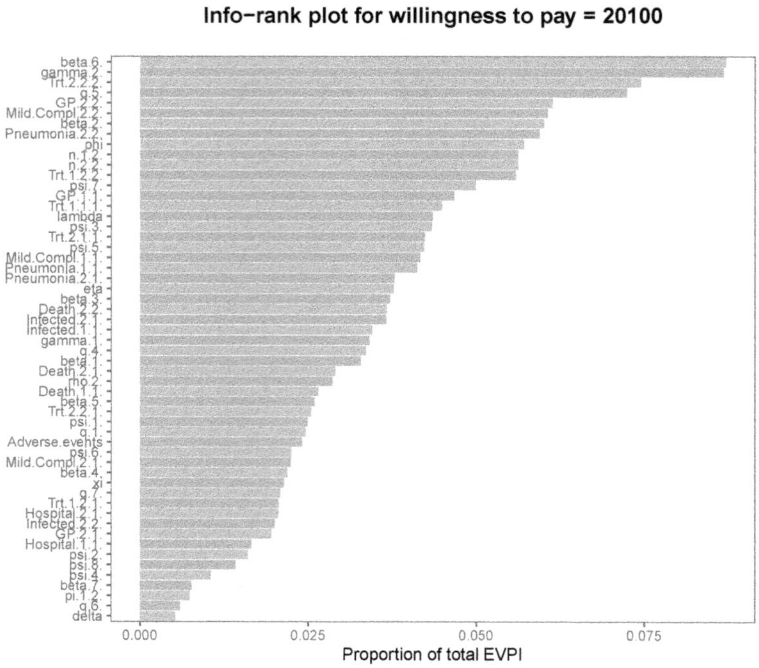

Figure 12.6: The analysis of the EVPPI for single parameters

low single EVPPI, only to interact strongly with another parameter – and thus their joint EVPPI might be very large.

12.5 Expected value of sample information

The final and most helpful measure of VoI is the *Expected Value of Sample Information* (EVSI). Here, the main idea is to relax the unrealistic assumption of perfect information even further and consider a situation in which we ask ourselves how much it is worth to get *some* sample information on specific parameters.

The main idea is visualised in Figure 12.7: the top panel is similar to Figure 4.1 and describes the current decision-making process. We collect data (potentially based on a variety of sources, such as literature review, clinical trials and expert opinion), with which we estimate a set of relevant parameters $\boldsymbol{\theta}$. These, in turn, inform the economic model, which is used to derive the optimal decision, based on current evidence and our model assumptions (see the discussion in Section 4.2).

The bottom panel of Figure 12.7 describes the "third option", i.e. the possibility that, instead of making a decision based on current evidence, we stop and collect new data. The current uncertainty on the model parameters (which is effectively a posterior distribution, based on the observed data) would be used as the prior before observing new data. We can define a sampling mechanism that determines the way in which a potential study would occur and if we actually obtain these new data, then we would update our current uncertainty on $\boldsymbol{\theta}$ into a posterior (given the new data $\boldsymbol{X}$).

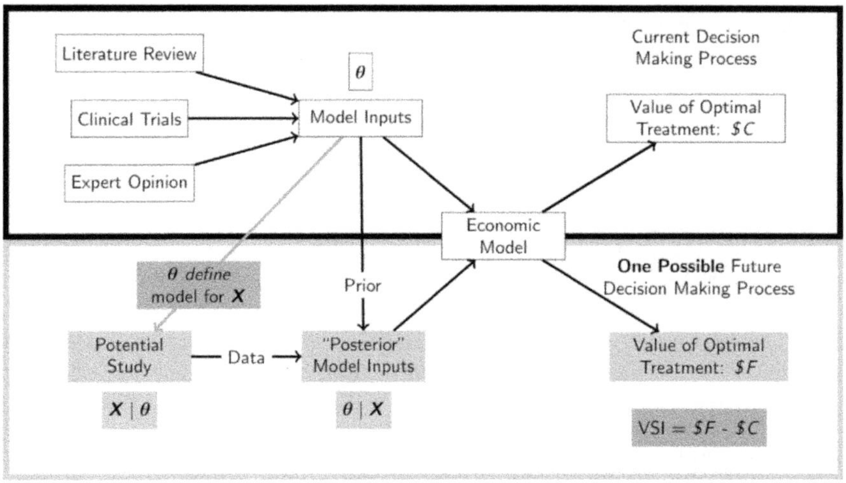

Figure 12.7: A schematic representation of the philosophy underpinning the analysis of the EVSI. Source: Heath et al. (2024)

Then we would feed these estimates onto the same economic model and with that obtain a revised decision analysis. The difference between the current value of the optimal treatment ($\$C$ in the top panel of Figure 12.7) and the revised possible future decision-making process ($\$F$ in the bottom panel of Figure 12.7) is the value of the sample information that we would have accrued.

Of course, we have not yet obtained the new study and therefore we must include the uncertainty generated by the sampling distribution of the data collection process and average over it to compute

$$\text{EVSI} = \text{E}_{\boldsymbol{X}} \left[\max_t \ \text{E}_{\boldsymbol{\theta}|\boldsymbol{X}} \left[\text{NB}_t(\boldsymbol{\theta}) \right] \right] - \max_t \text{E}_{\boldsymbol{\theta}} \left[\text{NB}_t(\boldsymbol{\theta}) \right], \tag{12.9}$$

where $\text{E}_{\boldsymbol{\theta}|\boldsymbol{X}} \left[\text{NB}_t(\boldsymbol{\theta}) \right]$ represents the value of the decision based on sample information $\boldsymbol{X}$ we may get to see (for a given study design) and, as usual $\text{E}_{\boldsymbol{\theta}} \left[\text{NB}_t(\boldsymbol{\theta}) \right]$ is the value of the decision made under current evidence.

In Equation 12.9, because the actual data collection has not happened yet, we must also include an outer expectation with respect to the sampling process $\text{E}_{\boldsymbol{X}}[\cdot]$ – this adds to the computational complexity to the point that the EVSI was largely just a theoretical concept until the advent of the modern computation techniques described above for the calculation of the EVPPI.

Heath et al. (2024) present detailed accounts of various methods can be used to estimate the value of Equation 12.9, given a specific design and a mechanism to describe the sample variability inherent in the potential collection of data $\boldsymbol{X}$. These include regression-based tools (effectively the same as in Section 12.4.2), methods that rely on importance sampling (Menzies, 2016) or Gaussian approximation (Jalal et al., 2015; Jalal and Alarid-Escudero, 2018) and moment matching (Heath et al., 2019). The `voi` package also includes a vignette with worked examples (available at `https://cran.r-project.org/web/packages/voi/vignettes/voi.html`).

Here, we do not concentrate on the technicalities; instead, we simply highlight the fact that working under an EVSI perspective is just a sensible way of planning future research: not only would we be assessing whether we have enough information in the current evidence in order to make a decision; we would only consider the value-for-money of a potential data collection and thus decide on key features such as design and sample size, in order to maximise the economic value of the new study and subsequent decision-making process.

Example 12.1. *Chemotherapy (adapted from Heath et al., 2024).* We consider here the Chemotherapy example, originally included in Baio et al. (2025a) and then expanded in Heath et al. (2024).

This is based on a Markov model describing the natural history of the disease for a cohort of cancer patients, for whom a specific form of chemotherapy is a viable therapeutic option. The EVSI is the expected value of a two-arm trial with a binary outcome of whether a patient experiences side-effects. The trial is only used to inform the log odds ratio of side effects between treatments and information about the baseline risk of side effects is ignored.

The details of the modelling structure are not too important, here, but they can be found in the `voi` vignette at `https://cran.r-project.org/web/packages/voi/vignettes/plots.html`, which also includes `R` code to generate the analyses and the plots.

Figure 12.8 shows the computed EVSI across a range of potential sample sizes, depending on different values for the underlying willingness-to-pay threshold (in a range from 0 to 50 000 monetary units).

Interestingly, the analysis of Figure 12.8 shows how the EVPI acts as an upper bound to the EVPPI, which in turn acts as an upper bound for the EVSI, when the sample size of the potential data increases sufficiently.

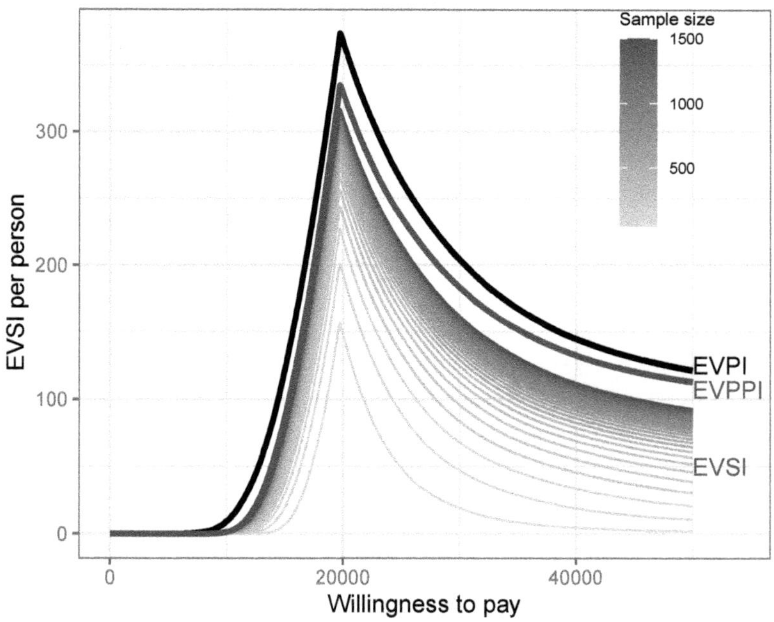

Figure 12.8: Analysis of the EVSI by willingness-to-pay threshold, over different assumed sample sizes. The EVSI peaks at around the break-even point (close to 20 000 monetary units) and it becomes increasingly small for larger values of the willingness-to-pay.

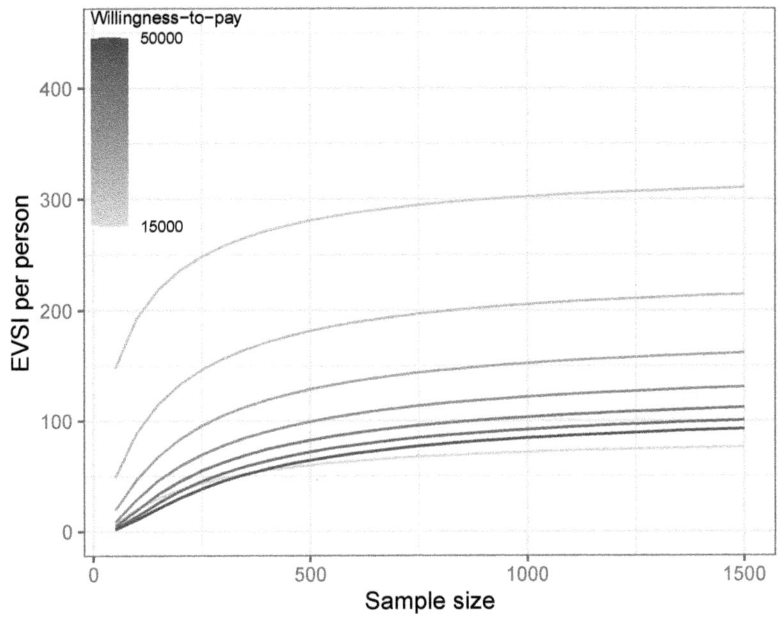

Figure 12.9: Analysis of the EVSI by sample size, over several willingness-to-pay thresholds. In this case, increasingly large sample sizes have marginally lower value as the curves tend to flatten out substantially.

The value of the data collection is marginally decreasing: after a while, there is no point in getting larger and larger sample sizes, as the curves are almost flat at around 1500, along the x–axis.

12.5.1 Expected net benefit of sampling

We can make better sense of the analysis of the EVSI by considering the actual economic value of a given study in terms of the *Expected Net Benefit of Sampling* (ENBS). This is defined as

$$\text{ENBS} = \text{EVSI} - \text{expected cost of the study}.$$

Here, by "cost of the study" we include the setup cost (e.g. to create the suitable infrastructure needed to deliver an intervention), the cost per individual necessary to buy the intervention (e.g. a given drug), as well as potential other items, including incentives to reduce drop-out. In addition, we typically want to scale this up to the intended target population for whom the technology under investigation will be used and the time horizon that we assume it will be active (e.g. before a new intervention is introduced and replaces the current one as the gold standard).

Of course, these may be complicated to estimate with precision – for instance, we may look into research pipelines to see how many studies are currently being conducted on a given pharmacological indication to get a sense of what the market might look like in the near future. Nevertheless, the ENBS framework forces us to think along those lines, which is helpful to anchor our analysis of the value-for-money of research and the future, potential introduction/reimbursement of a given technology in the real world.

Example 12.2. *Chemotherapy (continued): expected net benefit of sampling analysis.* Consider first a "standard" sample size calculation that would be performed to design the study. Recall that we are considering here a trial that will investigate the proportion of side effects observed under two interventions. The background probability in the "control" arm (standard of care) is set to $\theta_1 = 0.47$, from extensive background knowledge and in order to compute the required sample size, we need to make assumptions on the magnitude of the treatment effect (for the chemotherapy arm).

If we work in terms of OR and assume a substantial reduction in side effects for the chemotherapy, say

$$\text{OR} = \left(\frac{\theta_2}{1-\theta_2} \bigg/ \frac{\theta_1}{1-\theta_1} \right) = 0.55,$$

this also implies that the probability of side effects in the chemotherapy arm is

$$\theta_2 = \frac{\theta_1 \text{OR}}{1 - \theta_1 + (\theta_1 \text{OR})} \approx 0.37.$$

We can use standard power calculations and the following R code to produce the "power curve" depicted in Figure 12.10.

```
# Basic assumptions
theta1=0.47
OR=0.55
theta2=(theta1*OR)/(1-theta1+(theta1*OR))

# Standard sample size calculations
ssc=power.prop.test(
  p1=theta1,          # assumed proportion of side effects in the controls
  p2=theta2,          # assumed proportion of side effects in the treatment arm
  sig.level=0.05,     # significance level (to test p1=p2)
  n=seq(0,1500,10)  # grid of potential sample sizes
)
```

Typically, we select the sample size associated with a value of the power curve of at least some pre-specified threshold, often set at 0.8. In this case, following this rule, the trial would be designed to consider a sample size of $n = 190$ per arm – in Figure 12.10, this is the point along the x–axis in correspondence of which the power curve intercepts the threshold of 0.8, indicated by the dashed line.

If we perform the analysis based on the ENBS, instead, we obtain the results shown in Figure 12.11. Following the voi vignette, we stipulate that the costs of the study include a fixed setup cost, which we assume ranges between 5 000 000 and 10 000 000 monetary units (say, £), as well as a cost per individual, assumed to range between 14 000 and 21 000 monetary units. We also explicitly consider a target population of around 46 000 patients who would be affected by the change in practice from the standard of care to the chemotherapy and a time horizon of 10 years (over which we apply an annual discount rate of 3.5%) – all the details are described more thoroughly in Heath et al. (2024).

The analysis of Figure 12.11 shows clearly that the "standard" trial would not optimise the economic value of the study: for a sample size of $n = 190$ and assuming a willingness-to-pay threshold for the underlying economic analysis of $k = 20\,000$ monetary units, the overall ENBS is approximately 77 115 463. This is much lower than the maximum value in the

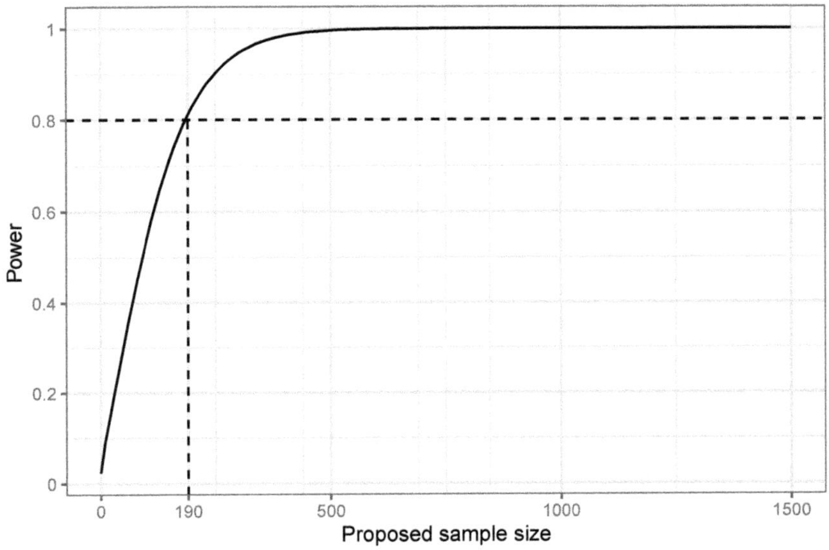

Figure 12.10: Power calculations for the proposed study. The power function reaches a value of 0.8 for around 190 patients per arm.

curve of Figure 12.11, which for a sample size of $n = 450$ reaches the maximum value of ENBS $= 84\,091\,443$.

Perhaps, we may not afford to recruit a total of 450 patients per arm, in our trial and thus we may need to settle for lower economic value. In any case, the analysis

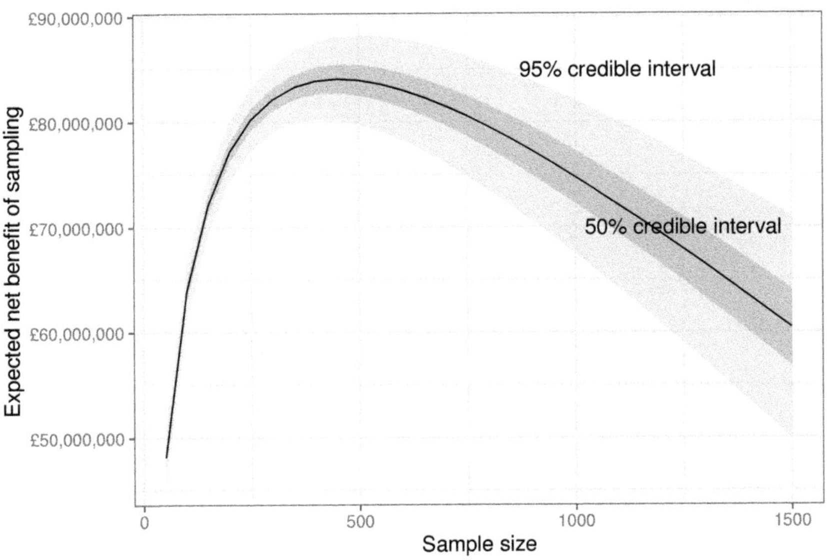

Figure 12.11: Expected Net Benefit of Sampling for the proposed study. Using this analysis, we are able to determine the actual estimated economic value of the data collection for different choices of the sample size. Increasingly large samples tend to produce decreasing marginal returns and a sample size of around 450 optimises the economic value of the study.

of the ENBS provides a more appropriate assessment of the value for money that we are implying with the specific study design and thus considerations of suitable compromise in terms of the sample size would be made on the relevant monetary scale.

12.6 Conclusions

Although VoI has not been fully included in the normal workflow and processes for HTA, there have been several instances in which regulators have started to open up to this methodology and its application for uncertainty analysis, research prioritisation and planning.

VoI has many important features, particularly within the HTA problem, notably the fact that all the design and analysis is grounded in the full economic evaluation. This has implications even just at the design of the study, because basing it on VoI would force the analyst to construct a model of analysis that closely aligns with it, thus rendering the full evaluation potentially more relevant.

References

Akaike, H., 1974. A new look at the statistical model identification. IEEE Transactions on Automatic Control 19, 716–723.

Alvares, D., Lázaro, E., Gómez-Rubio, V., Armero, C., 2021. Bayesian survival analysis with BUGS. Statistics in Medicine 40, 2975–3020.

Bailey, J., Webster, R., Hunter, R., Griffin, M., Freemantle, N., Rait, G., et al., 2016. The Men's Safer Sex project: intervention development and feasibility randomised controlled trial of an interactive digital intervention to increase condom use in men. Health Technology Assessment 20, 1.

Baio, G., 2025. Introduction to statistical modelling, in: Baio, G., Thom, H., Pechivanoglou, P. (Eds), R for Health Technology Assessment. Chapman and Hall/CRC.

Baio, G., 2020. survHE: survival analysis for health economic evaluation and cost-effectiveness modeling. Journal of Statistical Software 95, 1–47.

Baio, G., 2012. Bayesian Methods in Health Economics. CRC Press, Boca Raton, FL.

Baio, G., Heath, A., Berardi, A., Green, N., 2025a. Bayesian Cost-Effectiveness Analysis with the R Package BCEA, 2nd ed. Springer.

Baio, G., Thom, H., Pechlivanoglou, P. eds, 2025b. R for Health Technology Assessment. Chapman and Hall/CRC.

Barnsley, P., Towse, A., Sussex, J., et al., 2013. Critique of CHE research paper 81: Methods for the estimation of the NICE cost effectiveness threshold. Office of Health Economics Research Papers 81.

Bayes, T., 1763. Essay Towards Solving a Problem in the Doctrine of Chances. Philosophical Transactions of the Royal Society of London 53, 370–418.

Beeken, R., Leurent, B., Vickerstaff, V., Wilson, R., Croker, H., Morris, S., et al., 2017. A brief intervention for weight control based on habit-formation theory delivered through primary care: results from a randomised controlled trial. International Journal of Obesity 41, 246–254.

Benaglia, T., Jackson, C., Sharples, L.D., 2015. Survival extrapolation in the presence of cause specific hazards. Statistics in Medicine 34, 796–811.

Bernardo, J., Smith, A., 1999. Bayesian Theory. John Wiley and Sons, New York, NY.

Bertsch McGrayne, S., 2011. The Theory That Would Not Die: How Bayes' Rule Cracked the Enigma Code, Hunted Down Russian Submarines, and Emerged Triumphant from Two Centuries of Controversy. Yale University Press, New Haven, CT.

Betancourt, M., 2018. A Conceptual Introduction to Hamiltonian Monte Carlo. URL `https://arxiv.org/abs/1701.02434`

Black, W.C., 1990. The CE plane: A graphic representation of cost-effectiveness. Medical Decision Making 10, 212–214.

Blangiardo, M., Cameletti, M., 2015. Spatial and Spatio-temporal Bayesian Models with R-INLA. John Wiley and Sons, Chichester, UK.

Blangiardo, M., Cameletti, M., Baio, G., Rue, H., 2013. Spatial and spatio-temporal models with R-INLA. Spatial and Spatio-temporal Epidemiology 7, 39–55.

Box, G., 1979. Robustness in the strategy of scientific model building, in: Robustness in Statistics. Elsevier, pp. 201–236.

Brennan, A., Kharroubi, S., O'Hagan, A., Chilcott, J., 2007. Calculating partial expected value of perfect information via Monte Carlo sampling algorithms. Medical Decision Making 27, 448–470.

Briggs, A, Sculpher, M., Claxton, K., 2006. Decision Modelling for Health Economic Evaluation. Oxford University Press.

Brooks, S., Gelman, A., 1998. General methods for monitoring convergence of iterative simulations. Journal of Computational and Graphical Statistics 7, 434–455.

Brooks, S., Gelman, A., Jones, G., Meng, X., 2011. Handbook of Markov Chain Monte Carlo. Chapman and Hall/CRC.

Bürkner, P.C., 2017. brms: An R package for Bayesian multilevel models using Stan. Journal of Statistical Software 80, 1–28.

Burnham, K., Anderson, D., 2002. Model Selection and Multimodel Inference, 2nd ed. Springer.

Burnham, K., Anderson, D., 1998. Model Selection and Inference. Springer.

Campbell, H., Margossian, C., Jansen, J., Gustafson, P., 2026. Don't Disregard the Data for Lack of a Likelihood: Bayesian Synthetic Likelihood for Enhanced Multilevel Network Meta-Regression. URL https://arxiv.org/abs/2603.11019

Carlin, B., Herring, A., 2015. A conversation with Alan Gelfand. Statistical Science 413–422.

Caro, J., Ishak, J., 2010. No head-to-head trial? Simulate the missing arms. PharmacoEconomics 28, 957–967.

Carpenter, B., Gelman, A., Hoffman, M., Lee, D., Goodrich, B., Betancourt, M., et al., 2017. Stan: A probabilistic programming language. Journal of Statistical Software 76.

Carpenter, J., Bartlett, J., Morris, T., Wood, A., Quartagno, M., Kenward, M., 2023. Multiple Imputation and Its Application. John Wiley and Sons, Chichester, UK.

Chancellor, J.V., Hill, A.M., Sabin, C.A., Simpson, K.N., Youle, M., 1997. Modelling the cost effectiveness of lamivudine/zidovudine combination therapy in HIV infection. PharmacoEconomics 12, 54–66.

Che, Z., Green, N., Baio, G., 2023. Blended survival curves: A new approach to extrapolation for time-to-event outcomes from clinical trials in health technology assessment. Medical Decision Making 43, 299–310.

Chipman, H.A., George, E., McCulloch, R., 2010. BART: Bayesian additive regression trees. Annals of Applied Statistics 266–298.

Claxton, K., Lacey, L.F., Walker, S.G., 2000. Selecting treatments: A decision theoretic approach. Journal of the Royal Statistical Society: Series A 163, 211–225.

Claxton, K., Martin, S., Soares, M., Rice, N., Spackman, E., Hinde, S., et al., 2015. Implications for a policy threshold, in: Methods for the Estimation of the National Institute for Health and Care Excellence Cost-Effectiveness Threshold. NIHR Journals Library.

Claxton, K., Sculpher, M., 2025. Agreeing to the demands for higher branded drug prices in the UK will have significant negative effects on public health, social care and economic growth (Open Letter to the UK Prime Minister). Centre for Health Economics, University of York.

Cook, R., Forzani, L., 2008. Principal fitted components for dimension reduction in regression. Statistical Science 23, 485–501.

Cooper, N., Sutton, A., Abrams, K., Turner, D., Wailoo, A., 2004. Comprehensive decision analytical modelling in economic evaluation: A Bayesian approach. Health Economics 13, 203–226.

Cox, C., 2008. The generalized F distribution: an umbrella for parametric survival analysis. Statistics in Medicine 27, 4301–4312.

Cox, D., 1972. Regression models and life-tables. Journal of the Royal Statistical Society: Series B 34, 187–202.

Csárdi, G., Hester, J., Wickham, H., Chang, W., Morgan, M., Tenenbaum, D., 2024. remotes: R Package Installation from Remote Repositories, Including 'GitHub'. URL https://remotes.r-lib.org

Daniels, M., Hogan, J., 2008. Missing Data in Longitudinal Studies: Strategies for Bayesian Modeling and Sensitivity Analysis. Chapman and Hall/CRC.

Daniels, M., Xu, D., 2020. Bayesian Methods for Longitudinal Data with Missingness, in: Lesaffre, E., Baio, G., Boulanger, B. (Eds), Bayesian Methods in Pharmaceutical Research. Chapman and Hall/CRC.

De Angelis, R., Capocaccia, R., Hakulinen, T., Soderman, B., Verdecchia, A., 1999. Mixture models for cancer survival analysis: Application to population-based data with covariates. Statistics in Medicine 18, 441–454.

de Finetti, B., 1974. Theory of Probability. John Wiley and Sons, New York, NY.

Degeling, K., Clements, M., Koffijberg, E., O'Mahony, J., Sadatsafavi, M., Pechlivanoglou, P., 2025. Discrete Event Simulations in R, in: Baio, G., Thom, H., Pechivanoglou, P. (Eds), R for Health Technology Assessment. Chapman and Hall/CRC.

DeGroot, M., 1970. Optimal Statistical Decisions. John Wiley and Sons, New York, NY.

Demiris, N., Lunn, D., Sharples, L.D., 2015. Survival extrapolation using the poly-Weibull model. Statistical Methods in Medical Research 24, 287–301.

Dias, S., Ades, A., Welton, N., Jansen, J., Sutton, A., 2018. Network Meta-analysis for Decision-making. John Wiley and Sons, Chichester, UK.

Dias, S., Welton, N., Sutton, A., Caldwell, D., Lu, G., Ades, A., 2013. Evidence synthesis for decision making 4: Inconsistency in networks of evidence based on randomized controlled trials. Medical Decision Making 33, 641–656.

Diggle, P., Kenward, M., 1994. Informative drop-out in longitudinal data analysis. Journal of the Royal Statistical Society Series C 43, 49–73.

Donaldson, C., Farrar, S., Mapp, T., Walker, A., Macphee, S., 1997. Assessing community values in health care: Is the 'willingness to pay' method feasible? Health Care Analysis 5, 7–29.

Donegan, S., Williamson, P., D'Alessandro, U., Garner, P., Tudur Smith, C., 2013. Combining individual patient data and aggregate data in mixed treatment comparison meta-analysis: Individual patient data may be beneficial if only for a subset of trials. Statistics in Medicine 32, 914–930.

Drummond, M.F., Sculpher, M.J., Claxton, K., Stoddart, G.L., Torrance, G.W., 2015. Methods for the Economic Evaluation of Health Care Programmes. Oxford University Press.

Duane, S., Kennedy, A.D., Pendelton, B.J., Roweth, D., 1987. Hybrid Monte Carlo. Physics Letter B 195, 216–222.

Edney, L., Haji Ali Afzali, H., Cheng, T., Karnon, J., 2018. Estimating the reference incremental cost-effectiveness ratio for the Australian health system. PharmacoEconomics 36, 239–252.

Efron, B., Tibshirani, R., 1994. An introduction to the bootstrap. Chapman and Hall/CRC.

Fenwick, E., Claxton, K., Sculpher, M., 2001. Representing uncertainty: The role of cost-effectiveness acceptability curves. Health Economics 10, 779–787.

Fienberg, S., 2006. When Did Bayesian Inference Become Bayesian? Bayesian Analysis 1, 1–40.

Friedman, H.S., 2021. Ultimate Price: The Value We Place on Life. University of California Press.

Gabrio, A., 2024. missingHE: Missing Outcome Data in Health Economic Evaluation. URL https://cran.r-project.org/web/packages/missingHE

Gabrio, A., Daniels, M., Baio, G., 2020. A Bayesian parametric approach to handle missing longitudinal outcome data in trial-based health economic evaluations. Journal of the Royal Statistical Society Series A 183, 607–629.

Gabrio, A., Mason, A., Baio, G., 2019. A full Bayesian model to handle structural ones and missingness in economic evaluations from individual-level data. Statistics in Medicine 38, 1399–1420.

Gabrio, A., Mason, A., Leurent, B., Gomes, G., 2025. Missing Data, in: Baio, G., Thom, H., Pechivanoglou, P. (Eds), R for Health Technology Assessment. Chapman and Hall/CRC.

Gamerman, D., 1997. Markov Chain Monte Carlo. Chapman and Hall/CRC.

Gao, C., Heath, A., Baio, G., 2025. Regression augmented weighting adjustment for indirect comparisons in health decision modelling. Research Synthesis Methods 16, 900–921.

Gelfand, A., Smith, A., 1990. Sampling-based approaches to calculating marginal densities. Journal of the American Statistical Association 85, 398–409.

Gelman, A., 2006. Prior distributions for variance parameters in hierarchical models. Bayesian Analysis 515–533.

Gelman, A., Carlin, J.B., Stern, H.S., Dunson, D., Vehtari, A., Rubin, D., 2013. Bayesian Data Analysis, 3rd ed. Chapman and Hall/CRC, New York, NY.

Gelman, A., Hill, J., 2007. Data Analysis Using Regression and Multilevel/Hierarchical Models. Cambridge University Press, Cambridge, UK.

Gelman, A., Rubin, D., 1992. Inference from iterative simulation using multiple sequences. Statistical Science 7, 457–472.

Geman, S., Geman, D., 1984. Stochastic relaxation, Gibbs distributions, and the Bayesian restoration of images. IEEE Transactions on Pattern Analysis and Machine Intelligence 6, 721–741.

Gilks, W., Richardson, S., Spiegelhalter, D., 1996. Markov Chain Monte Carlo in Practice. Chapman and Hall/CRC.

Gómez-Rubio, V., 2020. Bayesian Inference with INLA. Chapman and Hall/CRC.

Goodman, S.N., 1999. Toward evidence-based medical statistics. 1: The P value fallacy. Annals of Internal Medicine 130, 995–1004.

Goudie, R., Turner, R., De Angelis, D., Thomas, A., 2020. MultiBUGS: a parallel implementation of the BUGS modelling framework for faster Bayesian inference. Journal of Statistical Software 95.

Grant, R., Di Tanna, G.L., 2025. Bayesian Meta-analysis: A Practical Introduction. CRC Press, Boca Raton, FL.

Green, N., Gao, C., Remiro Azócar, A., 2026. outstandR: Model-Based Standardisation for Indirect Treatment Comparison with Limited Subject-Level Data. URL https://StatisticsHealthEconomics.github.io/outstandR/

Green, N., Krijkamp, E., Thom, H., Dixon, P., 2025a. Decision Tree Models, in: Baio, G., Thom, H., Pechivanoglou, P. (Eds), R for Health Technology Assessment. Chapman and Hall/CRC.

Green, N., Kurt, M., Moshyk, A., Larkin, J., Baio, G., 2025b. A Bayesian hierarchical mixture cure modelling framework to utilize multiple survival datasets for long-term survivorship estimates: A case study from previously untreated metastatic melanoma. Statistics in Medicine 44, e70132.

Greenland, S., Pearl, J., Robins, J., 1999. Confounding and collapsibility in causal inference. Statistical Science 14, 29–46.

Guyot, P., Ades, A., Ouwens, M., Welton, N., 2012. Enhanced secondary analysis of survival data: reconstructing the data from published Kaplan-Meier survival curves. BMC Medical Research Methodology 12, 1–13.

Hallek, M., Fischer, K., Fingerle-Rowson, G., Fink, A., Busch, R., Mayer, J., et al., 2010. Addition of rituximab to fludarabine and cyclophosphamide in patients with chronic lymphocytic leukaemia: A randomised, open-label, phase 3 trial. The Lancet 376, 1164–1174.

Hardcastle, L., Livingstone, S., Baio, G., 2025. Averaging polyhazard models using piecewise deterministic Monte Carlo with applications to data with long-term survivors. Annals of Applied Statistics 19, 3179–3202.

Hasselblad, V., 1998. Meta-analysis of multitreatment studies. Medical Decision Making 18, 37–43.

Hastie, T., Tibishirani, R., 1990. Generalized Additive Models. CRC Press.

Hastings, W., 1970. Monte Carlo sampling methods using Markov chains and their applications. Biometrika 97–59.

Heath, A., Kunst, N., Jackson, C., 2024. Value of Information for Healthcare Decision-making. CRC Press.

Heath, A., Manolopoulou, I., Baio, G., 2019. Estimating the expected value of sample information across different sample sizes using moment matching and nonlinear regression. Medical Decision Making 39, 347–359.

Heath, A., Manolopoulou, I., Baio, G., 2016. Estimating the expected value of partial perfect information in health economic evaluations using integrated nested Laplace approximation. Statistics in Medicine 35, 4264–4280.

Hernán, M.A., 2010. The hazards of hazard ratios. Epidemiology 21, 13–15.

Hill, J., Linero, A., Murray, J., 2020. Bayesian additive regression trees: A review and look forward. Annual Review of Statistics and Its Application 7, 251–278.

Hoffman, M.D., Gelman, A., 2013. The No-U-Turn Sampler: Adaptively Setting Path Lengths in Hamiltonian Monte Carlo. Journal of Machine Learning Research 15, 1351–1385.

Howard, R., 1966. Information Value Theory, in: IEEE Transactions on System Science and Cybernetics. SCC-2, (1) 22-26.

Incerti, D., Jansen, J.P., 2021. hesim: Health Economic Simulation Modeling and Decision Analysis. URL `https://arxiv.org/abs/2102.09437`

Ishak, J., Proskorovsky, I., Benedict, A., 2015. Simulation and matching-based approaches for indirect comparison of treatments. PharmacoEconomics 33, 537–549.

Jackman, S., 2009. Bayesian Analysis for the Social Sciences. John Wiley and Sons, New York, NY.

Jackson, C., 2023. Survextrap: A package for flexible and transparent survival extrapolation. BMC Medical Research Methodology 23, 282.

Jackson, C., 2016. flexsurv: a platform for parametric survival modeling in R. Journal of Statistical Software 70.

Jackson, C., 2015. Slides for the Summer School 'Bayesian methods in health economics''. URL `https://gianluca.statistica.it/teaching/summer-school/`

Jackson, C., Heath, A., 2024. voi: Expected Value of Information. URL `https://cran.r-project.org/web/packages/voi`

Jackson, C.H., Thompson, S.G., Sharples, L.D., 2009. Accounting for uncertainty in health economic decision models by using model averaging. Journal of the Royal Statistical Society: Series A 172, 383–404.

Jackson, C., Latimer, N., Jansen, J., Pechlivanoglou, P., Baio, G., 2025. Introduction to survival analysis in HTA, in: Baio, G., Thom, H., Pechivanoglou, P. (Eds), R for Health Technology Assessment. Chapman and Hall/CRC.

Jackson, C., Sharples, L., Thompson, S., 2010. Survival models in health economic evaluations: Balancing fit and parsimony to improve prediction. The International Journal of Biostatistics 6.

Jalal, H., Alarid-Escudero, F., 2018. A gaussian approximation approach for value of information analysis. Medical Decision Making 38, 174–188.

Jalal, H., Goldhaber-Fiebert, J., Kuntz, K., 2015. Computing expected value of partial sample information from probabilistic sensitivity analysis using linear regression metamodeling. Medical Decision Making 35, 584–595.

Jansen, J.P., 2011. Network meta-analysis of survival data with fractional polynomials. BMC Medical Research Methodology 11, 1–14.

Jansen, J.P., Vieira, M., Cope, S., 2015. Network meta-analysis of longitudinal data using fractional polynomials. Statistics in Medicine 34, 2294–2311.

Jeffreys, H., 1961. Theory of Probability. Clarendon Press, Oxford, UK.

Joe, H., 2014. Dependence modeling with copulas. CRC Press, Boca Raton, FL.

Kaplan, E., Meier, P., 1958. Nonparametric estimation from incomplete observations. Journal of the American Statistical Association 53, 457–481.

Keng, M.J., Schlackow, I., Pullenayegum, E., 2025. Individual level data, in: Baio, G., Thom, H., Pechivanoglou, P. (Eds), R for Health Technology Assessment. Chapman and Hall/CRC.

Krainski, E., Gómez-Rubio, V., Bakka, H., Lenzi, A., Castro-Camilo, D., Simpson, D., et al., 2019. Advanced Spatial Modeling with Stochastic Partial Differential Equations Using R and INLA. Chapman and Hall/CRC.

Kruschke, J., 2015. Doing Bayesian Data Analysis: A Tutorial with R and JAGS and Stan, 2nd ed. Academic Press.

Laplace, P., 1812. Thorie analytique des probabilités. Veuve Courcier, Paris, France.

Laplace, P., 1774. Mémoires sur la probabilité des causes par les événemens. Mémoires de mathématique et de physique presentés à l'Académie royale des sciences, par divers sçavans & lûs dans ses assemblées 6, 621–656.

Latimer, N., 2011. NICE DSU Technical Support Document 14. Undertaking survival analysis for economic evaluations alongside clinical trials - extrapolation with patient-level data. URL `https://sheffield.ac.uk/media/34225/download?attachment`

Latimer, N., Henshall, C., Siebert, U., Bell, H., 2016. Treatment switching: Statistical and decision-making challenges and approaches. International Journal of Technology Assessment in Health Care 32, 160–166.

Latimer, N., Rutherford, M.J., 2024. Mixture and non-mixture cure models for health technology assessment: What you need to know. PharmacoEconomics 42, 1073–1090.

Lindgren, F., Rue, H., Lindström, J., 2011. An explicit link between Gaussian fields and Gaussian Markov random fields: the stochastic partial differential equation approach. Journal of the Royal Statistical Society: Series B 73, 423–498.

Lindley, D., 1972. Bayesian statistics: A review. SIAM.

Little, R., 1993. Pattern-mixture models for multivariate incomplete data. Journal of the American Statistical Association 88, 125–134.

Little, R., Rubin, D.B., 2019. Statistical Analysis with Missing Data. John Wiley and Sons, New York, NY.

Loomes, G., McKenzie, L., 1989. The use of QALYs in health care decision making. Social Science and Medicine 28, 299–308.

Lu, G., Ades, A., 2006. Assessing evidence inconsistency in mixed treatment comparisons. Journal of the American Statistical Association 101, 447–459.

Lu, G., Ades, A., 2004. Combination of direct and indirect evidence in mixed treatment comparisons. Statistics in Medicine 23, 3105–3124.

Luce, B.R., Drummond, M., Jönsson, B., Neumann, P.J., Schwartz, J.S., Siebert, U., et al., 2010. EBM, HTA, and CER: clearing the confusion. The Milbank Quarterly 88, 256–276.

Lunn, D., Jackson, C., Best, N., Thomas, A., Spiegelhalter, D., 2013. The BUGS Book. Chapman and Hall/CRC.

Lunn, D., Spiegelhalter, D., Thomas, A., Best, N., 2009. The BUGS project: Evolution, critique and future directions. Statistics in Medicine 28(25), 3049–3067.

Mamun, A.A., Peeters, A., Barendregt, J., Willekens, F., Nusselder, W., Bonneux, L., 2004. Smoking decreases the duration of life lived with and without cardiovascular disease: a life course analysis of the Framingham Heart Study. European Heart Journal 25, 409–415.

Martin, O., Kumar, R., Lao, J., 2021. Bayesian Modeling and Computation in Python. Chapman and Hall/CRC.

Mason, A., Gomes, M., Carpenter, J., Grieve, R., 2021. Flexible Bayesian longitudinal models for cost-effectiveness analyses with informative missing data. Health Economics 30, 3138–3158.

McCabe, C., Claxton, K., Culyer, A., 2008. The NICE cost-effectiveness threshold: what it is and what that means. PharmacoEconomics 26, 733–744.

McElreath, R., 2015. Statistical Rethinking: A Bayesian Course with Examples in R and Stan. Chapman and Hall/CRC, Boca Raton, FL.

Meng, X.-L., 1994. Multiple-imputation inferences with uncongenial sources of input. Statistical Science 538–558.

Menzies, N., 2016. An efficient estimator for the expected value of sample information. Medical Decision Making 36, 308–320.

Metropolis, N., Rosenbluth, A., Rosenbluth, M., Teller, A., Teller, E., 1953. Equation of state calculations by fast computing machines. The Journal of Chemical Physics 21, 1087–1092.

Milborrow, S., 2011. Earth: Multivariate adaptive regression splines. URL `https://cran.r-project.org/web/packages/earth`

Mullahy, J., 1986. Specification and testing of some modified count data models. Journal of Econometrics 33, 341–365.

Müller, K., Wickham, H., 2025. tibble: Simple Data Frames. URL `https://tibble.tidyverse.org/`

National Institute for Health and Care Excellence [NICE], 2025. Changes to NICE's cost-effectiveness thresholds confirmed. URL `https://www.nice.org.uk/news/articles/changes-to-nice-s-cost-effectiveness-thresholds-confirmed`

National Institute for Health and Care Excellence [NICE], 2016. The Social Care Guidance Manual. URL `https://www.nice.org.uk/process/pmg10`

National Institute for Health and Care Excellence [NICE], 2009. Rituximab for the first-line treatment of chronic lymphocytic leukaemia. URL `https://www.nice.org.uk/guidance/ta174/resources/rituximab-for-the-firstline-treatment-of-chronic-lymphocytic-leukaemia-pdf-82598435675845`

Neal, R., 2011. MCMC Using Hamiltonian Dynamics, in: Brooks, S., Gelman, A., Jones, G., Meng, X. (Eds), Handbook of Markov Chain Monte Carlo. Chapman and Hall/CRC.

Neumann, P.J., Cohen, J.T., 2018. QALYs in 2018—advantages and concerns. Journal of the American Medical Association 319, 2473–2474.

NIMBLE Development Team, 2016. NIMBLE: An R Package for Programming with BUGS models, Version 0.5-1. URL `http://r-nimble.org`

O'Mahony, J., Paulden, M., 2014. NICE's selective application of differential discounting: ambiguous, inconsistent, and unjustified. Value in Health 17, 493–496.

Ochalek, J., Wang, H., Gu, Y., Lomas, J., Cutler, H., Jin, C., 2020. Informing a cost-effectiveness threshold for health technology assessment in China: A marginal productivity approach. PharmacoEconomics 38, 1319–1331.

Office for National Statistics [ONS], 2024. Adult Smoking Habits in the UK: 2023. URL `https://www.ons.gov.uk/releases/adultsmokinghabitsintheuk2023`

Phillippo, D., 2024. multinma: Bayesian Network Meta-Analysis of Individual and Aggregate Data. URL `https://dmphillippo.github.io/multinma/`

Phillippo, D., Ades, A., Dias, S., Palmer, S., Abrams, K., Welton, N., 2018. Methods for population-adjusted indirect comparisons in health technology appraisal. Medical Decision Making 38, 200–211.

Phillippo, D., Ades, A., Palmer, S., Abrams, K., Welton, N., 2016. NICE DSU Technical Support Document 18. Methods for population-adjusted indirect comparisons in submissions to NICE. URL https://sheffield.ac.uk/media/34216/download?attachment

Phillippo, D., Dias, S., Ades, A., Belger, M., Brnabic, A., Schacht, A., et al., 2020. Multilevel network meta-regression for population-adjusted treatment comparisons. Journal of the Royal Statistical Society: Series A 183, 1189–1210.

Phillippo, D., Dias, S., Ades, A., Welton, N., 2023. Calibration of treatment effects in network meta-analysis using individual patient data. Statistics in Medicine 42, 2376–2397.

Phillippo, D., Dias, S., Welton, N., Ades, A., 2024. Multilevel network meta-regression for general likelihoods: Synthesis of individual and aggregate data with applications to survival analysis. URL https://arxiv.org/abs/2401.12640

Phillippo, D., Jansen, J., Remiro Azócar, A., Thom, H., 2025a. Population-Adjusted Indirect Comparisons, in: Baio, G., Thom, H., Pechivanoglou, P. (Eds), R for Health Technology Assessment. Chapman and Hall/CRC.

Phillippo, D., Remiro Azócar, A., Heath, A., Baio, G., Dias, S., Ades, A., et al., 2025b. Effect modification and non-collapsibility together may lead to conflicting treatment decisions: A review of marginal and conditional estimands and recommendations for decision-making. Research Synthesis Methods 1–27.

Plummer, M., 2023. rjags: Bayesian Graphical Models using MCMC. URL https://cran.r-project.org/web/packages/rjags

Plummer, M., 2010. JAGS: Just Another Gibbs Sampler. URL https://sourceforge.net/projects/mcmc-jags/files/Manuals/4.x/jags_user_manual.pdf/download

Plummer, M., 2008. Penalized loss functions for Bayesian model comparison. Biostatistics 9, 523–539.

Polack, F., Thomas, S., Kitchin, N., Absalon, J., Gurtman, A., Lockhart, S., et al., 2020. Safety and efficacy of the BNT162b2 mRNA Covid-19 vaccine. New England Journal of Medicine 383, 2603–2615.

Raftery, A., Lewis, S., 1995. The number of iterations, convergence diagnostics and generic Metropolis algorithms, in: Gilks, W., Spiegelhalter, D., Richardson, S. (Eds), Markov Chain Monte Carlo in Practice. Chapman and Hall/CRC.

Raftery, A., Lewis, S., 1992. [Practical Markov Chain Monte Carlo]: comment: one long run with diagnostics: implementation strategies for Markov Chain Monte Carlo. Statistical Science 7, 493–497.

Raiffa, H., 1968. Decision Analysis: Introductory Lectures on Choices under Uncertainty. Addison-Wesley.

Raiffa, H., Schlaifer, H., 1961. Applied Statistical Decision Theory. Harvard University Press, Boston, MA.

Ramsay, J., 1988. Monotone regression splines in action. Statistical Science 425–441.

Rawlins, M., Culyer, A., 2004. National Institute for Clinical Excellence and its value judgments. British Medical Journal 329, 224–227.

Remiro Azócar, A., 2025. Slides for the Summer School 'Bayesian methods in health economics'. URL https://gianluca.statistica.it/teaching/summer-school/

Remiro Azócar, A., Heath, A., Baio, G., 2024. Model-based standardization using multiple imputation. BMC Medical Research Methodology 24, 32.

Remiro Azócar, A., Heath, A., Baio, G., 2022. Parametric G-computation for compatible indirect treatment comparisons with limited individual patient data. Research Synthesis Methods 13, 716–744.

Remiro Azócar, A., Heath, A., Baio, G., 2021. Methods for population adjustment with limited access to individual patient data: A review and simulation study. Research Synthesis Methods 12, 750–775.

Robert, C., Casella, G., 2011. A short history of Markov Chain Monte Carlo: Subjective recollections from incomplete data. Statistical Science 26, 102–115.

Robert, C., Casella, G., 2010. Introducing Monte Carlo Methods with R. Springer Verlag, New York, NY.

Robert, C., Casella, G., 2004. Monte Carlo Statistical Methods, 2nd ed. Springer Verlag, New York, NY.

Robins, J., 1986. A new approach to causal inference in mortality studies with a sustained exposure period—application to control of the healthy worker survivor effect. Mathematical Modelling 7, 1393–1512.

Robins, J., Hernán, M., Brumback, B., 2000. Marginal structural models and causal inference in epidemiology. Epidemiology 11, 550–560.

Rosenbaum, P., Rubin, D., 1984. Reducing bias in observational studies using subclassification on the propensity score. Journal of the American Statistical Association 79, 516–524.

Rosenbaum, P., Rubin, D., 1983. The central role of the propensity score in observational studies for causal effects. Biometrika 70, 41–55.

Royston, P., Altman, D.G., 1994. Regression using fractional polynomials of continuous covariates: Parsimonious parametric modelling. Journal of the Royal Statistical Society Series C 43, 429–453.

Rubin, D., 1987. Multiple Imputation for Non-response in Surveys. Wiley.

Rubin, D., 1977. Formalizing subjective notions about the effect of nonrespondents in sample surveys. Journal of the American Statistical Association 72, 538–543.

Rubin, D., 1976. Inference and missing data. Biometrika 63, 581–592.

Rue, H., Martino, S., Chopin, N., 2009. Approximate Bayesian inference for latent Gaussian models by using integrated nested Laplace approximations. Journal of the Royal Statistical Society: Series B 71, 319–392.

Russo, P., Zanuzzi, M., Carletto, A., Sammarco, A., Romano, F., Manca, A., 2023. Role of economic evaluations on pricing of medicines reimbursed by the Italian National Health Service. PharmacoEconomics 41, 107–117.

Sampson, C., Zamora, B., Watson, S., Cairns, J., Chalkidou, K., Cubi-Molla, P., et al., 2022. Supply-side cost-effectiveness thresholds: Questions for evidence-based policy. Applied Health Economics and Health Policy 20, 651–667.

Saramago, P., Sutton, A., Cooper, N., Manca, A., 2012. Mixed treatment comparisons using aggregate and individual participant level data. Statistics in Medicine 31, 3516–3536.

Schneider, P., 2022. The QALY is ableist: on the unethical implications of health states worse than dead. Quality of Life Research 31, 1545–1552.

Schwarz, G., 1978. Estimating the dimension of a model. The Annals of Statistics 461–464.

Sharples, L.D., Demiris, N., 2020. Survival analysis and censored data, in: Bayesian Methods in Pharmaceutical Research. Chapman and Hall/CRC, pp. 207–222.

Signorovitch, J., Sikirica, V., Erder, M., Xie, J., Lu, M., Hodgkins, P., et al., 2012. Matching-adjusted indirect comparisons: A new tool for timely comparative effectiveness research. Value in Health 15, 940–947.

Signorovitch, J., Wu, E., Yu, A., Gerrits, C., Kantor, E., Bao, Y., et al., 2010. Comparative effectiveness without head-to-head trials: A method for matching-adjusted indirect comparisons applied to psoriasis treatment with adalimumab or etanercept. Pharmacoeconomics 28, 935–945.

Simpson, D., Rue, H., Riebler, A., Martins, T.G., Sørbye, S.H., 2017. Penalising model component complexity: A principled, practical approach to constructing priors. Statistical Science 32, 1–28.

Siverskog, J., Henriksson, M., 2019. Estimating the marginal cost of a life year in Sweden's public healthcare sector. The European Journal of Health Economics 20, 751–762.

Sklar, M., 1959. Fonctions de répartition à n dimensions et leurs marges, in: Annales de l'institut de Statistique de l'université de Paris. pp. 229–231.

Spiegelhalter, D., Abrams, K., Myles, J., 2004. Bayesian Approaches to Clinical Trials and Health-Care Evaluation. John Wiley and Sons, Chichester, UK.

Spiegelhalter, D., Best, N., Carlin, B., Van Der Linde, A., 2002a. Bayesian measures of model complexity and fit. Journal of the Royal Statistical Society: Series B 64, 583–639.

Spiegelhalter, D., Thomas, A., Best, N., 2002b. WinBUGS version 1.4. MRC Biostatistics Unit, Cambridge, UK.

Spiegelhalter, D., Thomas, A., Best, N., Gilks, W., 1996. BUGS 0.5: Bayesian inference using Gibbs sampling manual (version ii). MRC Biostatistics Unit, Institute of Public Health, Cambridge, UK 1–59.

Stadhouders, N., Koolman, X., Dijk, C. van, Jeurissen, P., Adang, E., 2019. The marginal benefits of healthcare spending in the Netherlands: Estimating cost-effectiveness thresholds using a translog production function. Health Economics 28, 1331–1344.

Stan development team, 2024. Stan Modeling Language Users Guide and Reference Manual. URL `https://mc-stan.org`

Stigler, S., 1982. Thomas Bayes's Bayesian inference. Journal of the Royal Statistical Society: Series A 145, 250–258.

Strong, M., 2018. Slides for the Summer School 'Bayesian methods in health economics'. URL `https://gianluca.statistica.it/teaching/summer-school/`

Strong, M., Oakley, J., Brennan, A., 2014. Estimating multiparameter partial expected value of perfect information from a probabilistic sensitivity analysis sample: A nonparametric regression approach. Medical Decision Making 34, 311–326.

Sturtz, S., Ligges, U., Gelman, A., 2019. R2OpenBUGS: a package for running OpenBUGS from R. URL `https://cran.r-project.org/web/packages/R2OpenBUGS`

Sturtz, S., Ligges, U., Gelman, A., 2005. R2WinBUGS: A package for running WinBUGS from R. Journal of Statistical Software 12, 1–16.

Su, Y., Yajima, M., 2010. R2jags User manual: A Package to call jags from R. URL `https://cran.r-project.org/web/packages/R2jags`

Sutton, A., Cooper, N., Jones, D., Lambert, P., Thompson, J., Abrams, K., 2008. Evidence synthesis as the key to more coherent and efficient research. BMC Medical Research Methodology 8, 3.

The EuroQol Group, 1990. EuroQol-a new facility for the measurement of health-related quality of life. Health Policy 16, 199–208.

Thom, H., Incerti, D., Jackson, C., Lamrock, F., Williams, C., 2025a. Continuous Time Multistate Models, in: Baio, G., Thom, H., Pechivanoglou, P. (Eds), R for Health Technology Assessment. Chapman and Hall/CRC.

Thom, H., Saramago, P., Soares, M., Krijkamp, E., Lamrock, F., 2025b. Cohort Markov models in discrete time, in: Baio, G., Thom, H., Pechivanoglou, P. (Eds), R for Health Technology Assessment. Chapman and Hall/CRC.

Thompson, S., Nixon, R., 2005. How sensitive are cost-effectiveness analysis to choice of parametric distributions? Medical Decision Making 14, 421–428.

Turner, D., Wailoo, A., Nicholson, K., Cooper, N., Sutton, A., Abrams, K., 2003. Systematic review and economic decision modelling for the prevention and treatment of influenza A and B: neuraminidase inhibitors for treatment. Health Technology Assessment 7.

Vallejo-Torres, L., García-Lorenzo, B., Serrano-Aguilar, P., 2018. Estimating a cost-effectiveness threshold for the Spanish NHS. Health Economics 27, 746–761.

van Baal, P., Perry-Duxbury, M., Bakx, P., Versteegh, M., Van Doorslaer, E., Brouwer, W., 2019. A cost-effectiveness threshold based on the marginal returns of cardiovascular hospital spending. Health Economics 28, 87–100.

van Buuren, S., 2018. Flexible Imputation of Missing Data, 2nd ed. Chapman and Hall/CRC, Boca Raton, FL, USA.

Van Hout, B.A., Al, M.J., Gordon, G.S., Rutten, F.F., 1994. Costs, effects and C/E-ratios alongside a clinical trial. Health Economics 3, 309–319.

Vanness, D.J., Lomas, J., Ahn, H., 2021. A health opportunity cost threshold for cost-effectiveness analysis in the United States. Annals of Internal Medicine 174, 25–32.

Vehtari, A., Gabry, J., Magnusson, M., Yao, Y., Bürkner, P., Paananen, T., et al., 2024. loo: Efficient leave-one-out cross-validation and WAIC for Bayesian models. URL `https://mc-stan.org/loo/`

Vehtari, A., Gelman, A., Gabry, J., 2017. Practical Bayesian model evaluation using leave-one-out cross-validation and WAIC. Statistics and Computing 27, 1413–1432.

Wabersich, D., Vandekerckhove, J., 2014. Extending JAGS: A tutorial on adding custom distributions to JAGS (with a diffusion model example). Behavior Research Methods 46, 15–28.

Wang, W., Yan, J., 2021. Shape-Restricted Regression Splines with R Package splines2. Journal of Data Science 19.

Wang, X., Yue, Y.R., Faraway, J., 2018. Bayesian regression modeling with INLA. Chapman and Hall/CRC.

Ware, J., Sherbourne, D., 1992. The MOS 36-item short-form health survey (SF-36). Conceptual Framework. Medical Care 30, 473–83.

Welton, N., 2018. Slides for the Summer School 'Bayesian methods in health economics'. URL `https://gianluca.statistica.it/teaching/summer-school/`

Welton, N., Sutton, A., Cooper, N., Abrams, K., Ades, A., 2012. Evidence Synthesis for Decision Making in Healthcare. John Wiley and Sons, Chichester, UK.

Wickham, H., 2016. ggplot2: Elegant Graphics for Data Analysis. Springer-Verlag, New York, NY.

Wickham, H., Averick, M., Bryan, J., Chang, W., D'Agostino McGowan, L., François, R., et al., 2019. Welcome to the tidyverse. Journal of Open Source Software 4, 1686.

Wickham, H., François, R., Henry, L., Müller, K., Vaughan, D., 2023. dplyr: A Grammar of Data Manipulation. URL `https://dplyr.tidyverse.org`

Willan, A., Briggs, A., 2006. The Statistical Analysis of Cost-effectiveness Data. John Wiley and Sons, Chichester, UK.

Williams, C., Lewsey, J., Briggs, A., Mackay, D., 2017a. Cost-effectiveness analysis in R using a multi-state modeling survival analysis framework: a tutorial. Medical Decision Making 37, 340–352.

Williams, C., Lewsey, J., Mackay, D., Briggs, A., 2017b. Estimation of survival probabilities for use in cost-effectiveness analyses: A comparison of a multi-state modeling survival analysis approach with partitioned survival and Markov decision-analytic modeling. Medical Decision Making 37, 427–439.

Williams, C., Rasmussen, E., 2006. Gaussian Processes for Machine Learning. MIT Press, Cambridge, MA.

Wood, S., 2017. Generalized Additive Models: An Introduction with R. Chapman and Hall/CRC.

Woods, B., Sideris, E., Palmer, S., Latimer, N., Soares, M., 2017. NICE DSU Technical Support Document 19. Partitioned survival analysis for decision modelling in health care: a critical review. URL `https://sheffield.ac.uk/media/34205/download?attachment`

Zellner, A., 1962. An efficient method of estimating seemingly unrelated regressions and tests for aggregation bias. Journal of the American Statistical Association 57, 348–368.

Zhang, J., Rios, J., Pechlivanoglou, T., Yang, A., Zhang, Q., Deris, D., et al., 2024. SurvdigitizeR: an algorithm for automated survival curve digitization. BMC Medical Research Methodology 24, 147.

Index

For Product Safety Concerns and Information please contact our EU
representative GPSR@taylorandfrancis.com
Taylor & Francis Verlag GmbH, Kaufingerstraße 24, 80331 München, Germany

www.ingramcontent.com/pod-product-compliance
Ingram Content Group UK Ltd.
Pitfield, Milton Keynes, MK11 3LW, UK
UKHW052218190926
475702UK00006B/1081

* 9 7 8 1 0 4 1 2 9 7 3 8 3 *